MELANCHOLIC HABITS

MELANCHOLIC HABITS

Burton's Anatomy & the Mind Sciences

Jennifer Radden

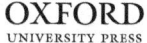

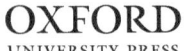
UNIVERSITY PRESS

Oxford University Press is a department of the University of Oxford. It furthers
the University's objective of excellence in research, scholarship, and education
by publishing worldwide. Oxford is a registered trade mark of Oxford University
Press in the UK and certain other countries.

Published in the United States of America by Oxford University Press
198 Madison Avenue, New York, NY 10016, United States of America.

© Oxford University Press 2017

All rights reserved. No part of this publication may be reproduced, stored in
a retrieval system, or transmitted, in any form or by any means, without the
prior permission in writing of Oxford University Press, or as expressly permitted
by law, by license, or under terms agreed with the appropriate reproduction
rights organization. Inquiries concerning reproduction outside the scope of the
above should be sent to the Rights Department, Oxford University Press, at the
address above.

You must not circulate this work in any other form
and you must impose this same condition on any acquirer.

Library of Congress Cataloging-in-Publication Data
Names: Radden, Jennifer, author.
Title: Melancholic habits : Burton's anatomy & the mind sciences /
Jennifer Radden.
Description: New York, NY : Oxford University Press, 2016. |
Includes bibliographical references and index.
Identifiers: LCCN 2016011949 | ISBN 9780199348190 (hardcover : alk. paper)
Subjects: LCSH: Melancholy. | Psychology. | Burton, Robert, 1577–1640.
Anatomy of melancholy. | Burton, Robert, 1577–1640. | Psychology.
Classification: LCC BF575.M44 R328 2016 | DDC 616.89—dc23
LC record available at https://lccn.loc.gov/2016011949

1 3 5 7 9 8 6 4 2

Printed by Sheridan Books, Inc., United States of America

This book is dedicated with love and admiration to Justyna Gudzowska, Lucian and Felix Keefe, Carlota Melo, and Gregory de Souza.

CONTENTS

Acknowledgments — ix

Introduction — 1

1. embodied mentality — 18
2. Imagination "queen of the mental powers" — 49
3. symptom, disease, cause — 82
4. between the confines of sense and reason — 118
5. the akratic melancholic — 150
6. when Reason is also corrupted — 180
7. who labors not of this disease? — 211

CONTENTS

8. remedies	243
9. from the *Anatomy* to the clinic and lab	273
References	*293*
Index of Names	*321*
Topical Index	*323*

ACKNOWLEDGMENTS

During its long gestation and through the completion of this book, many friends and colleagues have assisted me in innumerable ways, and I am grateful to every one of them. My particular thanks are due to those who read and commented on draft chapters: Pete Zachar, Somogy Varga, Barbara Houston, Jane Martin, Ann Diller, Beebe Nelson, Susan Fransoza, Serife Tekin, Ed Brown, Jeff Poland, John Sutton, Claire Pouncey, Alec Bodkin, and Georg Repnikov. Jenny Lloyd, Phil Gerrans, Angus Gowland, Amélie Rorty, and Dominic Murphy acted as valuable sounding-boards, and Frank Keefe provided editorial support through many changes and revisions. Also deserving my thanks are unnamed readers of my book proposal, who offered insightful suggestions and guidance. Audiences in Pittsburgh; Linkoping; Louvain; and Sydney, Melbourne, and Perth, provided valuable ideas and critiques. The Centre for the History of Emotions at the University of Western Australia afforded me a congenial perch as an academic visitor. And finally, along with his editorial wisdom on matters large and small, my patient editor Peter Ohlin allowed me the time I needed (while reminding me that I must stop eventually).

Introduction

Burton's *Anatomy of Melancholy* is a classic from English literature that has been almost entirely ignored by modern medical psychology. The present book is a selective and interpretive reading of the *Anatomy*. My aim is to test the durability of Burton's work as mind science using examples of its affinity with, and relevance for, present-day theorizing, findings, and controversies about the mind and its pathologies.

As a philosopher with an interest in aberrant mental states, I have long had a preoccupation with the concept of melancholy. And this interest has quickened in recent years due to a handful of transformative changes occurring within what can be called the mind sciences, those that include cognitive psychology, philosophy, neuroscience, and medical psychiatry. The first of these changes, affecting how mood disorders such as today's depression and anxiety are approached and can be studied, has been epistemological. The state of present-day knowledge and hypotheses about such disorders is a second. And their perceived worldwide increase to epidemic proportions is a third. As a result of such changes, Burton's analysis—long relegated to the status of dusty, antiquated humoral meanderings, unworthy of science or medicine—has become increasingly and newly relevant.

First, then: the emergence of cognitive psychology and neuroscience as disciplines has brought fresh paradigms affecting, and often unseating, traditional conceptions of mind, cognition, emotion, and mental health and disorder, and this is a pressing reason to reexamine Burton's ideas. Afforded by new ways of observing the brain as well as conceiving of the mind, this transformation has also brought welcome collaboration between psychology, medicine, and philosophy; their shared focus

INTRODUCTION

on mental states explains the label "mind sciences" for the disciplines involved.[1] Read selectively, Burton reveals a complex and sophisticated account of human psychology and the interaction between mind and body; he shares many of the presuppositions we associate with contemporary cognitivism, and he is alert to issues that are at the center of these recent perspectives and assumptions, including some that may have implications for the treatment of mood disorders in the clinic. Before the advent of cognitivism in psychology, and the development of neuroscience, Burton's ideas would have had little currency as science. Today, they are surprisingly, even strikingly, resonant with contemporary research on the mind and its pathologies.

Mental illnesses, their treatment, and the suffering associated with them are still incompletely understood, and these gaps in our understanding indicate a second obvious reason to read the *Anatomy*. The continuity between melancholy and today's mood disorders is debated, the parallels between them are incomplete, and no identity between the earlier and later disorders will be claimed in the following pages.[2] Regardless, though, and irrespective of the degree of those parallels, Burton's book addresses the same, or closely similar, unresolved issues over disordered feelings and emotions. Its ideas are couched in the language of humoral medicine and Aristotelian faculty psychology, yet the *Anatomy* contains insights, arguments, and observations of immediate relevance to debates that are ongoing—over depression and anxiety as disease, delusional thought, diagnosis, prediction, explanation, treatment, mental health and illness, and the social norms governing responses to human suffering. We can acknowledge the differences between seventeenth- and twenty-first-century forms of affective

---

1. Although he could hardly have anticipated the substance of these sciences, Coleridge uses "mind science" in rather the same way at the beginning of the nineteenth century. (See Holmes 2009.) Here, the expression is used broadly to include a range of research endeavors (laboratory sciences as well as neuropsychology and brain study) and clinically oriented practices (such as medical psychiatry) whose shared focus is the mind and mental functioning. That commonality of focus and purpose invites the label, especially when combined with the many collaborative efforts that now straddle and merge these separate fields.
2. See Radden 2000, 2003, 2009, 2013, Varga 2013, Berrios 1985, 2011.

disorder and still recognize these connections. We can certainly reject humoral medicine as anatomy and physiology without also ignoring the treatment recommendations for melancholy associated with it. And, unless human nature has changed more than seems likely, the phenomenological record—which is notably embellished, rich, and long-lived with disorders of affect—seems likely to aid our understanding of today's depression and anxiety.

A final reason to undertake this analysis today is that Burton saw melancholy everywhere he turned, judging it a disease of "Epidemicall" proportions, and these runaway melancholy *symptoms* are in some respects the primary subject of the *Anatomy*. We are similarly beset by reports of increasing, worldwide depressive disorder, as well as depressive symptoms accompanying a range of other ills including the posttraumatic stress diagnosed in returning warriors and all whose lives have been affected by war, want, and dislocation. Burton's recommendations were a response to what, construed in correspondingly broad terms, he also saw as a dangerously widespread and growing affliction. As we confront this more recent epidemic, we might hope to learn something from him.

At first, some of the *Anatomy*'s assumptions and emphases seem to do little more than foreshadow, or anticipate, aspects of today's models. They are of considerable interest as part of the history of medical science, but do not appear to bear directly on contemporary efforts in the mind sciences. Yet, there is more to this matter, I think it can be shown. Even what appear at first to be mere foreshadowings are through their implications linked in a range of ways to other ideas with present-day currency. The role of the imagination, and its importance within the affective life; the embodied mind; the multicausal, multidirectional looping interactions between conscious experience and bodily states; the place of emotion within all cognition; and representationalist assumptions are all in the *Anatomy*, as are ideas about self-control, self help, agency, and cognitive bias—to name some ideas key to the speculations, hypotheses, and findings of today's cognitive psychology and medical psychiatry. Uncovering and emphasizing these connections and considering implications they might hold for understanding and approaching today's mood disorders are central to the present endeavor.

INTRODUCTION

In addition to his broader theorizing, Burton offers explicit prescriptions about lifestyle, daily habits, and other measures aimed at preventing and avoiding, as well as assuaging, melancholy symptoms. These have more immediate and obvious application to the care of today's affective disorders. It is an eclectic treatment regimen—a total, symptom-prevention and -reduction program comprising a mix of behavioral, bodily, and psychological habits. All these are within the capabilities of the sufferer, and any but the most serious forms of entrenched disorder would likely be responsive to this regimen, Burton implies. When appropriately regulated, cognitive capacities, especially those involved in imagining, are presented as allowing us to avert, reduce, and often avoid, the symptoms of melancholy.

As an approach, this seems to have far-reaching societal, as well as clinical, implications. If practiced, such recommendations might alter the boundaries assigned to preventable disorder within today's understanding—with bearing on psychological suffering understood as an inescapable and nonpathological aspect of human nature. (This is the matter of "normal sadness" raised during recent revisions to the American Psychiatric Association's Diagnostic and Statistical Manuals in characterizing normal grieving processes.)

The *Anatomy* has received close attention from historians as well as those in literary studies.[3] The historical analyses, particularly, are invaluable in explaining the background and broader context of Burton's writing, including the religious and theological framework on which he depended. Because that framework is orthogonal to today's secular and scientific one, however, the discussion that follows is about what these scholars *have not attempted*: a demonstration of how, cast in naturalized language, Burton's rambling and eclectic text might speak to present-day scientific and clinical concerns.

Among Burton's theoretical ideas, I would note a handful of the most telling in this respect. There is the role of imagining (together with other functions assigned to the traditional, Aristotelian faculty

---

3. For important recent historical work, see Bamborough 1989–2000, Gowland 2006, 2007, 2014, Schmidt 2007, Lund 2010, 2015, Schmidt 2007, Bell 2014. Earlier studies include Babb 1959, Bamborough 1952, Evans 1972, and Fox 1976.

of Imagination, which include remembering and day-dreaming), arguably the *Anatomy*'s most innovative contribution. In normal and abnormal psychology alike, the centrality of the imagination arises from the *Anatomy*'s particular mixture of faculty psychology, emphasis on the passions and on the atypical case, and acknowledgment of the renaissance doctors' stress, tracing to Galenic medicine, on a damaged, deficient, or dysfunctional imagination as the locus of psychological disorder.[4]

Another feature distinguishing this work is its stress on *symptoms and natural history*, rather than categorical disease entities as they are today understood within the standard conceptions inherited from nineteenth-century medicine. In contrast to those, network models have recently been proposed as more applicable for mental disorder, and its emphasis on symptoms and natural history actually assigns the *Anatomy*'s account to a place among those. Related, and also challenging standard ideas, the *Anatomy* depicts remedies as nonspecific, multifactorial treatments with systemwide, holistic effects—in contrast to the remedies for disorders like depression associated with today's psychopharmacology, that rely on specific, "magic bullet" action.

A third feature of the *Anatomy* account with interest for the present day concerns the place of habit, and the relation between mild and more severe disorder. This relation is understood on a simple model influenced by the *habitus* of ancient medicine: Melancholy results from repeated patterns of thought and behavior that eventually become intractably entrenched. The more we carelessly give in to the lure of melancholy habits, the greater will be our risk of succumbing to the severe, chronic disorder that is difficult or even impossible to remedy, and beyond our own agency. This analysis of melancholy as habit, which can be reconstructed from within the pages of the *Anatomy*, seems to intimate how we might begin to think about other mood disorders, I suggest. Much writing about Burton's account applies to it the standard etiological analysis, known from most ordinary diseases encountered today: With that application the underlying disturbance of the black bile causally

---

4. Throughout this work, "normal" and "abnormal" are used statistically, as equivalents of "typical," and "atypical," and without normative implications.

explains melancholy's pathological status. By identifying the habituation model arising from the *Anatomy*'s conception of melancholy, I introduce an alternative reading of the work, however. If the claim that melancholy is a habit is drawn out and emphasized, then central aspects of Burton's analysis and recommendations appear in a different light. And this refashioning is a goal of the present effort.

NEGLECT OF THE *ANATOMY* BY PSYCHOLOGY

The reception to the *Anatomy of Melancholy* within psychology, philosophy, and psychiatric medicine has had its own curious history during the last hundred years. It has been dismissive, regarding Burton's project as doomed from the start. Philosophers of mind have rarely acknowledged Burton. There were meatier figures to concern themselves over from the seventeenth century, in Hobbes, Descartes, and Spinoza. Psychology has been similarly dismissive, leaving the *Anatomy* to the literary specialists and historians. Writing in 1959, Lawrence Babb devoted a chapter of his short volume on Burton to the matter of its science, concluding that it had "no genuine scientific value even in the writer's own time," since Burton was "essentially conservative, authoritarian, and backward-looking" (Babb 1959:72–3).

Babb is somewhat right in this characterization of Burton's approach, yet wrong to suppose his analysis exhausts what is there. In an earlier work it had been said of Burton, "he did not know how the mind works, but some of his guesses so strikingly foreshadow modern psychology that their long neglect must be regarded as one of the minor marvels of the history of thought" (Evans 1972:102). Written in consultation with the psychoanalyst George Mohr, Evans' own 1944 book offers now-dated, heavily psychoanalytic lore to explain and endorse a selection of Burtonian themes (as well as providing an analysis of our author's psyche). But in most cognitivism and neuroscience today, this, too, would be dismissed as testament to a want of knowledge about how the mind works. I no more share Evans' focus and assumptions than I agree with Babb's conclusion—and much present-day thinking about the mind and cognitive states would similarly dismiss Evans' psychoanalytic Burton. Yet Evans' work (now long out of print), is to my knowledge the only book-length discussion of these questions, and as he suggests, the *Anatomy has* been unwarrantedly ignored by those in mind sciences during the twentieth and twenty-first centuries. In a much-quoted remark from a 1914 *Yale Review,* Sir William Ostler names the *Anatomy of Melancholy* the greatest medical treatise ever written by a layman. The aim of the present work—again by a layperson—is to begin to redress the unwarranted neglect it has suffered.

THE MAN AND HIS BOOK

Robert Burton was an Oxford scholar and eclectic reader, thinker, and bibliophile, writing in the first half of the seventeenth century. (He lived between 1577 and 1640.) His interests and erudition led him from contemporary and ancient medicine and psychology, to philosophy, classical literature and philology, theology and religion. The first edition of the *Anatomy* of nine hundred pages that appeared in 1621 was followed by three ever-larger versions in Burton's lifetime (1624, 1628, 1632) and then by a posthumous one (1651). The causes and cures of melancholy are the respective topics of the First and Second "Partitions," or parts, of this very large work. They, particularly, bear on the present project and are our almost exclusive focus. (Religious and love melancholy, dealt with in the Third Partition, reflect Burton's more literary contributions, but are less relevant for us here.)

Burton was not the first to devote a full book to melancholy. The literary and dramatic focus on these states during the fifteenth and sixteenth centuries had been matched by scholarly interest.[5] And several well-known works from renaissance and early modern times are appealed to quite extensively in the *Anatomy. De vita libri tres* (Three Books on Life) (1489) by the Neoplatonist Marcilio Ficino (1433–1499) had extolled the link between intellectual genius and melancholy,

---

5. That literary and dramatic interest was extensive, of course, and powerfully entwined with these more medical and theological investigations. See Bamborough 1952.

INTRODUCTION

offering preventative measures and remedies.[6] Burton sees too many dangers in the scholar's life to entirely share Ficino's exultant attitude toward it, however, and although "Ficinus" is frequently acknowledged, the association between melancholy and inspiration is for the most part avoided.[7] The Low Countries physician Johann Weyer's 1562 *Di Praestigiis daemoum* (Of Deceiving Demons) was also well known to Burton. It held extensive implications for melancholy in its thesis that the power associated with witchcraft is better understood as the disturbed imagination of mental disorder than as demonic influence. (With this Burton concurred—although conceding a demonic influence effected through the imagination itself.) Melancholy was also dealt with in a popular medical volume by the French physician André Du Laurens (1558–1609) that included the subject as one of four separate dissertations.[8] Du Laurens, or "Laurentius," has been judged the major source for Burton's medical assertions, and Burton follows him in key definitions and fundamental assumptions.[9] Then there is *A Treatise of Melancholy* (1586) by the Englishman Timothy Bright, whose efforts to separate melancholy from sinful states, and elegant mind–body interactionism, find echoes and respectful acknowledgment throughout the *Anatomy*. Although not solely devoted to melancholy, also much used throughout the *Anatomy* were other general medical works, such as the influential *Praxeos Medicae* (1602) of Felix Plater.[10]

As these sources from nearer his own time indicate, Burton's preoccupation with melancholy in all its manifestations was not in itself particularly noteworthy. Since Elizabethan days this condition had become the affectation of rakes and the character trait of Shakespearian heroes.

---

6. This link between melancholy and genius was the inspiration for much sixteenth- and seventeenth-century writing (Kristellar 1988).
7. Exceptions occur: One is in the First Partition where, elaborating on the traits of the melancholy character, he includes "deepe reach, excellent apprehension, judicious, wise and witty" (I,3,1,2:391).
8. *Discours de la conservation de la veuë: des maladies melancoliques: des catarrhs, & de la vieillesse* (1594), translated in 1599 as: *A discourse of the preservation of sight, of melancholike diseases, of rheumes and of old age.*
9. Jackson 1986.
10. A Swiss physician, Plater or Platter (1536–1614) was a leading medical authority in his own day and widely read through the seventeenth century.

In addition, the renaissance humanists had expressed more tolerant attitudes toward mental aberration (including outright madness), rendering melancholy less remarkable. "I have not yet determined whether it be proper to include all the defects of sense and understanding under the common genius of madness," remarks Erasmus, before his famous enumeration of the follies, foolishness, and improprieties of his times. For folly, he goes on, is "so epidemical a distemper that it is hard to find any one man so uninfected as not to have sometimes a fit or two of some sort of frenzy" (Erasmus 2004:40–1).[11]

The renaissance revival of ancient medical focus on melancholy and madness, together with its popularity as a motif in literary and dramatic arts, served to "normalize" aberration, it is widely agreed. Even if not to the degree asserted by Michel Foucault, the lines between folly, sin, foolishness, and sheer delusion seem to have been blurred during those times.[12] As Erasmus suggests, and Burton agrees, avoiding all hint of melancholy would be impossible. Madness, and particularly melancholy, are akin to other forms of error. Rather than sharply separated from foolishness and error, they are our common, human lot. No one can be entirely free of madness and folly; moreover those errors and illusions we are able to correct seem to merge seamlessly into habituated states that are more severe, including some that those affected are powerless to deal with on their own.

Avoiding melancholy completely would be impossible for another reason, as well. For Burton, melancholy loosely understood includes entirely normal and quite unavoidable states of sadness, sorrow, fear, and worry. This feature of the *Anatomy* explains the confusingly broad use of the term "Melancholy." It is named for the black bilious fluid with which it is associated. And it refers to both affective states of disease and passing and entirely normal sadness, distresses, and fears. Only context, which includes the natural history or course of a given feeling, will indicate whether "melancholy" names a passing and insignificant mood or a habituated, chronic disorder. (As this suggests, more normal

---

11. Erasmus' *Praise of Folly* was first published in 1511 and is admired and regularly acknowledged by Burton.
12. Foucault 1965, Thiher 1999.

INTRODUCTION

and diseased states differ by degree.[13]) Although not distinctive to the period the way these other elements were, the doctrine of the four temperaments also carried strongly normalizing implications, it should be remembered. The inherent character type of *homo melancholicus* was an everyday variation, as normal as the next man.

While he may not otherwise differ from his renaissance medical and humanist contemporaries, Burton's success in normalizing melancholy sets his analysis apart from analyses within subsequent modern philosophy, where emphasis is often on disembodied reason, divorced from its corporeal container. (In his first *Meditation*, Descartes employs the laughable incomprehensibility of the madman as a foil against which we recognize rational thought and epistemic certainty. And such attitudes came to form a philosophical tradition of casting delusional thought as alterity, an attitude found even in our own times.[14]) Similarly, in modernist epistemological traditions, where ideal, and idealized, rationality is privileged, commonplace cognitive biases and other flaws in normal reasoning have regularly been overlooked. As a result, sane (and purportedly rational) thought processes are isolated and distanced from those associated with madness and delusion. By contrast with these philosophical traditions, Burton's starting points are not rational belief and certainty, but feelings and imaginings. Moreover, with his goal to compile all medical wisdom about melancholy as disease, it is primarily *aberrant feelings and imaginings*, not normal ones, that are the focus of his attention. Rather than placing disembodied reason at the center, his interest is in the intrinsically embodied and sensory passions and the Janus-faced faculty of imagination, with its special ability to affect the passions, and its always powerful, yet also dangerous, capabilities. Imagining—both appropriate and deficient—is at the core of things in the dynamic and ever-changing interaction between mind and body, and Burton's model grounds normal and abnormal mental life equally.

The relation between "madness" and "melancholy" in the *Anatomy* is confused by passages (in the jesting Letter to the Reader by Democritus

---

13. Whether states of outright madness lie on the same continuum is not so clear, it will become apparent in chapter 6. But see Bamborough 1989–2000:xxxiii.
14. See Radden 2011.

INTRODUCTION

Junior) where they are conflated. While still occurring as points on a continuum, because melancholy may through time become Madness, they are differentiated elsewhere in the text through contrasting definitions. (Only madness is vehement and violent; only melancholy is associated with sadness and unwarranted fear.) But Burton grants that some in the tradition of writing about melancholy fail to observe the distinction, and count all madness and melancholy but "one Disease."

The *Anatomy* is a unique and unusual book, as attested by its long popularity, and multiple editions. The extent to which it is an original treatise is more confusing, as Burton himself recognizes. "'Tis all mine and none mine," he says. He compares himself to the good housewife, who "out of divers fleeces weaves one peece of Cloath," or the Bee, which "gathers Wax and Hony out of many Flowers, and makes a new bundle of all." Though there were many "Giants of old in Physicke and Phylosophy," he concludes this passage,

> A Dwarfe standing on the shoulders of a Giant may see farther than a Giant himselfe; I may likely adde, alter, and see farther than my Predecessors. (I:12)

Perhaps Burton's amalgam of classical, medieval, and renaissance psychology was original in little more than its arrangement of inherited ideas into a "new bundle," as his comparisons with the good housewife and the bee, suggest. But it is a bundle that is different from what had come before, if so. Moreover, it is a bundle whose timing is noteworthy. Gathered at the very point when modern science and thought were emerging, Burton's bundle possesses a charge of unusual significance within intellectual history. He assembles and captures all that was known about melancholy in his day, omitting nothing. In this mixing of ancient ideas about the passions with renaissance psychology's emphasis on the imagination, I think it can be said that he sees "farther than his Predecessors." A parallel with Seneca invites itself here, the more so because Seneca ranks as Burton's favorite philosopher, and Burton appeals to his writing style to justify his own. It may be too strong to say of Burton, as has been said of Seneca, that if he did not himself create the ideas he transmitted, he did collect them, make them persuasive, and shape them into transmissible form.[15] Burton lacks Seneca's spare elegance, and others had written about melancholy as well, if not as copiously, before he did. Nonetheless, he stands as the last, and best, representative of a tradition that ends as the result of changes that, only a few years later, ushered in modern epistemology and psychology.

Not only Seneca but also other Stoic philosophers enjoyed a popularity during the renaissance that endured through the eighteenth century, and the second half of the sixteenth century had seen an increase in the translation, publication, and circulation of their works. We might wonder if Burton's neo-Stoicism, together with his Aristotelian psychology, are due for renewed attention today, as the assumptions of modern thought are challenged or left behind, and the new psychology of cognitivism upturns dualistic models of mind that have held sway since at least the eighteenth century. Such, at any rate, is the speculation and hope that fuels the chapters that follow.

A BOOK ABOUT A BOOK, PARTICULAR ISSUES

In several of its central assumptions Burton's analysis anticipates our contemporary models, yet he writes as a seventeenth-century clergyman. Revealing the relevance of the *Anatomy* for contemporary times thus involves a selection and interpretation of those of his ideas that fit the naturalistic language and presuppositions employed in science. This is no small task: as well as its nonscientific ideas, the work is notable for its digressions and prolixity, and Burton is not a neat, systematic, or consistent thinker in the style of the great modern philosophers of the seventeenth century such as Descartes and Spinoza. In selecting passages from the *Anatomy* with bearing on contemporary mind sciences, it will be necessary to disregard many of his claims and entirely bypass certain themes. As a Christian clergyman, Burton traces melancholy to original sin, for example, deeming repentance one remedy to ease melancholic

---

15. Hadas 1958:2.

INTRODUCTION

suffering. (It might well have been, of course, even if not for the reasons he supposed.)

There is also the matter of the *Anatomy*'s humoral language and assumptions. Although the early modern and modern era in western Europe saw the beginnings of science and medicine as we recognize them today, the *Anatomy* uses the language of ancient humoral theories, and the astrology and lore of renaissance humanism, as much as, or more than, scientific observation and method. Imbalances of the bodily humors not only explained temperament but also influenced health and disease, and as disease, the eponymous Melancholy is associated with the black bile. From beneath this humoral model can be reconstructed an elaborate and sophisticated analysis of the interaction between psychological and bodily states, but it is well concealed within the many references to the dark, cold, dry humor itself.

In addition to the challenge of reading through the humoral language and assumptions to find the conceptual structure beneath, and attributing to Burton a position of his own amid the plethora of others' opinions he cites, the present task is also magnified by the sometimes inconclusive or inconsistent, and often skeptical, attitudes expressed through the authorial voice of Democritus Junior adopted by Burton. These aspects of style impose such a hindrance that Burton's whole investigation has been judged "in essence infinitely complex, particular, and uncertain," and so, entirely skeptical (Gowland 2006:29)[16] It is a charge that seems very likely applicable to the *Anatomy* when taken as a whole. And, indeed, most twentieth-century commentators have made some version of the same complaint, acknowledging the work to be "chaotic and dispersive,"[17] its style giving rise to "confusion and obscurity,"[18] "disfiguring" the body of knowledge.[19]

But ours in what follows is a limited and interpretive reading. And despite the above impediments, the discussion here is driven by the

16. The addition of authorial opinion, the passage continues, "would be futile . . . the eclecticism of the era insurmountable except through recourse to some form of skepticism (Gowland 2006:29).
17. Tilmouth 2005:525.
18. Williams, H. 2003:35.
19. Williams, R. 2001.

conviction that opinions, positions, and assumptions *can* be uncovered beneath the often deliberately inconclusive surface, and that a selective reading reveals a coherent theoretical whole. In adopting this position, I thus accept Christopher Tilmouth's endorsement of a "core consistency" within the *Anatomy*, at whose heart there is " a corpus of knowledge the unity of which has been underestimated," and a "half submerged foundation" that forms a rational account of melancholy (Tilmouth 2005:525). It is not as orderly perhaps, or as complete, as we could wish. Nonetheless, extricated from much of the rest of the work, and detached from its religious assumptions, humoral language, and evidently mistaken biology, the restructured *Anatomy* exhibits consistent and coherent themes and presuppositions. Moreover, combined with a shrewd understanding of human nature, and recognition of some of the implications of these for the treatment of melancholy, it affords us insights of considerable interest for our contemporary preoccupations.

The interconnections between Burton's ideas that form this "half submerged foundation" came to me belatedly, after reading the *Anatomy* for twenty years. My epiphany was about the extensive implications of his frequent references to the habitual, or chronic nature of melancholy. A chronic disease has a natural history; a natural history emphasizes ongoing symptoms, and symptom sequences, over initiating causes. Presuppositions about disease from the etiological lens through which we are inclined to view the *Anatomy* suddenly fell away, with this realization. A habit of Melancholy, as Burton puts it, is just that: an entrenched set of thought patterns and emotional habits, incurred and consolidated, over time. And there lies the force of my title: Burton invites us to understand melancholy as no more, and no less, than habit.

Extricating Burton's ideas from his religious and humoral assumptions, and jesting style, represents a challenge for the present project. The choice of text from which to work is quite another, since aside from the bowdlerized versions that found their way into print after Burton's death, the *Anatomy* came out in several differing editions during his lifetime as the result of his additions, changes, and tinkerings. His own copies of each version contain further handwritten annotations and notes, moreover, not always reflected in the printed texts. Scholars have carefully identified features distinguishing the respective editions in the published sequence, at least, undertaking the monumental task of collating each of the six seventeenth-century versions.[20] Guided by their efforts, I here use the Third Edition (1628), on the grounds they offer for their choice: Unlike the other editions, the third was proof-corrected by Burton, and it is the first edition to represent the work in near-final form. Whatever additions and elaborations alter the later editions, the basic analyses, particularly, remain unchanged.[21] A newer version of the *Anatomy* is in preparation revising some points of emphasis in light of Burton's extensive later annotations to his own copies. But my arguments here are reliant on the Faulkner, Kiessling, and Blair version from which all quotations are taken, and sometimes, they may be specific to it.

Passages are quoted in their original form; when spelling and vocabulary might be unfamiliar, I have added the spelling or meaning in square brackets within the text. Burton's own italics are kept, indicating his personal translations, as are his capitalizations, and my own italics for emphasis are in each case noted. Citations provide page numbers to this edition as well as Partitions shown with Roman numbers, followed by Sections, Members, and Subsections indicated with Arabic ones. Capitalization is used more liberally in the *Anatomy* than is customary in today's English, and I have omitted it, although selectively. (Imagination is capitalized, for example, when it contrasts with the rather narrower conception of present-day usage.) And finally, references to "Burtonian Melancholy," indicate when specificity is called for, such as where there is divergence from other analyses in the canon of writing about melancholy.

ARGUMENTATIVE SEQUENCE

The overall strategy is roughly as follows. The first seven chapters provide an explication of Burtonian science and psychology, normal (mainly in chapters 1 and 2) and then abnormal (in chapters 3–7). These chapters

---

20. Faulkner, Kiessling, and Blair 1989–2000.
21. Indeed, the medical aspects of the *Anatomy* changed little after the First Edition, it has been pointed out (Fox 1976).

INTRODUCTION

indicate, and illustrate by appeal to our contemporary research, those aspects of the *Anatomy* model of mind, or we might say *cognitive architecture*, with application to today's new science about mind. That model is dominated by relations between three "faculties," or functions: the imagination, reason, and the passions, and it is the interaction between and within these three to which Burton appeals in his most perspicuous accounts of the causes and remedies for melancholy symptoms. (The work of neuroscientists Antonio Damasio and Joseph LeDoux, is employed to illustrate the similarities between Burton's account and contemporary models, for example, to the extent that it stresses the involvement of affective states in all cognition, and the complex interactions between affective and felt states and other brain activities.) The larger context here includes the person's soul, that inviolate metaphysical entity whose existence and unchanging nature Burton never doubts or questions. It also includes that soul's corporeal vessel, whose humoral "temperature" ceaselessly alters, and is altered by, the mental faculties. The present volume separates and explains Burtonian ideas about each of the imagination, reason, and the passions in relation to their normal and aberrant functioning, pointing to their implications within the extensive set of preventive and therapeutic measures and regimens proposed in the Second Partition. The dangers around inappropriate uses of the imagination place everyone at risk of succumbing to habitual, and next to untreatable, melancholy. But the *Anatomy* can nevertheless be seen to separate the less advanced tendencies we have some power to avert and control, from the habituated, chronic condition, and each form taken by melancholy is dealt with here. Out of this theorizing and basic cognitive architecture come the broad principles underlying Burton's prescriptions for the prevention and treatment of melancholy. They are the subject of chapter 8. Then, finally, some of the implications of these principles for the understanding and treatment of today's mood disorder, particularly symptoms of depression and anxiety, are illustrated in a concluding ninth chapter.

    The argumentative sequence traces that of the *Anatomy* itself. From the earlier explication of more general ideas about the mind, normal and aberrant, in the First Partition are derived the treatment recommendations, or "cures," in the Second. The present book also moves from

INTRODUCTION

broad architecture to remedies before addressing some implications for contemporary times. The similarities between Burton's account and contemporary models and analyses are emphasized here—with the supposition that if these contemporary models have currency, then Burton's very similar system invites our attention. And if the basic model deserves our attention, then the many remedial measures for melancholy Burton infers from it may as well. Indeed, they may carry implications for the understanding and treatment of today's mood disorders—even if, as will become apparent throughout the chapters to follow, it is at most by relationships of analogy, rather than identity, that Burtonian Melancholy is linked to such conditions.

Chapter 1

embodied mentality

Because they are not essential to the embodied mind and interactionism constituting cognitive architecture in the *Anatomy*, the black bile and its metaphors are briefly introduced here and then set to one side.[1] By contrast with them, the *Anatomy*'s faculty psychology, and the classical and renaissance ideas Burton follows in describing how bodily states affect and are affected by thoughts, imaginings, and feelings, have more telling parallels in today's sciences of mind. Rather than eclipsed, these faculty categories form the basis of modern philosophy and cognitive psychology alike, as they have always done folk psychology. They have sometimes undergone small shifts of meaning (as we see in chapter 4, with the reduction of "passions" to "emotions"), but for the most part the broad categories of perception, memory, feeling, imagination, and the like remain for us, as they were for Burton, the structure on which our understanding of human psychology is built. In addition, although his dualistic account of the mind and its workings was not of the naturalistic kind we find in contemporary science, those mental workings were firmly, inextricably, and interactively *embodied*. In this respect, its particular form of dualist interactionism leaves the *Anatomy* system surprisingly compatible with the materialistic systems of modern, mental science.

---

1. In choosing to bypass all but the broadest aspects of Burton's humoral system, I do not mean to disparage present-day efforts to explore and vindicate other humorally based anatomy and physiology, such as that employed by Burton's close contemporary Descartes. (See Cottingham 1998, and essays in Gaukroger, Schuster, and Sutton 2000.)

BLACK BILE AND ITS METAPHORS

Found in later writings from the Hippocratic corpus, and acknowledged by works attributed to Aristotle, humoral lore had been maintained and developed by Galen (in the second century CE); preserved and elaborated by scholars such as Avicenna, Rufus, and Rhazes; and faithfully reproduced until Burton's day.[2] One or another humoral fluid, or a distinctive combination of them, predominated in each person as a relatively stable humoral "complexion." When excessive, overly heated, or otherwise affected, these were associated with disorder and even madness. Among the several diseases of the black bile known through the long tradition of medical lore, the eponymous Melancholy was a condition whose characteristic symptoms included unwarrantedly dispirited and mistakenly apprehensive affective states. Moreover, within a powerful network of meanings and metaphors, the coldness, dryness, and darkness of the humor were linked with other things also possessed of those same qualities. The melancholic's perceived swarthiness and darkened skin color were thus emblematic, reflecting the commonality of all dark things; and through an association tying overheated ("adusted") black bile to smoke-like fumes, his delusions resulted through the obscuring effect on reasoning.[3,4] The four humors of blood, phlegm, black and yellow bile also corresponded to a character typology that had prevailed since medieval times.[5] In any given person, lasting temperamental traits reflected the particular, relatively stable, arrangement of humors. And in Burton's day the humoral categories of melancholic, phlegmatic, choleric, and sanguine corresponded to recognized types,

---

2. Unified, aligned with Aristotelian natural philosophy, and systematized, it was to some extent projected back onto Hippocratic thought, it has been argued. See Bell 2014, chapter 1.
3. Bodies widely affected by melancholy, Burton says, "are most part blacke, the melancholy juice is *redundant all over*, hirsute they are, and leane, they have broad veines, their blood is grosse and thicke" (I,3,2,3:413).
4. For a discussion of increased reliance on this "mechanics of qualities," providing "a qualitative coherence with its own laws of transmission, development, and transformation," see Foucault 1965:121.
5. On the origins of these normal differentiations based on temperament, see Bell 2014, chapter 1.

familiar from literary and pictorial traditions as well as medical typologies.[6] These inborn, temperamental variations are frequently acknowledged in the *Anatomy*. (One cause of melancholy, is "our temperature, in the whole or part, which wee receive from our parents" [I,2,1,6:205], for example.) Imperceptible animal spirits circulated and mixed with inhaled air through hollow nerves to produce these bodily and mental changes, altering the body's temperature and humidity, and conveying messages from the soul to the heart, brain and other bodily parts. The humoral terms "temperature" and "complexion" indicated the *overall* relation between the four humors in the body, determined by the balance of the four qualities of hot, cold, wet, and dry. There were compound in-temperatures, in which two of these qualities (such as the cold dryness of melancholy) predominated, as well as states where one humor and its characteristic qualities prevailed over the rest.

Burton's admiration for Galen is unwavering. (By comparison with other medical authorities, he judges Galen "the common master of them all, from whose fountain they fetch water" [II,2,6,1:100].) And the Galenic medicine guiding most of Burton's recommendations and remedies for avoiding and averting melancholy was essentially concerned with balance and imbalance between these qualities, understood in systemwide terms. A state of imbalance or *diskrasia* was one of ill health, and one of *krasia*, health, to be sought through adherence to the daily (*dietary*) *regimen* involving the regulation of movement, rest, eating, breathing, evacuation, and the passions—a regimen as much related to moral as to bodily health, for this was holistic medicine at its most thoroughgoing.

By the early seventeenth century, the findings of Versalius, Paré, and Fallopio, and later Boyle and Harvey, had challenged details of Galenic anatomy, and the powerful hold of humoral assumptions on the cultural imagination was gradually loosening.[7] Burton is situated at a critical point in this momentous transformation that ushered in modern, empirically grounded scientific thought. Some of the new work was known to

---

6. The way the psychological type of the melancholy man took hold on the popular and literary mind in Elizabethan times is described by Bamborough (1952).
7. See Wear 1985, Jackson 1986, Schmidtt and Skinner 1988, Porter 2006, Arikha 2007.

him. So was the rejection of humoral medicine by contemporaries such as Paracelsus, and the efforts of the less Galenic and more empirically minded medical men (the "Empirics"). Commentators have generally judged Burton to maintain the older, Galenic traditions, unaware of, or ignoring, the intimations of the more empirically based modern biological science around him.[8] (The evidence is somewhat inconclusive over the extent to which he might have been able to insulate himself from these new discoveries.[9]) But "black bile" lingered within a powerful set of metaphors.[10] Indeed, humoral categories and ideas remain with us still in conceptions of temperament, and ideas about psychic and bodily balance and imbalance.[11] So the intent of descriptions and explanations such as Burton's, during this time of transition from more to less literal usage, cannot be entirely resolved.

That the *Anatomy* contains reference to the humors as robust causes of melancholy is not in question. Humoral changes sometimes initiate and explain the disturbed affections and ideas fostering melancholy and constituting melancholy symptoms. But causation also flows from mind to body—in which case, change does not originate with them. Burton's dualistic form of interactionism precludes any fixed, unidirectional causal sequence leading unfailingly from bodily to affective states. Nothing is fixed. Melancholy is marked by incessant multicausal and

---

8. See, for instance, Babb 1959, Jackson 1986.
9. There is no reference to Harvey's work on the circulation of the blood, for example, even though Harvey had repeated his yearly lecture about it at the Royal College of Physicians from 1616 and published his findings in 1628. And in general, Burton's interest in the new anatomy was limited, by contrast with his mathematical and astronomical knowledge and interests. In his defense, it has been pointed out that 1640, the year of his death, marked "a watershed, with the earlier part of the century as a kind of preparation for the advances that were to come later" (Bamborough 1989–2000:xviii). Whether, in the small circle at Oxford, Burton could have remained largely unaware of those preparations, seems doubtful, if perhaps not impossible.
10. Porter 2006:136–48, Jackson 1986, Bamborough 1989–2000.
11. "We talk quite naturally of a happy temperament, or a bad temper; of a jovial or saturnine disposition; of animal spirits or a heart moved by passion" (Bamborough 1952:145). And: "A mood is an *humeur* in French and an *umore* in Italian; and English-speakers still have to humor the whims of a temperamental colleague, face a Monday with ill-humor, and remain good humored throughout the week" (Arikha 2007:xix).

bidirectional change.[12] Causes became symptoms, and symptoms subsequent causes, the whole system too elusive to be "anatomized" with any precision—and this dynamic itself arguably leaves Burton's adherence to humoral physiology tepid at best.

Further hints that Burton recognizes the limits of humoral explanation include the gentle skepticism he often expresses toward previous medical lore. This becomes sharper when he dismisses as insignificant the different types of melancholy classified on a humoral basis, scoffing that these types are inseparable in practice.[13] As if indifferent to such details, he reports learned disagreements over minutiae of the humoral system without offering a concluding opinion of his own. And similarly, those who rejected humoral medicine, including the more empirically minded "Empirics," are acknowledged without any accompanying dissent. Finally though, however loosely, literally, or seriously Burton may have taken these humoral descriptions, his faculty psychology survives unaltered today and it is more important for our purposes.

CLASSICAL LEGACIES AND THE CANON ON MELANCHOLY

Little is entirely new in the elements making up Burton's model of mind. He builds on Aristotelian faculty psychology and employs categories familiar from the Galenic medicine of his day, together with their interpretation in renaissance writing from the sixteenth century. So it is differences of emphasis and implication, rather than of fundamentals, that for the most part distinguish his analyses from those of earlier traditions, or from the work of his nearer contemporaries it closely resembles. Originality was not Burton's goal, as we have seen. "'Tis all

---

12. When they do bring about change, humoral states are offered as explanatorily sufficient, in contrast to the effects of astrological influences, for example. As "causes" the stars are said to "incline" but not "compel"—and that gently, so that their influence can be resisted (I,2,1,4:199).
13. How difficult a thing it is, he says, "to treat of severall kindes apart; to make any certainty or distinction among so many casualties, distractions, when seldom two men shall be like affected *per omnia*" (I,1,3,4:171).

mine *and none mine*," he is happy to admit of his great compendium.[14] Yet his starting point with atypical affective states and the consequent depiction of the mind's embodiment, together with his form of interactionism, his emphasis on imagination, and his preoccupation with the abnormal case, all combine to suggest a model of mind that contrasts notably with ideas expressed by his near-contemporary Descartes, particularly. And it is the more striking because it so neatly fits present-day cognitivism and many recent findings from neuroscience.

Of the classical legacies in the *Anatomy*, the commonly held psychological assumptions derived from Aristotle and Aristotelianism are focused on normal mental processes. These are divided according to functional units or faculties. (The faculties are in turn assigned to bodily locations and functions.[15]) Within the sensible or sensitive soul, as distinct from its rational and vegetable aspects, the apprehensive faculty, which allows us to perceive all sensible things, comprises two parts: the (outward) five senses and three inward ones of common sense, memory, and imagination, or phantasy. (Phantasy is not distinguished from imagination, at least by Burton, and is sometimes also rendered as "fancy.") This trio of common sense, imagination, and memory supplies the content with which the higher faculties of reason (the understanding and will) engage.

The intermediate, inward senses of imagination and memory, as Burton explains in his account, have as their objects not only

> things present, but ... the sensible Species of things to Come, Past, Absent, such as were before in the Sense. (I,1,2,7:152)

14. I:11. On this issue of attribution, he continues, "the matter is theirs most part, and yet mine."
15. Burton complies with the standard anatomy: The vegetative powers are associated with the liver, served by the veins and auxiliary members such as the bladder and genitals. The emotive functions of the sensitive soul reside in the heart, served by the arteries, while its faculties of cognition and voluntary motion are in the brain, served by the nerves, the sense organs, and the muscles. There, common sense and imagination lie in the anterior cerebral ventricle, fantasy and estimation in the middle ventricle, and memory in the posterior one. All these organs rely for their operations on the animal spirits, produced from blood and disseminated throughout the body. See Kristellar 1988:469–71.

As its presence alongside other outer senses indicates—as does, indeed, its etymology—the Imagination involves sensory capabilities as well as ones that are more intellectual or "cognitive" in the narrow sense, because it produces images. In an account to which we will return, Burton describes imagination as

> an inner sense which doth more fully examine the Species perceaved by common sense ... and keeps them longer, recalling them to mind againe, or *making new of his owne*. (I,1,2,7:152, emphasis added)

Rather than our contemporary notion of common sense, suggesting reasonableness, Burton adheres to the Aristotelian idea of a sensory capacity that serves a binding function, coordinating the separate sights, sounds, tastes, smells, and feelings offered by the five outward senses and apprehending the "common sensible" qualities (such as size and shape) known through more than one sense.[16] Common sense is thus, in his words,

> judge and moderator of the rest, by whom we discern all differences of objects. (I,1,2,7:152)

The coordinated functions of common sense and imagination go this way, then: The sight, texture, and taste of honey are unified or bound together by the common sense; the imagination allows us to think about it as a whole, even substituting some element—envisioning it as different in color or viscosity, for example, or applying other, past tastes of honey recalled from memory for comparison with this one. Scholars sometimes interpret Aristotle's common sense to be bound up, or identical, with the imagination (*phantasia*) responsible for imagery. When it functions in perception, it is appropriately called the common sense; when producing images in remembering or imagining, it is called the

---

16. Versions of the challenge presented, to which such binding is the Aristotelian solution, are known within contemporary consciousness studies as the Binding Problem and are widely agreed to remain without a satisfactory resolution (Flanagan 1998).

imagination.[17] Burton's references to the common sense do not consistently acknowledge this separation into perceptual and nonperceptual roles, yet nor does he conflate the two. As in much of his discussion of the imagination, he seems, rather, to be guided by Du Laurens, whose use is similarly encompassing.

Understanding and will are each intricately involved in melancholy. To acquire knowledge, the understanding must assess the evidence of the senses already organized by the common sense, evaluate the creations of imagination, and elicit appropriate memories. The will also plays a critical part. We are free to disregard the dictates of the understanding, although we ought to follow them. In the simplest and clearest instance, such displays of willfulness are evident when we wantonly give in to bodily appetites or strong passions. The *akratic* is one whose inclinations continually defy reason, and sometimes overwhelm it this way. And Burton also depicts a struggle against less carnal inclinations in similar terms, we'll see: Melancholy arises from a failure to curb an imagination that, without being valuably productive, has become overly intense, powerful, or fecund.

Attitudes toward the imagination in the psychology of the renaissance era were at best ambivalent, as this suggests. The imagination's first and more innocuous function is to examine and evaluate what is presented through common sense. But it is also inclined to resist the higher faculties. Misapprehensions, "opinions," or "fancy" are the outcomes of this resistance. So, in extreme cases, is floridly delusional thinking, as well as every degree of self deception short of that. The imagination dominates this way due to its power to arouse the passions, when the body is drawn to a pleasurable object or inclined to avoid a source of pain or distress. In these renaissance ideas, Reason's role was "supervisory," and the Imagination was "a suspect faculty, only to be tolerated if kept in its proper place" (Bamborough 1952:37–40).

Arguably, Burton's emphasis on, and admiration for, the power of the imagination places him at some distance from this rather condemnatory assessment by earlier thinkers (although he slips closer toward

---

17. Shields 2008.

it here and there in the *Anatomy*). He was surrounded by the positive benefits of imaginative capabilities in the wealth of past knowledge he so valued, and the great accumulation of literary and dramatic works from classical and renaissance times. Even if he were to have ignored the role of imagining in the emerging and important scientific speculations of contemporaries nearer his own time, we might suppose, these other contributions could hardly have failed to impress him.[18] And in fact he does emphatically credit the imaginative origins of science and mathematics.[19] Convinced of the unmatched power of the imagination to affect the humors and the passions with changes that were as often beneficial in their consequences as not, Burton represents the imagination in impressive, at times even resplendent, terms, in spite of all its dangers.

The importance of the will and self-control in this account is evident. And attitudes toward deterministic materialism separated Burton's ideas from those of some of his near contemporaries in relation to these claims. Du Laurens leaves little room for the will or the soul (to which he pays brief lip service), while Bright decries such godlessness, establishing a sharp division between the material and the divine, and positioning himself in contrast to some men who have mistakenly judged human vices "nought else but a fault of humour."[20] Burton was closer to Bright here; the soul and will are each, and equally, indispensable.[21] In spite of his admiration for their other ideas, the Stoics were mistaken in their failure to acknowledge the soul and free will, he asserts.[22] Moreover,

---

18. We know much of what Burton read. See Kiessling 1988.
19. At I:2,3,2:251, for example.
20. In the full passage from his Dedicatory Epistle, Bright observes that some people have been caused to judge "more basely of the soule, then agreeth with pietie or nature, & have accompted all manner affection thereof, to be subject to the physicians hand, not considering herein any thing divine, and above the ordinarie events, & natural course of things: but have esteemed the vertues them selves, yea religio, no other thing but as the body hath bin tempered, and on the other side, vice, prophanenes, & neglect of religion and honesty, to have bin nought else but a fault of humour" (Bright 1586: fol I,iiv). In this, as in other areas, Bright offers the crisper analysis.
21. Bright was particularly intent on separating melancholy suffering from the suffering of an afflicted conscience, and Burton respects his reasoning, while pointing out in his discussion of religious melancholy that "melancholy alone . . . may be sometimes a sufficient cause of this terror of conscience" (III:4,2,3:412).
22. I,1,2,11:160.

his insistence that, when addressed early, melancholy can be relieved, or even averted, by its sufferer's own efforts, was evidence of Burton's unshakably libertarian convictions. (Although there seems no reason to doubt his sincerity, those convictions left his account of causes and cures conveniently immune from the deterministic taint associated with renaissance medicine.)

On the tripartite division between the Rational, Sensitive (or Sensible), and Vegetative (or Vegetable) soul, we come now to the Rational Soul, of which the understanding and will are instruments.[23,24] As a religious entity the Rational soul will play little part in our analyses. (Burton himself endorses the opinion that the rational soul remains "a *pleasant, but a doubtfull subject*"[25]) Our interest is in its instruments (understanding and will) and in the Sensitive soul, or faculty. (The language here can be confusing, Burton notes. Some philosophers have spoken of one soul divided into three faculties, he explains, while others make three distinct souls [I,1,2,5:147].) But to recognize the embodiment of all mental processes, expressed in the incessant, multistranded causal interaction between the Passions, Imagination, and Reason, and to acknowledge the Rational Soul's additional, elevated detachment from these activities, we need to remember its properties of immortality, immateriality, and indivisibility.[26] Health and illness were often ascribed to the (Rational) soul, but because of these properties such attributions could only be understood figuratively. Its

---

23. Within this transcendent arena, Aquinas had linked Aristotelian faculty psychology with Galenic medicine to divide the immaterial, rational soul into vital (or irascible) and vegetative (concupiscible) elements marking human tendencies. The concupiscible or coveting soul was activated with desire or aversion without reference to circumstances, while the irascible or invading soul saw obstacles or effort in the achievement of respectively reaching, or avoiding, desirable or aversive objects. Burton acknowledges this contrast, although he employs it minimally, in one passage emphasizing the equal need for moderation in both appetites (I,2,3,11:380). See also I,2,3,11:280, I,2,3,3:255.
24. The Greek word *psuche* is safely rendered "mind" and encompasses feelings as well as the narrowly *cognitive* or intellectual states set in contrast to affective ones. Into Latin, *psuche* becomes *animus*. And although *animus* sometimes corresponds to the purely intellectual *mens*, for the Stoics, for example, to whose work on the passions Burton is most indebted, it includes emotions and appetites (Nussbaum 1994:317).
25. I,1,2,8:155.
26. Kocher 1953, Gowland 2007, 2013.

agreed-on indivisibility prevented the soul from actually sickening or being directly affected by the bodily constitution in any literal sense at all.[27] As instruments of the soul, the understanding and will could be so affected, but the soul could not.

The will is a powerful capacity. The sensual appetite cannot but desire objects that are convenient goods, Burton explains: We are "ruled and directed by sense," whereas we are "carried by reason" when directed by the rational appetite.[28] And our human tendency is to be willful this way: Egged on by our natural concupiscence, as he puts it, we cannot resist

> our heart is evil, the seat of our affections, captivates, and enforceth our will. So that in voluntary things we are averse to God and goodnesse . . . *bad by nature,* by ignorance worse, by Art, Discipline, Custome, we get many bad Habits, suffering them to domineer and tyrannize over us. (I,1,2,11:160, emphasis added)

That these wrongful tendencies are unavoidable and common, Burton confirms repeatedly; vicious habits ensue "*because we give so much way to our Appetite, and follow our inclination,* like so many beasts" (I,1,2,11:161, emphasis added).

Understanding the soul and its attributes is unsurpassingly difficult, Burton explains. For

> the Essence and particular knowledge, of all other things it is most hard . . . to discerne, as Aristotle himselfe, Tully, Picus Mirandula, Tolet and other Neoteric [new] Philosophers confesse. *Wee can understand all things by her, but what shee is we cannot apprehend.* (I,1,2,5:147)[29]

---

27. Bright, too, emphasizes that the substance and qualities of the soul are quite unalterable, and not able to be in any way affected by bodily properties or material circumstances (Bright 1586:39–40).
28. "Some [actions of the Will are] . . . freely performed by himself, although the Stoicks absolutely deny it, and will have all things inevitably done by Destiny, imposing a fatall necessity upon us, which we may not resist" (I,1,2,11:160).
29. Tully was still thought separate from Cicero in Burton's time.

Particularly defying human understanding is the relationship within the parts of the soul:

> The common division of the Soule, is into three principall faculties; *Vegetall, Sensitive,* and *Rationall,* which make three distinct kinde of living Creatures: *Vegetall* Plants, Sensible *Beasts, Rationall* Men. How these principall faculties are distinguished and connected ... is beyond humane capacitie.... The inferior may be alone, but the superior cannot subsist without the other; so *sensible* includes *Vegitall, Rationall* both, which are contained in it (saith *Aristotle*) ... as a Triangle in a Quadrangle. (I,1,2,5:148)

While there was agreement that it depended on the body for its knowledge of the external world, the soul's existence in relation to the body in renaissance metaphysics had been vaguely, and variously, construed.[30] Generally held, at least, was that certain of its Sensitive faculties, such as imagination, somehow reached beyond the bodily ("sensible includes Vegitall and Rationall both"), and that the Rational soul possessed knowledge not derived from sense. Burton cites past authorities, including Bright, to explain how, being material, the body "worketh upon the immateriall soule," in the manner, as we might think of it, of one substance on another. (It is sometimes misleadingly implied that earlier forms were not substance dualisms; often they were, but the conception of substance was altered and refined with Descartes' analysis.[31]) Instead, the relation of immaterial soul to material body was conceived in Aristotelian terms. In an inextricable union, the soul is the *form* of the body. Burton's simple metaphors in the following passage reflect his efforts to convey this Aristotelian legacy. As the Heart, humours, and spirits, he observes, are purer, or impurer,

> so ... the Minde ... equally suffers, as a Lute out of tune, if one string, or one organ be distempered, all the rest miscarry.

---

30. See Bamborough 1952, essays in Wright and Potter 2000, and Gowland 2007.
31. His efforts in other writing have left Descartes' dualism a puzzling and ambiguous subject (Lokhorst 2015).

The Body is the soul's house (*domicilium animae*), he goes on, and just as a torch gives a better light,

> according to *the matter it is made of*: so the soul performs all her actions, better or worse, as her organs are disposed. As wine tastes of the cask where it is kept, so the Soule receaves a tincture from the Body, *through which it works*. (I,2,5,1:373 emphases added)

Soul and body are here inseparable, the soul working through its (or "her") material dwelling, and reliant on that structure for its effectiveness.

Aristotelian categories and Galenic humoral medicine had been endorsed and employed by scholars and doctors alike through the renaissance, although there was also some unorthodoxy.[32] But in these ideas, Burton is to a great extent a man of his background in classical culture. That he read the ancients themselves, as well as their medieval and renaissance interpreters is evident. He wrote in English rather than Latin only reluctantly.[33] But he provides many of his own translations and accommodates every one of the classical thinkers in his deluge of citations and references (including some so obscure they mean little within present-day learning[34]). Scholars of Burton differ in the emphasis placed on one such influence and another.[35] Yet with his aim to gather and present all comers, our author is so eclectic, generous, and respectful in his acknowledgments that these differences need not detain us.

The classical sources for the *Anatomy* derive from two traditions, we have seen: Aristotelian assumptions about normal mental processes and faculties, and ancient ideas about melancholy as disease. Originating with Hippocratic writing, systematized by Galen, and embellished and

---

32. See Wear, French, and Lonie 1985.
33. "It is not mine intent to prostitute my Muse in English" he explains; he would have used Latin "if I could have got it printed" (I,16,9–18).
34. His reference to characters from the comedies of Terence such as Gnathoes (III,1,2,3:23), once familiar to all educated readers, is an obvious example, but hardly the most obscure.
35. For emphasis on the *Anatomy*'s "markedly Galenist preoccupation," see Tilmouth 2005:535.

faithfully reproduced through medieval and renaissance times, the latter ideas concerned aberrant passions, particularly unwarranted sadness and fear ("without cause") as medical symptoms.

The effect of this dual legacy from ancient writing on Burton's work is profound. Burton is directed from the start toward the atypical case: Melancholy is the subject of his whole book, and in those classical medical traditions, melancholy is primarily disease, for all its other elaboration and applications to normal states. Characteristic symptoms of that disease, moreover, are aberrant *feelings* ("affections" or "Passions"). Thus, for Burton the Sensible soul, with its feelings and imaginings, rather than the more intellectional Rational soul, is at the center of his analysis. Unlike Reason, the Passions emanate from a bridging or hybrid place: They lie, as he says, "between the confines of Sense and Reason" (1:2,3,3:255). This hybrid and bridging function of the passions, traditionally associated with the heart, is also conveyed by references to the location of other functions:

> The rationall resides in the Braine, the other in the Liver . . . the heart is diversly affected of both, and *carried a thousand ways* by consent. The sensitive faculty most part over-rules reason, the Soule is carried hood-winked, & the understanding captive like a beast. (III,1,2,1:16, emphasis added)

His version of mind-body dualism, as a consequence, is the most holistic one possible.[36] His adherence to Hellenistic and Christian ideas ensures that Burton often seems to fear and disparage feelings and passions as much as do more intellectualistic traditions. The passions are dangerous, both in their irrationality and in their sinfulness, he makes clear. Yet the task he sets himself is to gather and lay out in encyclopedic breadth the collected knowledge of Melancholy as disease. That task leaves him

---

36. Burton was well aware of materialistic reductionism. On this matter, like that of the will, and its freedom, however, he adhered to conventional Christian doctrine. (He does differ from the Church on the fate of those, like his beloved Seneca, who are materialistic atheists. "Many worthy Greekes & Romans, good morall honest men, that kept the law of nature, did to others as they would be done to themselves, are as certainly saved" (III,4,2,6:437).

no choice but to acknowledge the sensory and bodily aspect of the states of imagination and feeling making up the Sensitive or Sensible Soul, that so obviously straddle mind and body. In its embodiment, the relation of thoughts and feelings, mind and body, differs in this respect from the interactionism of the better-known, and more influential, dualistic traditions associated with modern philosophy and psychology as they emerged through later eras.

BURTONIAN DUALISM, EMBODIMENT, AND INTERACTIONISM

The soul has two distinct roles in the scheme of things accepted by Burton and most of his contemporaries. It is an organizing principle coordinating the body and the mind and its faculties through the use of the instruments of understanding and will; it is also an immortal entity (a pre-Cartesian substance) persisting after the demise of its bodily container.[37,38] At least through Burton's time, these roles were combined without apparent tension, seeming entirely compatible.[39] Similarly, although the body and soul were recognized to possess distinguishing attributes, the soul's coordinating role in the mutually interactive relationship with the body ensured a practical inseparability. Thus,

> the Body works upon the minde, by his bad humours, troubling the Spirits, sending frosse fumes into the Braine; and so per consequens disturbing the Soule, and all the faculties of it . . . : so, on the other side, the minde most effectually works upon the Body. (I,2,3,1:247)

---

37. From ancient times to the early modern period, the soul "was believed to be integrally linked to the human body as the locus or cause of its vital and cognitive activities [. . . [as well as] . . . the vehicle . . . of personal immortality" (Michael 2000:147).
38. This separation has been divided into substance and functional dualisms: only the former maintained that soul and body were substances of entirely different and incompatible natures (Wright, J. 2000). Burton was no mere functional dualist, however.
39. See Michael, and other essays in Wright and Potter 2000.

In addition to Christian ideas about the soul, philosophical traditions tracing to Plato's writing were familiar, and debated, among renaissance and early modern thinkers.[40] As the above passage indicates, the *Anatomy* analysis seems to integrate the tripartite soul within the unity of mind and body. The soul is naturally tied to the body through the body's vegetative and sensitive attributes and activities, and interconnected through the shared, nonsensory and more intellectual capabilities associated with imagination and the common sense.

With the emergence of modern thought in Burton's own seventeenth century, the separation of the mind from its body received a concise and robust formulation by Descartes. As Christians, Burton and Descartes each accepted the soul as an entity destined for immortal life, in addition to an organizing principle uniting bodily and mental functions. Nonetheless, the precision Descartes bestowed on these ideas in some of his early writing diverges radically from the Burtonian model. (It was a precision so extreme as to be belied by his other writing, indeed.[41]) Descartes was at the forefront of the new science of the seventeenth century, and in many respects his work is antithetical to Burton's backward-looking, Aristotelian compendium. Compared with some Cartesian writing about the relation between mind and body however, Burton's account may be more amenable to the particular combination of ideas and presuppositions making up today's mind sciences.[42]

Descartes scholars point to inconsistencies, subtleties, and developments in his thinking about these relations.[43] Most obviously, writing of the passions in 1649, Descartes offers an account not substantially different from Burton's. But it has been pointed out that even in his earliest formulations, "thoughts" (*pensées*) for Descartes do not quite map onto what we would today regard as the contents of consciousness. And his

---

40. For these details, see essays in Wright and Potter 2000.
41. See Sutton 2000.
42. Of the particular harmony in much renaissance thinking on these matters, it has even been observed that both the quasi-bodily sensitive soul and the human mind can be said to "think," inviting a conclusion entirely compatible with today's cognitivism: They function together "as an information processing system" (Michael 2000:169).
43. For inconsistencies, see Robinson 2012; for subtleties and developments, see essays in Graukroger, Schuster, and Sutton 2000.

formulations reveal a recognition that sensations and feelings are anomalous.[44] Nonetheless as dualistic strands of modern philosophy and psychology during the eighteenth, nineteenth, and twentieth centuries, these characterizations came to prevail in the terms laid out in the 1641 *Meditations Concerning First Philosophy*. Of the two substances, mental and physical, the essence of body was extension, the essence of mind, thought. Thought in turn was defined in terms of what we can know through self-awareness. A thinking being is one "which doubts, which understands, which conceives, which affirms, which denies, which wills, which rejects, which imagines also, and which perceives," Descartes writes in the *Meditations* (Descartes 1960:85). What is *unthinking* is *matter*, by definition; and what is *thinking* is *mind*.[45]

For Burton, no such bifurcation between the thinking and unthinking, or conscious and unconscious, could be possible. The immortal soul

---

44. In Descartes' defense, Cottingham points out that even his early "official position" does not do justice to ways Descartes elsewhere qualified his stark dualism, with references to the "union" between soul and body. About sensation, for example, Descartes adds, "we perceive that sensation such as pain are not pure thoughts of a mind distinct from a body, but confused perceptions of a mind really united to a body" (from a private correspondence of 1542, quoted in Cottingham 1998:83). In reply to queries by Princess Elizabeth dated May 1643, he offers a tripartite division, comprising body, soul, and the union of the body and soul together, "on which depends our notions of the soul's power to move the body, and the body's power to act on the soul and cause its *sensations and passions*" (quoted in Cottingham 1998:85, emphasis added). And by the time he is writing the *Passions of the Soul* later that decade, Descartes speaks in Article 212 of the pleasures "common" to soul and body (Descartes 1961:210). Cottingham also challenges as a misreading the interpretation that the operations of the passions are transparent to their subject, explaining that for Descartes, "the causal genesis and subsequent occurrence of the passions is intimately linked to corporeal events in ways which often make the force of the resultant emotion opaque to reason" (Cottingham 1998:92). Questioned by Princess Elizabeth about the "substantial union" between mental and physical, Descartes acknowledges that some forms of human awareness (in sensations and emotions) "must not be referred either to the mind alone or to the body alone" (quoted in Cottingham 1998:85).
45. If, as John Sutton complains, in a "curious consensus" across analytic history of philosophy, medical anthropology, feminist theory, dynamicist cognitive science, and phenomenology, Descartes has become the "anti-magus, stripping nature and the body of all power and activity," so that his objectification of the body is "but one symptom of the mechanistic violation of an earlier enchanted world," then passages such as these in the *Meditations*, for all that they may misrepresent his position, are to blame. See Sutton 2000:697.

transcends and can be divorced from the bodily and mental, but body and mind are entwined. In a relationship that eludes precise definition, the passions and imagination are the site of this union. Each partakes of both the sensory and the intellectual. Employing a figure of speech from earlier writing on the passions by Thomas Wright, Burton speaks of our being "drowned in corporeall organs of Sense" (I,2,3,3:255). With his stringent division, Descartes may have been able to rid his *Meditations* system of "the middling, corporeal soul," as it has been put (Arikha 2007:221). But his particular preoccupations prevent Burton from doing so.[46]

THE IMAGINATION, REASON, AND THE PASSIONS

While it is also reflected in the work of some of his contemporaries, the roles assigned to the imagination constitute one of Burton's more singular contributions from the standpoint of contemporary mind sciences, and its place in Burton's scheme of things is the subject of the next chapter. The special bidirectional causal relationship linking the imagination and the passions explains this focus, together with the place of the imagination in classical, medieval, and renaissance accounts of psychic disorder: First and foremost, it is disordered imagination.

Burton's account of the normal functioning of the faculty of Imagination reflects Aristotle and medieval and renaissance Aristotelianism, as we saw, while allusions to the disordered imagination show the influence of the classical medical canon that he cites so extensively, as well the writing of the renaissance doctors. And the capabilities of the normal imagination hold the key to the disordered one. If this faculty is allowed to run free and goes unchecked—out of negligence, or a willful enjoyment of the fancies, delights and comforts it affords when it creates mental pictures in the absence of an object of sense impression—the imagination may eventually lead to serious

---

46. With his premodern cognitive architecture, Burton is unlikely to have recognized the contrast between conscious and unconscious mental states at all, this suggests.

illness. Haunted by the idea of the terror and distress such imaginary objects could produce and the multiplying fears they engender, Burton returns to these dangers again and again. His awareness that melancholy is "self-propagating and . . . terrifyingly tenacious" explains what has been described as a recurrent fear that "man's descent into disease may be unavoidable" (Tilmouth 2005:526).[47] Yet the imagination is as much solution as problem, since melancholy's causes and cures are each, and equally, attributable to it. The imagination will "work upon itself," to bring, or exacerbate, symptoms; but in comparable, or even greater, measure, it can also be employed to avoid, alleviate, and quell those symptoms.

Its relationship to the passions (or what we loosely call feelings or emotions) explains this power. From the Greek *pathé*, passions or affections are states *undergone*, in contrast to actions. The primary passions, appetites and fears, correspond to attraction and aversion, bringing pleasure and pain (or distress), respectively. The most important passions Burton describes as love, joy, desire, hatred, sorrow, and fear. The mind is endlessly affected, and disturbed, by these perturbations. They "trouble the phantasy," serving as a prompt for imaginative activity. And any of these feelings—but particularly fear and sadness or sorrow—when inappropriate to their object, or entertained too intensely, or long, can incite melancholy.[48]

The passions are ever present, and always dangerous. People often find themselves powerless in the face of their passions, "slaves to their several lusts and appetites"; of this Burton is not in doubt. There may be "some few discreet men" who can govern themselves, he admits, but most

---

47. These repetitive fears have been regarded as motivating the whole project, Burton's copious writing and prolixity a "frantic effort to . . . prove that mankind can be exempt from melancholy by demonstrating that he still retains a critical perspective over it . . . the means by which Burton tries to overwrite an anxiety about the uncontrollable expansiveness of his subject" (Tilmouth 2005:543).
48. Love also has its special role as instigator and symptom of melancholy, explored in the more literary Third Partition of the *Anatomy*, but it will not be dealt with in the present work.

suffer themselves wholly to be led by sense; and are so farre from repressing rebellious inclinations, that they give all encouragement to them ... they follow on, wheresoever their unbridled Affections will transport them, and doe more out of custome, selfe-will, than out of Reason. (I:2,3,4:256)

With these cares and perturbations, such men "continually macerate their soules" (I,2,3,4:256). What's more, the passions affect bodily states. They endanger health in other ways as well, but heat, cold, moisture and dryness being the qualities associated with the four humors, alterations in them are the primary emphasis. Thus, for example, anger

> heats the blood and vitall spirits, Sorrow on the other side refrigerates the body, and extinguisheth natural heat, overthrowes appetite, hinders concoction, dries up the temperature, and perverts the understanding. Feare dissolves the spirits, infects the heart, attenuates the soule. (II,2,6,1:100)

As well as causing a person to sweat, blush, tremble, blanch, and stagger, for example, the passions alter the temperature of the whole body, they cause the heart to expand, contract, and become heavy, and interfere with digestion. Examples are common, says Burton, of how sorrow causes "melancholy, desperation, and sometimes death it selfe" (I:2,3,4:258). Equally, the body can affect the passions, symptoms proceeding "from the Temperature, itself, and the Organicall parts, as Head, Liver, Spleene, Meseraicke veines, Heart, Wombe, stomacke, &c. and most especially from distemperature of Spirits" (I,3,1,3:397).

"IMAGINATIO... MISINFORMING THE HEART"

The relationship between feelings and other mental states and processes in this model involves complex, multicausal, multidirectional systems linking bodily to subjective states, with feedback from thought to feeling, and feeling to thought, themselves affected at every turn by changes in the humoral and other bodily states that mirror, but also sometimes alter, each mental element. The following description makes clear how imagination affects the passions and disturbs the humors:

> To our imagination commeth, by the outward sense or memory, some object to be knowne . . . which he mis-conceiving or amplifying, forthwith communicates to the Heart, the seat of all affections. The pure spirits flocke from the Braine to the Heart, by certaine secret channels, and signifie what good or bad object was presented; which immediately bends it selfe to persecute, or avoid it; and withall, draweth with it other humours to help it: so in pleasure, concurre great store of purer spirits; in sadnesse, much melancholy blood; in ire, choler. If Imagination be very apprehensive, intent, and violent, it sends great store of spirits to, or from the heart, and makes a deeper impression, and greater tumult, as the humours in the Body be likewise prepared, and the temperature it selfe ill or well disposed, the passions are longer and stronger. So that the first steppe and fountaine of all our grievances in this kinde, is . . . *Imaginatio*, which misinforming the Heart, causeth all these distemperatures, alteration and confusion of spirits and humors. (I,2,3,1:249)[49]

Whether stimulated by memory, imagination, or some immediate perception, a thought or representation occurs and is registered—but also, at the very start, interpreted, even distorted or misconstrued. This interpretation involves evaluative appraisal, and an emotional valence

---

49. Burton borrows from Thomas Wright's 1601 *Passions of the Mind in General* in other places as well, and the above account adopts not only Wright's causal analysis but also his words and phrases, without acknowledgment. Wright's wording is as follows: "First, then, to our imagination cometh by sense or memory some object to be known, convenient or disconvenient to Nature; the which being known . . . in the imagination, which resideth in the former part of the brain . . . , presently the purer spirits flock from the brain by certain secret channels to the heart, where they pitch at the door, signifying what an object was presented, convenient or disconvenient for it. The heart immediately bendeth either to prosecute it or to eschew it, and the better to effect that affection draweth other humours to help him; and so in pleasure concur great store of pure spirits; in pain and sadness, much melancholy blood" (T.Wright 1986:123).

or attitude: it incites approach or avoidance. Such information is conveyed to the heart by the animal spirits, and in response, the heart changes in size, expanding when the information has a positive valence. The stronger the imagination the more intense and disruptive are the person's affective attitudes about the thought, with their accompanying humoral and other bodily changes and action tendencies. Because of its special power to ignite emotions that in turn engender further bodily changes, the imagination can be seen to initiate these sequences. Burton goes on here to emphasize that it is thus the imagination, rather than any "distemperature of the body" that is the *cause* of melancholy – although other passages make clear that humoral states and tendencies, temporary and inborn, as well as additional bodily conditions, may also initiate such changes.

So this is a multicausal analysis, reflecting multidirectional sequences uniting the bodily with cognition through affective states. We return to Burton's complex system in chapter 3, when we see its implications for identifying the model of disease underlying this collection of ideas.

Notable in the account are several features, the most obvious being the centrality of the passions in affecting and reflecting bodily states, and mediating between the intellect—particularly the imagination, so attuned to affective responses—and the body. A second feature is the role of the imagination in affecting both feelings and bodily states. (Its special role in instigating and curing melancholy is discussed in later chapters.) Another is the way every representation or representational object is subject to immediate evaluation (by the heart) as appealing or aversive. And finally, although the anatomy of Burton's time had acknowledged the brain as the locus of executive functioning, the integration of mind with the corporeal is a whole-body affair, not limited to the brain. Humoral anatomy involved every bodily organ, as well as the animal spirits circulating, and mediating, between them. This is a view of cognition, albeit not one expressly articulated, where representation is distributed.[50]

50. Theories of "embodied cognition" similarly emphasize the causal and physically constitutive role in cognitive processing played by parts of the body other than the brain (Varela, Thompson, and Rosch 1991, Wilson and Foglia 2011, Gallagher and Zahavi

We also see contemporary intimations in the notion of representation involved in this transfer of information or "communication" by which the heart is "misinformed." When he speaks of "some object to be known," Burton's representational object carries no suggestion that these are nonbodily items, or the products, or exclusive objects, of conscious awareness. They are simply information, and entirely neutral as to either their ontological status or their status vis-à-vis the subject's awareness of them.

The *Anatomy*'s bare "cognitive" unconscious mind avoids the epistemic transparency often attributed to Cartesianism, where our thoughts are supposed fully available to us through no more than an act of attention.[51,52] And the heart itself, to which representations are communicated, illustrates further contrasts with Cartesianism. Primarily, and literally, we will be inclined to say, the heart is a bodily organ. Yet as the "seat" or center of the affective states, it is one deeply identified with those states, so that it is more than brute, unthinking matter. *I know, and feel, it in my heart,* we still say, but for Burton, the heart participates more directly in the knowing and feeling; somehow, more than metaphorically, it, too, knows and feels. This is not mind-body reductionism: Burton never doubts the duality of soul and body, for all that his soul is firmly embodied.[53] Yet the description approaches a more literal

---

2013). The assumption that cognitive processing occurs exclusively in the brain has been unseated by empirical studies of embodied experience (Wilson and Foglia 2011). While in some ways the *Anatomy*'s broadly Aristotelian account resembles models of cognition where discrete, internal representations are realized in underlying, functionally separated modules and highly specific brain mechanisms, the closer resemblance may be the dynamic interplay depicted by embodied cognitive science between neural and nonneural processes, and the convergence of cognition, bodily experience, and the larger social environment.

51. See Gardner 1993:207, Tauber 2010:146–7.
52. Again focusing on Descartes' later writing on the passions, Cottingham points out that with acknowledgement that we are embodied creatures must have come recognition that our emotional life has "serious and pervasive opacity," and cannot all be available to awareness (Cottingham 1998:93).
53. For a defense of Burton against interpretations that would expunge his dualism and *reduce* the mental to the bodily, see Gowland 2013. There was psychological materialism, but only as a complement to the equally important somatic spiritualism, as Gowland puts it, describing the ineluctably embodied dualism reflecting Burton's Aristotelian ideas.

interpretation. Cognitive linguistics asserts that human sense-making is underwritten by such metaphors, cognitive structures and processes that, emerging from our bodily and perceptual interaction with the world, influence inferences and judgments (Lakoff and Johnson 1999). And the Burtonian heart appears to work as a metaphor with just such extra metaphorical effects. Infamously, the pineal gland was the site of mind–body interaction for Descartes. It was an impossible choice, but so would any organ or any mental state have been, according to the carefully defined binaries by which, at least on the "official" doctrine announced in the *Meditations*, the mind and it alone was that which thinks, and the body that which is extended. By contrast, when the imagination "misinforms" the heart in the interaction Burton describes, he is saved, and we are caught, within such a web of associations that an entirely literal reading eludes us. On this point, Burton's confusing and perhaps ill-worked-out scheme may have anticipated the changes brought by cognitivist psychology's stripped-down conception of representation more successfully than the dualism derived from Descartes' *Meditations*.[54]

To illustrate where aspects of the *Anatomy* can be found in today's mind sciences, we may start with the centrality of the passions in affecting and reflecting bodily states, and mediating between the intellect and the bodily, described in the passage quoted on page 38. This observation is a commonplace today. It is neatly captured in an observation by the contemporary neuroscientist Antonio Damasio. The fabric of our minds and of our behavior, Damasio says, "is woven around continuous cycles of emotions followed by feelings that become known and beget new emotions, a running polyphony that underscores and punctuates specific thoughts in our minds and actions in our behavior" (2010:43).

The analogy between Burton's representations and the informational items in cognitive science can be illustrated using Joseph LeDoux's

---

54. At the "information-processing" level of cognitive science, within which most scientific hypotheses of cognitive psychology, traditional artificial intelligence, and connectionism are formulated, a person's cognitive properties (cognition broadly understood, that is) are theorized as a computational and representational system, where representations are symbolic structures with quasi-linguistic and combinatorial properties that act as vehicles of content. See Von Eckardt 2012.

well-known exploration of the relationship between the amygdala and the frontal lobes during states of fear. Fear is an apt example for us, since unwarranted and inappropriate fear constitute one of the two most common symptoms of melancholy described in the *Anatomy*. LeDoux is dealing with more universal states of fear, however: those we share with other creatures such as the laboratory rats he studied. And in this case, the trigger for the fear is some observed dangerous object in the external world, affecting sensory receptors—not an imaginary item, since we cannot find out what rats imagine if they do at all.[55] After sensory awareness of a dangerous or fearsome object is registered, Le Doux has shown how the amygdala, located in the medial temporal lobe, immediately gets involved, triggering a range of neural systems including a process of evaluation (as fearsome, dangerous, or safe), that is distinct from, and may precede, the eventual cortical activity allowing us to recognize and identify the feeling of fear and its object.[56] A "defensive motivational circuit" is initially generated, with direct input from the amygdala to the cortical areas, brain arousal, body feedback, and initiation of goal-directed behavior. That whole state may then be accompanied by *felt states of fear*, but the mechanisms of defensive motivational states are not those that generate the feelings themselves. Feelings of fear require more: the integration of thoughts and memories. This leads LeDoux to warn that the hardwired survival circuits responsible for defensive motivational states are not to be confused with the brain circuits that generate our conscious feelings of fear. (And that said, as we will see below, emotions may also arise from cognitive processes in a top-down fashion, without the involvement of motive state ingredients.[57])

BURTON, LEDOUX, AND DAMASIO

As the above passage from Damasio indicates, there are additional parallels between Damasio's analysis of the mind–body interactions and

---

55. Le Doux 2015.
56. Le Doux 1996, 2000, 2015.
57. LeDoux 2015.

the neural basis of feelings.[58] Other contemporary models would have served. I chose Damasio's because first, it recognizes the role of affective states in all cognition, and second, it offers a picture close to Burton's of the normal processes involved when feelings and affective disturbances are experienced. Damasio's account is also Jamesian (which Burton's is not). Feelings are construed as the felt end products of largely unfelt bodily processes, their objects include bodily sensations, and the whole system yields a sense of self. So, similarities with Burton's account lie not with the *outcome* of the processes involved, but only with the processes themselves.[59]

Four similarities between Damasio's and the *Anatomy* accounts are readily identifiable. The first we saw: Like Burton, Damasio accords a central place to affective states of feeling and emotion; they are core features of mental life, required alike for all higher cognition, decision-making, language, and social cognition. Second, they are tied to the systems of reward and punishment. In Damasio's words, "Emotions are the dutiful offspring of the value principle" (2010:115). These systems are neural for Damasio, located in the insular cortex, amygdala, and ventromedial prefrontal cortex; and for Burton, as we saw, their locus is the heart (with all the ambiguity that claim entails). The inevitable link with attraction and aversion then, not their location, constitutes the parallel.

Third, Damasio recognizes and stresses the tie between emotions and images, and thus the activities Burton identifies as the functions of the imagination. These both constitute the initial data to start the cascade of events resulting in emotions and feelings, and acknowledge the power of "imaginary" states to evoke emotions, through what are called "as if" loops. These "as if" loops occur in two ways, Damasio explains. Sometimes the body landscape is changed as the result of solely bodily signals; but by an alternative mechanism (the "as if body loop") the representation (of body-related changes) is "created directly in sensory body maps, under the control of other neural sites, for instance in the prefrontal cortices. It is as if the body had really been changed, *but it has*

---

58. These are recounted in two works: Damasio 1999 and 2012.
59. These outcomes have been subject to considerable criticism. See, for example, Block 2010.

not. "As if body loop" mechanism bypasses the body proper, partially or entirely." These "as if" mechanisms are important not only for emotion and feeling but also for "a class of cognitive processes *one might designate 'internal simulation'*" (Damasio 1999:281, emphasis added). Fitting his neo-Jamesian notion that the objects of emotions and feelings include bodily states and maps, Damasio depicts the representations acquired through this second route as "as if" *body* loops. And with the idea that the sole object of simulated representations was bodily states, Burton would have disagreed.[60] But as simulated representations that are in these cases the products of the prefrontal cortices, "as if loops" can be nothing other than Burtonian imaginings, and correspond, as we will see in the chapter following, to the simulated products of the attentional network known as the default network system. For the *Anatomy*, so focused on the products of the imagination in their tendency to unsettle and alter the passions, this acknowledgment of the part played by merely simulated ideas points to an important added parallel between these two accounts.

Fourth, like Burton, Damasio portrays affective states as emerging out of an elaborate, looping exchange between different systems (the "emotion-feeling cycle"), which begins with a stimulus from outside the mind, through sensory perception, or from within it, as in a memory, or an entirely imaginary object. It is processed in the visual cortices, and ends with a felt state accompanied by "the representation of the object that caused the emotion in the first place"—an awareness of bodily sensations, as well as of psychic feelings.

To assess the value of these loose equations between Burton's and Damasio's accounts, we need to stop for a moment on language, for Damasio's is not quite Burton's or that of our everyday speech, and it has its own peculiarities. First, the term "action," usually reserved for events occurring due to human intention, is employed indifferently by Damasio for conscious, mental events, and bodily ones that take place beneath conscious awareness. Also, Damasio makes a distinction, consistently recognized in neither everyday language nor the philosophy of

---

60. The representational content of Damasio's "as if loops" has been criticized more recently as well. See Ratcliffe 2008.

mind, between emotions and feelings. Emotions are defined as "automated programs of actions" (read "events") together with "certain modes of cognition." (His notion of the automated programs refers to the preestablished cognitive and attitudinal "set," within which any new data must be accommodated.) Thus, when images of objects (real or imagined) affect several emotion-triggering brain regions or functions, chemical and endocrinal changes are produced. Then, after a millisecond delay, "certain thoughts come to mind"—the thoughts that are the conscious emotion. Feelings, by contrast, are understood to be perceptions of what happens in our body *and mind* "when we're emoting." They are close to William James' notion of emotions, as Damasio recognizes, although he wants to add to James' account. Not only the "perceptual readout of the bodily state" (James' idea) and a preset cognitive component (that is the "automated program" introduced above) must be included, but also "the representation of the object that caused the emotion in the first place" (Damasio 1999:127). (This feature of Damasio's account of feelings has been the subject of criticism; however Burton's casual and all-encompassing conception of the passions prevents us from assigning him a place within these debates.[61]) So one aspect of this contrast between emotions and feelings is that for Damasio emotions (together with the representations that they comprise) take place beneath conscious awareness, whereas feelings—since *unfelt feelings* seems a contradictory category—are conscious states. LeDoux encounters a similar issue of vocabulary, it should be added. Even the term "emotion" is so inextricably entwined with conscious feelings, he concludes, that to use it in any other way invites confusion: Instead he will speak of the fearful states he describes as "the mental states that people experience when they face situations in which survival is challenged or enhanced" (LeDoux 2015:98).

Apart from Damasio's separation of feelings and emotions, which Burton could have accommodated, and about which the *Anatomy* remains uncommitted, there is at first sight one significant difference between its multidirectional looping effects and Damasio's model.

---

61. For criticisms of Damasio on feelings see Ratcliffe 2008:108–10.

A millisecond delay between the initial stimulus and the felt state, together with the language of "cascade," indicate that Damasio's is a unidirectional causal flow. First comes the stimulus, then the brain and bodily events ("actions"), and finally the conscious cognitive states and feelings. By contrast, Burton's causal flow is multidirectional, from mind to body as well as body to mind. Yet even this inconsistency proves less than it at first seems. Damasio also emphasizes the effects that take place when "as if" loops occur as the result of *simulated* ideas or representations that produce the same reactions, similarly initiating unidirectional "cascades." Not only outer perception but also internally directed thoughts generate such causal sequences, those thoughts often triggering further thoughts in elaborate feedback systems. Apparently confirming this idea in later work (2010), Damasio acknowledges that new thoughts are prompted by the emotion *as it emerges.*

So here is a description that matches the multidirectional causal loops described by Burton. Of "thoughts prompted by the ongoing emotion," Damasio explains,

> [some thoughts] . . . are components of the emotion program, evoked as the emotion unfolds so that the cognitive context is in keeping with the emotion. *Other thoughts, however,* rather than being stereotypical components of the emotion program, *are late cognitive reactions to the emotion under way. The images evoked by these reactions end up being part of the feeling percept* along with the representation of the object that caused the emotion in the first place, the cognitive component of the emotion program, and the perceptual readout of the body state. (2010:127, emphasis added)

Once the emotion event is begun, this implies, it is altered not merely by the neurobiology that makes it possible, but by attitudes toward it that take place in the conscious mind. In this way, there will be involved a form of feedback loop.

LeDoux's analysis of the sequence between initial stimulus and felt state is similarly unidirectional in what he takes to be the prototypical bottom-up cases of fear, those that are adaptations we share with other primates. But there are also top-down fears that more closely correspond to Damasio's "late cognitive reactions to the emotions under way." LeDoux allows that while emotions resulting from nonconscious motive states emerge into consciousness in bottom-up fashion, they can also be built from cognitive processes in a top-down way without the involvement of motive state ingredients. Compassion, pride, and shame are named as examples of such feelings, arising, as he says, from an assessment of our circumstances. And even fears, if they are intellectual (his examples include the fear of failing in life), might eventually depend on top-down processes, rather than in every case emerging as a result of external stimuli (LeDoux 2015).

The sequences involved in Damasio's "late cognitive reactions to the emotion under way," and the processes generating LeDoux's top-down emotions, seem very similar. And each would be compatible with the whirl of feeling, thinking, and imagining making up Burtonian feedback loops. Many of the *Anatomy*'s references to looping effects are invoked to explain the repetition associated with entrenched melancholia, when these systems are imbalanced, rather than the ordinary course of mental life depicted by Damasio and implied by LeDoux's animal studies. But Burton's normal psychology is not different: Normal states also "beget one another and tread in a ring," as he says of sorrow and melancholy (I,2,3,4:256). All feelings are affected by the workings of the imagination, whether these are defective or normal interactions, and all imagining similarly prompts feelings.

Unlike Burton, Damasio limits his focus to normal emotions and feelings.[62] Yet the ingredients he describes may also accommodate the imbalanced and dysfunctionally habituated frames of mind that Burton explores in depicting how disordered imagination and feeling, and careless and self-indulgent cognitive habits, together yield the recalcitrant moods and fears afflicting the melancholic. LeDoux more explicitly acknowledges abnormal states. The mechanisms underlying the genesis and maintenance of aberrant and pathological fear and anxiety, he conjectures, will also lie with implicit and nonconscious states: "hyper responsiveness to threat stimuli due to overactive defensive survival and motivational circuits" (LeDoux 2015:104).

---

62. He also studies deficit and abnormality, although cases from the neurological clinic, not the psychiatric one, have been the basis of his inferences about normal functioning.

Burton's attention is primarily directed toward where these interactive systems fail. There, imagination (too intense and prodigious) and the will (too weak) result not merely in the disruptions and looping systems that, as he says, are our human lot, but in the chronic melancholic's endless, habituated miseries. Nonetheless, the broad similarities uniting Burton's analysis with these contemporary ones are evident.

Tracing to Aristotle, and to medieval and renaissance Aristotelianism, Burton's faculty psychology frames the embodied mind. But his starting point is also the long canon of medical writing about melancholy. Together these two sources shape his mind–body interactionism, which differs significantly from the versions of substance dualism that came to dominate modern philosophy and psychology until the last decades of the twentieth century. Some of these differences make Burton's model of mind more fitting than the later ones for cognitivist models. Moreover, as the work of the neuroscientists Damasio and LeDoux introduced here illustrates, there are similarities between Burton's account and contemporary neuroscience—both as they stress the involvement of affective states in all cognition and in the complex interactions between felt states and brain activities. If these contemporary models have currency, then Burton's very similar system may warrant our attention.

That sorrow and grief can be cause and symptom of melancholy explains one part of the causal order depicted in the *Anatomy*, as we'll see. And sometimes, if the sorrow "takes root" or finds a ready temperament, the body's (humoral) temperature will foster new sadness in an endless circle. This apparently happens when an earlier distress has permanently altered the person, introducing what might be deemed a persisting enhanced risk factor. (One sufferer is described whose earlier melancholy left him prone to subsequent attacks incurred by only "the smallest occasion of sorrow" [I,2,3,4:258].) More commonly though, Burton depicts melancholy symptoms as the sole result of the whirling mix of feelings and humoral temperatures allied with a dangerously powerful or insufficiently disciplined imagination, that have been allowed to grow, incrementally, into a habit.

Chapter 2

Imagination "queen of the mental powers"

The centrality of the Imagination and imagining for Burton's analysis of Melancholy are boldly and unequivocally stated in several passages. "I may certainly conclude," one of these begins,

> [that] this strong conceit or imagination, is *astrum hominis*, the rudder of this our ship, which reason should steire, but overborne by phantasie, cannot manage, and so suffers it selfe and this whole vessel of ours to be overruled, and often overturned. (I,2,3,2:254)

As the rudder of our vessel, imagination and imagining join thought and feeling within the hectic, multicausal and multidirectional interactive network making up Burton's normal and abnormal psychology alike. In this chapter we consider the first of these, the ways in which Burton's expansive and powerful faculty of imagination functions in all of us, including its particular role and potential to influence healing and self-care. Burton's intense focus on the imagination finds parallels throughout the mind sciences, particularly in their recognition of the centrality of default network systems as part of normal cognition, in a range of parallels with the category of simulation, and in findings from the science of expectation anticipated in the *Anatomy*'s focus on the use of the imagination for self-healing.

ANCIENT AND MEDIEVAL SOURCES

Although derived from a composite of received ideas, appeals to the imagination in the *Anatomy* can lay claim to real originality. That composite includes three, in particular. First, as the Passions, feelings are the central focus of the canon on melancholy that Burton derives from ancient medical lore, and feelings in turn bear a special relationship to the imagination: Each is somehow prone to affect the other in an unending causal sequence. In addition, the *Anatomy* account develops and consolidates the role of imagining as depicted in earlier renaissance medical works, where the ancient stress on the disordered imagination of mental disorder is emphasized and elaborated. In medieval lore the melancholic imagination is a point of vulnerability to demonic influence, and even when that idea had been naturalized, the imagining faculty remains at the center in depictions of disturbed and abnormal psychic life. And finally, the activity of imagining also holds a special place, we'll see, because it is integrated into the remedial and preventive efforts that form the practical side of the *Anatomy*. In conditions whose characteristic symptoms are aberrant mood states and imaginings, our imagination is our best means of regulating our feelings. These ideas about the imagination's normal functioning each have descendants within today's mind sciences. Some of the assumptions, categories, and concepts employed today, as well as recent findings made possible by new ways to observe the brain, are illustrated in this chapter while the disordered imagination is dealt with in chapters 5 and 6.

The litany of causes of melancholy among the daily habits involving diet, air, rest, and the like is interrupted in the *Anatomy* for a full subsection devoted to the "Force of Imagination," this "brief Digression" justified because imagination "hath so great a stroke in producing this maladie [Melancholy], and is so powerfull of it selfe" (I,2,3,2:249). Its power to heal, as well as concern over the disturbed imagination, and the runaway, delusional notions and imaginings of those who are severely afflicted with melancholy, together accord this faculty its dominant place in Burton's "anatomizing." But understood first as a normal capability, the imagination is presented as a faculty with widely varying, powerful effects in any person. In some, these *become*, and in most if not all they *threaten to become*, harmfully disordered. Of the unhealthy kind of imagination, Burton says,

> the first step and fountain of all our grievances is a disordered imagination, which, misinforming the heart, causeth all these distemperatures, alteration and confusion of spirits and humours. (I,2,3,1:249)

Through this dangerous faculty, our feelings become disturbed—disturbance further reflected in humoral imbalance and other bodily disorder. Thus, imagining, at once admirable and dangerous, is the key element in the dynamic interaction between mind and body. Janus-faced, it permits Burton's model to encompass in equal measure not only the sensory and the intellectual—from its place within the sensitive (sensible) soul—but also normal and abnormal mental life.

Ideas about the imagination (or phantasy) from Aristotle remained almost unchanged when adopted by the medieval thinkers, including the Persian and Arab physicians like Avicenna and Rhazes, whom Burton appeals to so liberally.[1] His favorites, the Hellenistic philosophers, were the exception in this orthodoxy. Diverging from Aristotle's *phantasia*, their notions reflected the atomism associated with Lucretius (c. 99–50 BCE), whose poem *De Rerum Natura* describes the constant motion among the clusters of atoms constituting objects in the world around us. The surface atoms are *eidola* or *simulacra* that, faithful to the form of the objects from which they emanate, cause images of the things we perceive.[2] If the *Anatomy* can be said to reflect any influence

---

1. In the First Partition alone, Avicenna is cited almost as frequently as Aristotle, and Rhazes is cited more. After the twelfth century CE, Aristotelianism had become the dominant philosophy of the Western world. Even with the turn against Aristotelian ideas accompanying the emergence of modern science, Aristotle's views about imagery continued to be influential. The impact on later thinkers of Aristotle's account of cognition in general, and of imagery and imagination in particular, it has been stressed, was enormous, and extended far beyond those who were avowed Aristotelians to thinkers like Hobbes and Descartes (Thomas 2014).
2. As well as *De Rerum Natura*, where they are found in Book IV, 54–238, these ideas are also in Epicurus, *Letter to Herodotus*.

of the flying simulacra, it is not in an imagistic conception of imagining, for Burton is not wedded to these analogies with visual impressions and images. It is rather seen in the ceaseless movement, wherein atoms collide, re-form, and intermingle in an endless, dizzying vortex. Similar incessant movement occurs in Burton's model of mind, seemingly more dynamic than Aristotle's, where imaginings affect thought, feeling, and humoral temperature in a confusion of ever-changing rearrangements. Despite his affinity for the Hellenistic philosophers, however, Burton for the most part adheres to the older ideas, wherein Imagination is one of the three inward parts of the apprehensive faculty comprising the sensible soul. These ideas themselves are not always entirely clear, and Burton's account inherits their obscurity.

Aside from Aristotle and Aristotelianism, renaissance medical thinking also provides an important source for the *Anatomy* discussions, particularly the work of Du Laurens, and to a lesser extent that of Weyer, Plater, and their contemporaries. Du Laurens, like Burton, stresses that the imagination is inevitably disturbed in melancholia, whereas reason may, but need not, be damaged or defective, a distinction quite widely accepted among the renaissance accounts of melancholy.[3,4] (It is part of the analysis provided by both Weyer and Bright, for example.) Burton in one passage actually separates "diseases of Imagination" from "diseases of Reason itself" (I,1,1,3:131).[5] So imagining might be seen implicated in Melancholy in two separable ways. It is the commonest initial cause

---

3. "All melancholike persons have their imagination troubled . . . they have also very often their reason corrupted" (Du Laurens 1599:87).
4. For example, the English physician Andrew Boorde (1490–1549) in his 1547 work *The Breviarie of Health* writes, "This sicknes is named the melancholy madness which is a sicknes full of fantasies, thinking to here or to see that thing that is not heard nor seene, and a man hauing this madness, shal thinke in himself that thing that can never be, for some bee so fantasticall that they will thinke themselfe God or as good, on such lyke thinges pertaining to presumption or to desperation to be dampned, the one hauing this sicknes doth not go so farre the one way, but the other doth dispayre as much the other way" (Boorde 1547: fol 78r).
5. Out of diseases of the Head, he explains, "I will single such as properly belong to the Phantasie, or Imagination, or Reason it selfe, which Laurentius calls the diseases of the mind" (I,1,1,3:131). His diction is confusing, but that last plural suggests a separation between diseases of the imagination and those affecting reasoning.

of melancholy symptoms and, as a faculty, the locus of the defect characterizing them. An overfecund imagination can bring about the subsequent "corruption" of the faculty, when it ceases to function as it should in some more extreme and chronic way.

Also shared with the renaissance doctors is the emphasis on how these melancholy symptoms vary from person to person, as well as from time to time within any given person.[6] Like Du Laurens, Burton enumerates at length the variety of individual delusions that result from a troubled imagination. It is an enumeration largely reproducing earlier medical lore, where the fear of having swallowed a serpent, the notion one is a fragile container that might be dropped or broken, and belief one is dead were much-quoted, stock examples, apparently far removed from clinical observation. They can be found in Plater as well, with little variation. And Burton shamelessly resorts to all the same tales, with and without attribution.

Although agreeing that melancholy reflects a disturbed imagination, Du Laurens' account differs from that of the *Anatomy*'s. For him, melancholy symptoms are primarily attributed to disturbances in the humoral states themselves (the cold, dry black bile), when these *in turn* affect the faculties of the mind, continually presenting the imagination with "blacke forms and strange visions," as he puts it.[7] This is a significant difference. Du Laurens allows the humors to cause the distorted and troubled imaginings, while for Burton, as we saw in chapter 1, imagination "hath so great a stroke in producing this maladie" it usually *initiates* the causal chain, as the *"first step* and fountain of all our grievances." (I,2,3,1:249, emphasis added).

---

6. "The imagination of melancholike men bringeth forth such diversitie of effects, according to the difference of the matters whereabouts it is occupied, as that a man shall scarse find five or sixe among ten thousand, which dote after one and the same maner" (Du Laurens 1599:96).
7. Du Laurens 1599:91. His position is somewhat ambiguous, however. Hints that the imagination may be the sort of initial prompt Burton describes (the "first step and fountain") may lie in the suggestion that not "the disposition of the bodie" but the "maner of living, and of such studies as they bee most addicted unto," explains the condition of melancholy folk, and in the notion (attributed to Plato) that "the greatest part of the mischiefs that fall upon the bodie, doe come from the minde" (Du Laurens 1599:98, 107).

Bright emphatically denies this order of things: The passion "is not moved by an adversity present or imminent" but is solely caused by the humor, in being "without externall occasion." Perhaps to secure the contrast between melancholy suffering *without cause* and the sense of sin ("the greatest cause that worketh misery upon men"), this leads Bright to emphasize the distinction. Melancholy ("this passion") is solely caused by the humor, "polluting both the substance, and spirites of the braine, causeth it without externall occasion, to forge monstrous fictions" (Bright 1995:99). Burton's insistence that imagination was at the beginning of the sequence resulting in melancholy is repeated, with considerable emphasis.[8] (Occasional allusions are also made to the role of the Devil, and to the place of original sin, in this causal sequence. Burton accepts that the Devil at least works through, or by way of, the imagination, however.[9])

The prominence accorded to the imagination is particularly notable, but far from exclusive to Burton's account. The salience of this faculty is a mark of the early modern period. And emphasis on the normal imagination was matched, if not exceeded, by a great fascination with the diseased imagination.[10] Once known as "queen of the mental powers," and long thought at the root of the disordered mind, the imagination's importance eventually declined—but not until after Burton's time.[11] His was the Age of the Imagination. This prominence derived in part from the occultism and astrological ideas of the sixteenth century. In the writings of Paracelsus and Ficino and their followers, the customary view of imagination as a bridge between material things and the immaterial soul permitted the immaterial soul to affect the material world through occult means. Were the effects of the imagination a merely natural pathology, it

---

8. On this matter, Plater is closer to Burton in acknowledging exogenous as well as endogenous causes (he names receiving a fright, and the death of loved ones, as causes).
9. Another renaissance authority, Biarmannus (1595–1620), is quoted with approval: "[The Devil] *beginnes first with the phantasie, & moves that so strongly, that no reason is able to resist*. Now the *Phantasie* he moves by mediation of humours: although many Physitians are of opinion that the Divell can alter the minde, and produce the disease himselfe" (I,2,1,2:193).
10. Haskell 2011:4–6.
11. See Berrios 2011:xiv. This decline led to a crisis for psychiatry, it has been argued: With it, new explanations for mental disorder needed to be sought (Berrios 2011).

was asked, or were preternatural or supernatural factors involved?[12,13] Burton acknowledges such ideas, remaining noncommittal although not dismissive. He is wary, as the widespread controversies surrounding them would have required him to be, historians have pointed out. And this may partly explain the carefully skeptical attitude he conveys.

Added emphasis on the corruption of the imagination in aberrant mental states, as we saw, also reflected a long association, originating with classical writing but reinvigorated through medieval Christian thought. As the devil's bath (*Balneum Diaboli*), the free play of the melancholy imagination was the point of moral vulnerability: "the Divell spying his opportunity of such humours drives [the melancholy sufferer] . . . many times to despaire, fury, rage &c. mingling himself amongst those humours" (I,2,1,2:193). (Because such considerations can have no place in modern science, these alleged causes can be dispensed with in the present analysis.)

As well as a source of mental disorder, the imagination is a faculty of almost unequaled importance, power, and value, and here too, Burton mirrors the attitudes widespread in his own times.[14] The "wonderful effects and power" of a "strong conceit" are lauded.[15] And he is alert to the countless creative efforts, momentary and sustained, important and unimportant, from daydreams to artistic and scientific works of genius, that stem from the imagination. (Du Laurens is similarly laudatory.[16]) The striking capacities and prodigious effects of this faculty are

12. Gowland 2006:90–91.
13. Occultist alternatives to the conventional Galenic theory available from the mid-sixteenth century onward included the ideas of Neoplatonism, with its confusing array of spirits intermediate between God and man: "multitudinous orders of creatures airy and semi-divine," to which astral powers were attributed. Opinions as to whether they were corporeal or incorporeal, mortal or immortal, and the extent of their power, however, varied widely (Kocher 1953:119). Burton knew of these ideas through thinkers like Ficino and Paracelsus, who, while explaining melancholy as an excess of "vital spirit" in the brain, also invoked the influence of planets and supernatural spirits. (For a discussion of these theories, see Gowland 2006.)
14. See Haskell (2011), who links the prominence of imagination to the decline of Aristotelianism.
15. I,2,3,2:250.
16. Of the imagination, he says, "I have set it in rank amongst the excellentest and noblest powers of the mind. The Arabians have so highly recommended it, that they have verily believed, that the mind by virtue of the imagination could work miracles, pearce the heavens, command the elements, lay plain the huge mountains, and make mountains of the plain ground . . . that which is called imagination is the first faculty or power of the mind" (Du Laurens 1599:75–6).

a recurrent theme. "How many Chimaeras, Anticks, golden mountains and Castles in the Aire doe they build unto themselves?" Burton asks, answering:

> I appeale to Painters, Mechanicians, *Mathematicians*. (I,2,3,2:251)

In Poets and Painters, it is noted, Imagination "forcibly workes, as appeares by their severall fictions, Antickes, Images" (I,1,2,7:152).

Some of these creative products come from continual and strong meditation; others indicate a faculty that is deficient, damaged, or disordered. Imagination is eminent in all people, as he says, yet

> most especially it rageth in melancholy persons, in keeping the species of objects so long, mistaking, amplifying them by continuall and strong meditation, untill at length it produceth reall effects, causeth this and many other maladies. (I,2,3,2:250)

In fact, the Imagination can be said to play no less than four different parts within the Burtonian mental economy. There are: (i) the imaginative capabilities so unsurpassingly valuable in scientific, scholarly, and artistic matters; (ii) the useful imagination that can be employed to balance and regulate our passions; (iii) the prodigious but damaged imagination associated with frankly delusional thinking; and (iv) the initially enjoyable but dangerous tendencies toward idle daydreaming and rumination that may lead to severe, chronic melancholy, but are at first within our power to curb.

DEFINITION

Imagination is defined as

> an inner sense, which doth more fully examine the species perceaved by common sense, of *things present or absent*, and keepes

them longer, recalling them to mind, again, or *making new of his owne*. (I,1,2,7:152, emphasis added)

The phrase "things ... absent" is elaborated: "things to come, past, absent, such as were before in the sense." In addition to objects that are as we say "imaginary"—counterfactual or nonexistent—then, the objects of hope or expectation are products of the imagination, as are those of remembering.[17] Dreams and nightmares are explained by nothing more than insignificant bodily machinations: a "concourse of bad humours." When we sleep, also, he explains,

> this faculty is free, & many times conceaves strange, stupend [stupendous], absurd shapes, as in sick men we commonly observe. (I,1,2,7:152)

Unfettered, and disordered, imagination thus produces dreams and delusional states, respectively. The acknowledgment of the parallels between dreaming and delusions follows a long tradition, to which we return in chapter 6. But that aside, there is much in this brief definition that helps us understand Burton's faculty of the imagination. It is a conception with considerable similarities to our contemporary folk psychological ideas and even to the more "propositional" imagination associated with the cognitive turn in psychology, where imaginings are more often portrayed in terms of "data" than sensory images. The early modern imagination has been described as "first and foremost an image-producing factory" (Haskell 2011:6). But Burton's account is eclectic, and his occasional use of "representation" in this context roughly matches, and accommodates, the term of art it has become.[18] The many examples of the mistaken ideas and notions entertained by melancholy sufferers make evident that not only sensory, image-based

---

17. The same range of capabilities is attributed to imagination by Du Laurens.
18. See Von Eckhert 2012.

imaginings but also less sensory propositional ones are encompassed by his conception.[19] Nor does he employ the distinction between "productive" imagination, and that which is merely mimetic, or "reproductive," important in eighteenth-century writing; his is a capacity that is both creative and mimetic.

Several features of Burton's definition confirm these parallels with today's ideas about imagining as it is understood in normal cognitive functioning. There is a great deal of contemporary interest in and research about the imagination that bears on this definition as well, mirroring the central place Burton assigns to it in all mental processing. In order to see these parallels, we need to recognize what is little more than a shift in vocabulary: Today's *simulation* is a descendant category. Simulating and imagining are used as equivalents in the mind sciences. Like imagining, "simulating" encompasses the activities associated with *pretending*. (Within the study of social cognition, the activity of simulation has a narrower, although consistent, focus in being particularly identified with imagining oneself in another person's situation.) Imagination and simulation are used as rough equivalents in what follows, then, and enable us to see several features of Burton's definition shared with present day accounts of imagining and simulating.

(i) Burton's account emphasizes the freedom of the imagination in that we can imagine (or simulate) almost anything, including all manner of absurd notions: Thus unconstrained, imagining takes counterfactual and nonexistent objects ("things absent"), allowing us to shift independently each separate element or variable making up an image or idea in order to envision alternatives, actual and merely possible. While still subject to orderly chains of inference, normal exercises of the imagination, at least, are freely and willfully engaged in. Unlike believing, imagination is "at the whim of our intentions," as it has been put. "We typically decide when to engage in an imaginative episode, and in many ways we can also control the particular

---

19. For the view that the primary way to look at imagination is as an image producer, see Brann 1991, McGinn 2004.

contents that we imagine." Moreover, although flexible in some ways as a result of this freedom, imagination often follows orderly inference chains, so that when, for example, "I read that Wilbur is a pig, I infer (in imagination) that Wilbur is a mammal" (Nichols 2006:7). The phenomenology of such willful imagining frequently includes a sense of agency—of directing, even creating, our own thoughts.[20] This sensed freedom to imagine admits of qualifications in nondeliberate, spontaneous imaginings, both welcome and unwelcome.[21] In the case of unbidden thoughts, or the unwelcome memories or "flashbacks" suffered by trauma victims, this sense of agency is absent. The *Anatomy* also acknowledges something close to these in the repetitive, unwelcome, and seemingly unfree thoughts that come to afflict the melancholic, as we'll see.

(ii) Remembered objects are not experienced as freely chosen in quite the same way as those we experience in moments of deliberate reverie either, yet *forms of remembering are included in Burton's capacious definition*. Like its descendent conception of simulation, imagination is understood very broadly in the *Anatomy*. Not only remembering, and the "castles in the air" and false, impossible, improbable, and counterfactual ideas, but also conjectures, speculations, daydreams, and "conceits" are part of its functioning. So are dreams and nightmares, mental images (broadly understood to include not only visual images and sounds but also imagined sensations of touch, taste, and smell), artistic and intellectual creations, fantasies, and hypotheses.

Traditional faculty psychology separates remembering from imagining, and processes of memory have often been distinguished from imagining within modern psychology and philosophy, based partly on the kind of phenomenological differences noted in (i). But the inclusion of remembering as part of imagining is independently noteworthy. Spurred by recent observations within science, the inclusion of remembering among the functions of the imagination has begun to make a new

---

20. For a description of that sense of agency, see Pacherie 2010, Gallagher 2012.
21. Walton 1990.

kind of sense. Imaginative constructions of hypothetical events or scenarios share neural pathways with the activities involved in remembering the past, for example.[22] Indeed, whether temporality plays the part long thought to distinguish remembering the past from envisioning the future, or conceiving of any other hypothetical state, has itself come under new scrutiny as the result of advances in our ability to observe brain functioning. On the "nontemporal perspective," the activity previously attributed to simulating future events, it has been asserted, is better characterized as simulating *imagined* events, thus serving to emphasize the link between memory and imagination or simulation.[23] In support of this nontemporal perspective, activation of the same network systems has been observed not only when people remember (the past) but also when they simulate the future. Moreover, almost identical patterns of network activity occur, for example, when subjects have been asked to imagine merely hypothetical events that did not, but *might have occurred* in the past, as appear when they recall actual events.[24] In further support of Burton's capacious category of imagination, what's more, this activation of the same network also occurs in related forms of mental simulation (taking the perspective of others, spatial navigation, and imagining novel scenes).[25] Phenomenological differences between imagining, simulating, and remembering, such as those noted above, have been found to make use of the same cognitive substrates, although in subtly different ways.[26] More generally, though, Burton's inclusion of remembering

---

22. Schacter et al. 2012. "a common . . . network, commonly referred to as the default network . . . underlies both remembering and imagining" (Schacter et al. 2012:677). See Schacter et al. 2007, Buckner and Carroll 2007.
23. Schacter et al. 2012.
24. Addis et al. 2009. When participants imagined both future and past events in order to disambiguate whether future-event-specific activity found in previous studies was related specifically to *prospection* or a general demand of *imagining* episodic events, two subsystems were observed within the core network, one associated with imagining both future and past events, suggesting that "regions previously associated with future events, such as anterior hippocampus, medial prefrontal cortex and inferior frontal gyrus, support processes general to imagining events rather than specific to prospection" (Addis et al. 2009:2222).
25. See Buckner and Carroll 2007, Spreng et al. 2009, Hassabis et al. 2007.
26. Anderson et al. 2012.

among the functions of the faculty of the imagination finds considerable confirmation in these recent findings from neuroscience.

The broad category is consonant with many present-day observations pointing to cognitive capacities whose outcomes we might have hitherto regarded as stemming from separate mental activities. A notable example is known as "scene construction," an activity hypothesized as required for both memory and imagination (simulation). Scene construction involves retrieving and integrating perceptual, semantic, and contextual information and framing it within a coherent spatial context.[27] Like the Burtonian imagination, scene construction is also a hybrid, comprising imaging, imagining or simulation, and memory.

Burton's category of imagination, and the similarly broad simulation, each include entertaining mental images. Gone are the days when the fact that mental images were difficult to accommodate within a scientific conception of mind led to attempts to explain away their existence, and the phenomenon of imagining *excluded* such "ontologically dubious entities" (Kind 2001:85).[28] Present-day research postulates that tokens of a single distinct cognitive attitude account for both imaginative speculations and mental images.[29] The visual cortex is activated when one creates a visual image just as when one sees something in the outer world, for example.[30] More generally, recent neuroscience has vindicated imaging, and shown the important role it plays in cognition. Scans have established that the same areas and systems implicated when real touch, smell, or sight are involved are also affected when images of these experiences are entertained.[31] As a result of brain anatomy and

---

27. See Hassabis and Maguire 2007, 2009, Summerfield et al. 2010.
28. Kind's attention is particularly on, as she says, "putting the image back in imagination," when the formation of images is not only one form of imagining, as Burton supposed, but also essential to it. This specificity thus leaves her work without immediate relevance to our discussion.
29. A growing trend has been observed toward positing that "there exists one ... DCA (Distinct Cognitive Attitude), tokens of which play the role played by imaginative thoughts and mental images" (Schroeder and Matheson 2006:24).
30. Kosslyn et al. 1999.
31. See Yoo et al. 2003 for touch, Bensafi et al. 2003 for smell, Laeng and Teodorescu 2001, for sight; also Madan and Singhal 2012.

function, it has been observed, emotions will likely evoke images, and the images that form will in turn affect emotions.[32] Not only constructing but also viewing actual (nonmental) images, it should be added, is similarly associated with strong emotional responses.[33]

Imagery-based accounts of imagination were long presupposed in spiritual exercises employing guided imaging to bring about affective states.[34] By contrast, attention to imaging has come late to science and psychology.[35] New technologies, particularly the ability to scan brains, combined with the voluntary nature of controlled imaging, have made guided imaging an ideal subject for the brain sciences. Burton only understood the second of these elements, yet his inclusion of imaging as part of the function of the imagination leaves his account consistent with these present-day developments.

(iii) Although our imaginings and simulations sometimes prompt or direct action, they are often motivationally inert and do not play the regular "behavior-guiding" role associated with beliefs. For example, neither young children engaging in fantasy play, nor adults reading fiction, fantasizing, or daydreaming are typically inclined to act on their imaginings at all.[36] Burton captures this aimless aspect of imagining

---

32. Recent work on affect and imagery includes Holmes, Lang, and Deeprose 2009, Holmes 2013, Murphy et al. 2015, Blackwell et al. 2013, and Moscovitch et al. 2013. One such study confirms that mental images are both "more emotionally arousing and more likely to be confused with real events than are verbal descriptions" (Matthews 2013:229). See also Pictet et al. 2011, Perecman 2012, Segal et al. 2012. Similarly, forming an image of an emotional scenario has been shown to be accompanied by bodily signs of the emotion envisaged (Winkelman et al. 2015).
33. Perecman 2012, and Segal et al. 2012.
34. See St. Ignatius 1964, and for that history, Hadot 1995.
35. The controlled use of images to ease pain symptoms in several different disorders, including depression, dates only to the last decades of the twentieth century. The Center for Mind-Body Medicine, founded by doctors at Massachusetts General Hospital in the 1990s, is one center for this practice. The success of *guided imaging*, where the subject is asked to envision or otherwise invoke an image using the sense modalities of touch, smell, or sight, lies with its proven effects on stress levels, immune system functioning, and mood. An account of this practice is found in Gordon 2008. For anatomical and neuroscience explanations of the particular causal relationships linking image and feeling, see Brown 2008, Crowther 1983, Yoo et al. 2005, Bakke et al. 2002, Stetter and Kupper 2002, Collins and Dunn 2005.
36. Nichols 2006:7.

when he refers, as we still do today, to thoughts, fantasies and conceits as *idle*. And this idleness, as we will see, is as dangerous for him as the idleness of listless physical inertia.

(iv) The mental activities making up Burton's eclectic category of imagination involve attention that is for the most part inwardly directed. When we daydream, just as when we dream while asleep, our attention is toward the objects of our thought or images, not the world around us. This feature locates his category within the "default" network system in the brain, identified within recent work, that is defined by patterns of rest, or deactivation, during goal-directed tasks. (Once focus is directed away from outward, goal-directed tasks to inner activities, it has been pointed out, this definition is less useful, since thoughts can be inner-focused yet goal-directed (mental arithmetic, for example).)[37,38] The category derives from the observation that two inversely related and coregulated attentional brain networks are distinguishable, the one characterized by states directed toward external stimuli and focused on goal-directed, outward activity, and the other freer, internally directed, and less stimulus dependent.[39] The "resting" or "task negative" system has been widely assigned the title of "default network."[40] The ensuing thoughts are said to be "decoupled," "task-unrelated," and may involve the "mental time travel" associated with remembering the past and envisioning the future. The speculating, conceiving, imagining, and daydreaming attributed to the faculty of the imagination in the *Anatomy* are seemingly all examples of the default mode of functioning.

The idle thoughts and "conceits" of the *Anatomy* are also instances of the cognitive states identified as "mind wandering." As examples of

---

37. Rather than operating in isolation, the default network contributes to several active forms of internally directed cognition, thus comprising multiple interacting subsystems (Andrews-Hanna, Smallwood, and Spreng 2014).
38. The evidence for this analysis emerged from neuroimaging studies. During passive rest conditions, compared with attention-demanding or goal directed cognitive tasks, levels of activation were observed in regions including the medial temporal and frontal lobes, posterior cingulate and retrosplenial cortex, and lateral parietal and temporal areas showing increased activation (Buckner et al. 2008, Andrews-Hanna 2012, Schacter et al. 2012).
39. Raichle et al. 2001, Seeley et al. 2007, Schacter et al. 2012, Gerrans 2014.
40. Buckner and Vincent 2007, Immordino-Yang et al. 2012, Schacter et al. 2012.

default system functioning, mind-wandering states have been similarly defined, in terms of mental decoupling from stimulus events in the external environment. Their neural signatures are also a disruption, and reduction, in both sensory and cognitive level processing of external stimuli. Default systems, and their manifestations in such mind-wandering states, it seems to be agreed, are entirely normal and extremely common. (Estimates from experience sampling studies of normal people indicate that from one-third to a half of daily life is spent engaged in this kind of default mode mind-wandering.[41]) They are also indispensable to more goal-directed cognitive functioning, despite being in certain respects antithetical to such processing. The adaptive value of these default network activities has been recognized, both as a system supporting and cooperating with other systems, and for its distinctive aspects. The default network undergirds goal-directed autobiographical planning, for example, by cooperating with the frontoparietal control network, which appears capable of flexibly coupling with distinct networks as tasks demand.[42] Although internally directed rather than focused on external stimuli, the default system thus cooperates with executive control systems as it regulates inner states.[43] Other advantages cited of default network mind-wandering include its provision of incubation intervals for generating creative solutions, rehearsals for future behavior, or a restorative period after the taxing demands of attention.[44] (The default system has evolved to allow humans to simulate experiences in the absence of an eliciting stimulus, it has been conjectured. Released from the stimulus-bound present, "we can review previous possible scenarios and experience characteristic emotions before committing to action" [Gerrans 2014:67].)

(v) Burton's faculty psychology ensures that the mental functions undertaken by the imagination are sui generis. And similarly, in many contemporary models, imagining, or simulating, presupposes

---

41. Kam and Handy 2013:13.
42. Schacter at el. 2012:686, Andrews-Hanna et al. 2010, Spreng et al. 2010.
43. Andrews-Hanna, Smallwood, and Spreng 2014. But see also McVay and Kane 2010, Walkins 2008.
44. Kam and Handy 2013, Burman et.al. 2008.

functionalist thinking where the mind comprises discrete modules and separate cognitive states such as beliefs, desires, and imaginings are distinguished functionally in terms of their differing causal interactions with the outside world and other mental states.[45] Imaginings are thus not reducible to the cognitive activity of believing, despite the shared intentional structure between imaginings and beliefs allowing them to each take objects (often the same ones). Both as faculty psychology and as Fodorian functionalist modularity models, this system has its critics. Amelie Rorty has decried the tradition of postulating and reifying imagination as a special faculty, pointing out the open-ended range of cognitive and rhetorical skills and activities customarily included in practical imaginative thinking, for example.[46] Our loose notion of *thinking*, she illustrates, is capacious enough to include more than we would usually judge merely *imagining*. And, indeed, brain-imaging studies indicate that although they may be default system activities, the imaginary or imagined engage the same processes in the brain as other forms of cognition.[47]

For Burton, however, imagining remains significantly distinct in allowing him to follow a long tradition, particularly emphasized within the medical writing of his renaissance peers in supposing that the symptoms of disorder inevitably affect the imagination while only sometimes affecting (other) reasoning capabilities as well. When (in chapter 6) we explore the frankly delusional material described by Burton, we will see the import of this within contemporary models of psychopathology. (According to some theories of delusion, for example, an ability to *distinguish* these two functions of believing and imagining is an aspect

---

45. Fodor 1975, Schroeder and Matheson 2006.
46. See Rorty 2010:425–44.
47. There is no distinct anatomical region of the brain used for representing the merely imaginary, it has been pointed out: "nor is there a distinct set of nerve fibers carrying information exclusively about the merely imaginary; nor does there seem to be a special affective or, for that matter, motor region designated for receiving input about the merely imaginary.... All simulacra [imaginings] are represented much as real things would be, by the same unimodal and multimodal representational structures" (Schroeder and Matheson 2006:28).

of normal cognitive functioning that is lost in the person entertaining delusions.)

(vi) The relation between imagination and the affective Passions reveals a final similarity with present-day accounts. In the unceasing dynamic Burton depicts between imagining, feeling, and thinking, thoughts—with objects as often imaginary as real, and resulting from imagining—produce feelings, while feelings in turn bring, and generate, thoughts and imaginings. And once some stimulus occurs, as we saw in chapter 1, data are conveyed to the emotion centers that, when activated, bring about the effects in affective and bodily responses that we associated with felt emotions, while these in turn prompt further imaginings, comparable to Damasio's "as if loops," in an incessant round of psychic rearrangements.[48]

The interaction between imagining and feeling so emphasized in the *Anatomy* has not always been acknowledged in psychology or philosophy since Burton's time. The unsteady course of Imagination from its seventeenth-century enthronement as queen of the mental powers, through its eclipse at the hands of the Empiricists like Hume, to its eventual revival through Kant and the Idealists to twentieth-century phenomenology, is too long a story to be told here.[49] So is the way, within the philosophy of mind, the general link between imagination and emotion was long sidelined by the particular set of puzzles surrounding aesthetic responses, where imagined fictional characters and scenarios elicit inexplicably normal emotional responses.[50] Yet the power of the fictional to evoke feelings is only a special case—albeit a puzzling one—of the power of the imagination to do so.[51] Emotionally charged relations to

---

48. One such interaction has been hypothesized this way: "the subject suffers from an emotional disturbance centering on anxiety or thwarted desires. This emotion stimulates the imagination, producing images of persecution or wish fulfillment. These images feed back to the emotions and inflame them further. A feedback effect ensues. The images come to be *believed* by the subject; hence the conviction of persecution or of grandeur. The essence of this simple model is that the delusional beliefs are generated by the imagination system, driven by the affective system" (McGinn 2004:113–4). This account relies on an imagistic example, but nonetheless offers a plausible sequence.
49. But see Haskell 2011 and Lennon 2015.
50. Berrios 2011, Walton 2000.
51. Schroeder and Matheson 2006:22, Lennon 2015.

what is "only" imagined are constitutive of *all ordinary mental life*, in experiences like remembering past events (with regret, remorse, or nostalgia), speculating on what might have been (with horror, or relief), and envisioning future states of affairs with hope, excitement, or dread. In fact, comparatively little of one's emotional attention, Richard Moran has reminded us, concerns objects "in the actual here and now," and relief, regret, remorse, and nostalgia are "among the paradigm cases of emotional response" (Moran 1994:78).[52] The earlier neglect of the ties between imagining and feeling has changed. The link between affective and imaginative (simulation) states, in particular, has been confirmed in numerous studies. In "priming" studies, for example, expectancies wrought by mental imagery (of a fearful face) produce subsequent perceptual distortion, having primed the brain for misperception.[53] In another demonstration, from guided imaging, it has been shown that differently imagined scenarios produce different affective responses.[54] Indeed, as simulation, the activities included in the Burtonian imagination enter into innumerable contemporary discussions and research endeavors, so much so that its differing definitions, classifications, and emphases leave imagination (simulation) an unwieldy category.

Six features were loosely separated here: the unconstrained nature of imagining vis-á-vis its objects; the broad range of activities it encompasses, including remembering and image-forming; its motivational indifference; its status as less stimulus dependent than the brain's other attentional network, suggesting parallels with the default network system that includes mind-wandering states; its status as irreducibly distinct from other mental activities such as believing; and finally, its close interaction with affective states. These aspects of Burtonian imagining all foreshadow contemporary analyses of the activities known as simulation, some strikingly. At the least, we can say, they leave the *Anatomy* conception compatible with much in today's mind science.

---

52. See also Schroeder and Matheson: "That the imagination produces strong feelings in most of us is *just as evident* as that fictions do" (2006:22, emphasis added).
53. Diekhof et al., 2011.
54. Izard 1991, Harris 2000, Schroeder and Matheson 2006.

REGULATING THE IMAGINATION

Employed to further the sciences or the arts, the capacity to imagine is indispensible—as it is when, whether willfully or inadvertently, it furthers the interests of healing. The task of regulating how much and over what objects imagining is to be permitted or even encouraged is assigned to Reason in the *Anatomy*, and the appropriateness of engaging in useful or productive imagining will depend on its effects. But Reason's supervisory and adjudicative role is complicated by the sheer pleasure derived from entertaining "fond conceits," or phantasies. The source of this idea may be Du Laurens, of whom Burton offers the following version in his own paraphrase:

> the Imagination inwardly or outwardly moved, represents to the understanding, not inticements only; to favour the passion, or dislike, but a very intensive pleasure followes the passion, or displeasure, and *the will and reason are captivated by delighting in it.* (I,3,3,1:421, emphasis added)

The will and reason are captivated by imagining; they delight in it.[55] And because imagining is often a pleasurable activity, there are strong parallels between the temptations it offers and the thrall of other vices. For Burton fantasizing is a compelling, addictive, and sensual, almost sensuous leaning. It seems to invite *akratic* states, as we'll see in chapter 5. Pleasant chimeras and fantasies are produced by our imaginations, however, providing the initial lure that only later turns into unpleasant, and eventually agonizingly painful, fears, suspicions, and misapprehensions.

The idea of melancholy as temptation is returned to throughout the *Anatomy*.[56] On the delights of "pleasing his mind with fond imaginings,"

---

55. Psychologists have designed experiments to confirm the pleasurability of imagining. Given the choice of achieving a desirable outcome immediately, or deferring it for a week, subjects chose to defer, thus increasing the anticipatory pleasure (Elster and Loewenstein 1992).

56. But he also knew his Milton:
 . . . uncouth cell,
 Where brooding darkness spreads his jealous wings,
 And the night-raven sings.
 Il Penseroso

Burton cannot say enough. Yet he also sounds repeated, somber warnings. Indulging these fond imaginings is almost irresistibly tempting, but dangerous. This is an inclination that must be vigilantly controlled through direct efforts of will, and the employment of Reason. Reason should exercise control—and *can*. "Rule thyself ... with reason," he admonishes,

> wean thyself from ... fond conceits, vain fears, strong imaginations, restless thoughts. *Thou mayest do it ... we may frame ourselves as we will* ... Doe that voluntarily ... which thou canst doe ... *thou maist refraine if thou wilt,* and master thine affections. (II,2,6,1:103, emphasis added)

By the use of distraction, and by deflating excessive, biased, and overblown ideas that would invoke unbalanced and excessive feelings, the imagination can divert and quell the passions. We thus possess a means of managing these tendencies, Burton promises.

MIND TO BODY EFFECTS

In another feature of the Burtonian imagination rendering it compatible with contemporary cognitive psychology the imagination affects the body as much, and as directly, as the mind. How does this happen? As well as through the passions, which are both altered by and alter it, the imagination affects the bodily constitution directly because it is a partly sensory capability:

> Imagination enforceth spirits, which by *an admirable league of nature*, compel the nerves to obey, and they our severall limes [limbs]. (II,2,6,1:104)

The activities that compel the nerves and limbs to obey are not, and cannot be, conscious. Despite his dualism, Burton's account adheres to what has today been called an unconscious that is "cognitive" or "adaptive."[57] In contrast to the Freudian unconscious, items in the cognitive or adaptive unconscious are permanently unavailable to conscious awareness. We lack direct access to many higher-order mental processes, such as the way selection, interpretation, and the evaluation of incoming information are achieved. From the point of view of cognitive science, an internal state responsible for the causation of behavior is, as David Chalmers has put it, "equally mental whether it is conscious or not" (Chalmers 1996:11).[58] Mentality is unrelated to consciousness. Similarly, the workings of the imagination in the conscious mind are not at all privileged by Burton over the mysterious way imaginings bring about bodily effects. It is though some "admirable league of nature" *we do not understand*, by which these mind to body effects occur. Announcing this causal sequence, Burton reminds his readers of unexceptional examples of the imagination affecting the body, with which they could all concur: some people, he says,

> will laugh, weepe, sigh, groane, blush, tremble, sweat at such things are suggested to them by their imagination. (I,2,3,2:252)

About some of the alleged effects of the imagination on bodily states, he is more circumspect. The common medieval belief that a pregnant woman seeing a terrible sight will produce a monstrous offspring, for example, is noted several times in the *Anatomy*.[59,60] And Montaigne describes such phenomena, entirely without qualification: *"we know by experience* that women transmit marks of their fancies to the bodies of the children they carry in their womb."[61] Burton recounts these folk

---

57. The adaptive unconscious has been defined as mental processing that, while inaccessible to consciousness, influences judgements, feelings, or behavior (Wilson 2002:23).
58. See also Clark 1997.
59. In one story, a concubine of Pope Nicholas III, "by seeing a Beare, was brought to bed of a monster" (I,2,3,2:251).
60. Although the mother's imagination was never considered the only possible cause of monstrosity, it has been shown, it nevertheless haunted centuries of medical research (Huet 1993:6–7).
61. Montaigne 2003:75, emphasis added. Burton cites "Montaigne the Frenchman in his Essays," in several places, although not on matters of any great significance.

tales with similar gusto, yet he arguably conveys an attitude toward their veracity that is slightly less sure.⁶²

In a more confident tone, he asserts that at least some illnesses—and particularly melancholy symptoms themselves—are exacerbated or alleviated by efforts of imagination, and here Burton apparently speaks from something approaching actual observation. The healing effects of talismans and charms are admitted, for example, with the explanation:

> hee doth the best cures, according to Hippocrates, in whom most trust (I,2,3,2:254).⁶³

In a rare, personal reference, he also recounts a visit to his parents' house in Leicestershire. There, despite his mother's fame for "good cures upon diverse poore folks . . . otherwise destitute of helpe," he at first doubted the effectiveness of the amulet she offered these sufferers made of "a Spider, in a nut-shell lapped in silke." The amulet seemed "most absurd and ridiculous, I could see no warrant for it," he admits. After reading that such devices were recommended by the ancients, however, he reconsidered:

> I beganne to . . . give more credit to Amulets, when I saw it in some parties answere to experience. (II,5,1,5:254–5)

Burton is particularly intrigued by the power of expectation in healing. The imagination will "work upon itself," to cause or exacerbate

---

62. "*If we may believe* Bale," he begins one tale (I,2,3,2:251, emphasis added), perhaps suggesting that we may not.
63. For the same reason, an Empiricke, "oftentimes, and a silly Chirurgian [surgeon], doth more strange cures, than a rationall Physitian," he goes on. In letters to Princess Elizabeth of Bohemia during the 1640s, Descartes similarly insists that by directing and controlling our imagination, we can bring about bodily changes affecting the course of a disease: By concentrating on objects that could furnish contentment and joy, the imagination alone "would be capable of restoring health" (Descartes 1991:249–50).

symptoms, even achieving something like social contagion: if another man is seen who is

> sick of some feareful disease, [men's] apprehension and feare is so strong in this kind, that they will have the same Disease.

Yet the imagination is equally capable of bringing about the alleviation of symptoms, he notes in the same passage: Sometimes, nothing more than "a strong conceit or apprehension ... will take away Diseases" (1,2,3,2: 252).

The Imagination works each way:

> As Imagination, feare, griefe, cause such passions, so conceipts alone, rectified by good hope, counsel, &c. are able againe to helpe: and 'tis incredible how much they can do in such a case. (II,2,6,2:110)

Recognition of expectation as a source of self-healing can be found in the writings of Greek, Persian, and Arabic doctors as well as the renaissance humanists, such as Montaigne (as Burton acknowledges). While far from original to the *Anatomy*, this stress on the power of expectation in healing is nonetheless one of its hallmarks.

As Montaigne also knew, these changes wrought by the imagination work through its effect on the passions. In passions and affections, Burton explains, the imagination "shewes [shows] its strange and evident effects." The imagination is the endless goad to the passions, inciting, altering, and sometimes quelling them. This intimate link between imagining and affections is a theme running throughout these discussions. For,

> what will not a fearfull man conceave in the darke; what strange forms of Bugbeares, Divels, Witches, Goblins? (I,2,3,2:251)

Here, fear generates imaginary horrors. But the effect runs each way: Imaginings similarly trigger feelings. Ask a man to walk across a board over dry land, then over the same board placed at some height,

Burton observes: The fearful frame of mind, and giddiness, produced in the second case are entirely the result of the imagination.[64]

Medical treatments in the early seventeenth century commonly included the outright deception of patients.[65] Although Burton regards these as remedies of last resort, they form part of his case in support of the power of the imagination in healing. When other means fail, he notes, and only then, "it will not be amisse" to take such action, deceiving patients with "some fained lye, strange newes, witty device, artificiall invention." He has read, he says, "a multitude of examples of Melancholy men cured by such artificiall inventions." Among others, the case of a man is described who supposed his nose so big that

> he should dash it against the wall if he stirred; his Physitian tooke a great peece of flesh, and holding it in his hand, pinched him by the nose, making him believe that flesh was cut from it. (II,2,6,2:112)

This kind of deception may have been effective, as Burton concedes. It is entirely incompatible with contemporary ethics. Yet, he is right: It does provide support for the power he accords the imagination.

BURTON'S CREDULITY

The issue of Burton's credulity touches on the historical place of the *Anatomy* in relation to empirically grounded modern science. By the early seventeenth century, skeptical attitudes had begun to challenge many of the popular superstitions from earlier eras, when it had been readily accepted that witches' spells soured the milk and ruined the crops. Fostered by Neoplatonist ideas about occult happenings, however, not only demonic and magical influences but also other unseen forces were said to bring changes in the material world around us.[66]

---

64. Although today's science might doubt this analysis of depth perception, his challenge is to those who deride the effects of the imagination here (I,2,3,2:253).
65. See Macdonald 1981:153–4.
66. Even those skeptical about witchcraft, for example, accepted the possibility of action at a distance. Thus the most ardent defenders of the power of imagination, it has been

Some assertions in the *Anatomy* apparently echo the older credulity, and it is as credulous, and hopelessly unscientific, that Burton has often been treated by those writing about him in our present times, most notably Babb.[67] His credulity deserves better, however. He *is* credulous, it is true—but with some warrant when it comes to the capabilities attributed to this remarkable faculty of the imagination. Moreover, although perhaps merely because he must steer through scholarly controversies over occult causes, he does stay gently skeptical about some of the less plausible cases he describes. Learned attitudes toward nonnatural effects had importantly changed in the renaissance, it is true. From being cast as external, and demonic, the sources of some untoward, apparently magical effects had come to be seen as internal and psychological, with accompanying shifts toward increasingly humane and secular attitudes. This more modern view, exemplified in the writings of Weyer, Burton sometimes adopts. Yet these were matters of confusion and controversy, and he is neither consistent nor clear. Backed by a whole raft of thinkers including Wierus (Weyer) and Paracelsus and unidentified "many Phylosophers," he discounts magical explanations of how old women can "bewitch" children, for example, only to introduce what seems today an equally implausible explanation involving action at a distance, "the forcible imagination of the one party moves and alters the spirits of the other" (I,2,3,2:254). Even among empirically minded medical writers, it was an era of occult thinking, historians point out, in which there was belief in a "sympathy" (*consensus*) that would allow one corrupt substance to affect another. Also, as part of the sensitive soul,

---

observed, included both the most and least credulous, the latter accepting the imagination as "a credible and natural explanation for some of the more far-fetched claims of popular magic and religion" (Huet 1993:14).

67. Of Burton, Babb says, "[he] . . . does not understand the fundamental importance of the experimental method. There is no evidence in the *Anatomy* that Burton himself ever conducted an experiment. . . . Apparently it never occurs to him that firsthand observation and experience might be necessary to scientific competence. . . . [He] lacks . . . the experimental curiosity but also the critical skepticism which the true scientific thinker must have" (Babb 1959:71–2). Science in Burton's time was not really a science at all in the modern sense of an "experimental and inductive study of nature which is systematic and highly exact" (Babb 1959:58–9). This accusation that Burton made no contribution to science has been repeated since then, it should be added. See Lyons 1971.

the imagination bridged material and immaterial parts of the person, particularly inviting its use as an instrument of the devil.[68]

About claims made on behalf of the imagination Burton shows himself aware of the naysayers—and of the imperatives of systematic, empirical proof, admitting that "Many will not belleeve such stories to be true, but laugh commonly, and deride when they heare of them" (I,2,3,2:253). He had also read Reginald Scot, the ultimate skeptic when it came to demonology and witchcraft.[69] Many times, the appearances of sorcery and witchcraft were achieved through deceit (legerdemain), Burton acknowledges Scot to have shown.[70] And he often remembers to distance himself from the old wives' tales he reports.

In defense of Burton's nascent empiricism, it must also be pointed out that although he may be mistaken in some of the actual instances he cites with confidence, his belief that the imagination can effect and affect bodily responses is not entirely, or in principle, mistaken. By challenging the general possibility that the imagination brings about bodily changes, thoroughgoing Empiricists such as Scot (as indeed critics writing later, such as Babb), are left to explain a range of findings about mind–body interactions, such as placebo effects, which as we will see later in this chapter, have today acquired considerable empirical confirmation. In recognizing the general principle that imagination can affect bodily states, Burton was closer to our contemporary findings than to those who derided the very possibility of psychological effects on the body. What is more, in an era when medical remedies were very limited in their potential, so that the effectiveness of most would have rested on

---

68. See Gowland 2007:50–56, 85–97. Burton's own discussion of these demonic influences (in "Digression of the Nature of Spirits, bad Angels or Divels") is confusing, and does not directly concern us here. About his apparent prevarications over occultism, we can accept Gowland's conclusion that he "did not settle on either supernatural or rationalist-sceptical grounds. Ultimately he insisted only on the indisputably orthodox point that any cases where melancholy could be said without doubt to be supernaturally induced were to be traced ultimately to divine permission" (Gowland 2007:87).
69. Scot (1538–1599), whom Burton describes as "our country-man Scot" (I,2,1,3:196), had published *Discovery of Witchcraft* in 1584. Of poor melancholike women, it is there explained, "melancholie abounding in their head, and occupieng their braine, hath deprived or rather depraved their judgments, and all their senses" (Scot 1584:52).
70. I,3,3,1:425.

enlisting the self-healing power of expectations, a degree of credulity would have been somewhat persuasive. The evidence supporting psychosomatic healing was more salient than it has become in succeeding centuries, overtaken by the success of physical medicine's fail-safe, targeted cures. At least in common estimation, this salience left the epistemic status of such healing relatively enhanced, it has been suggested.[71] If any remedy might succeed, the best bet was one that rested on the power of the self-healing imagination.

With regard to mind-to-body effects, Burton clearly recognizes that whether these occur in specific instances finally awaits empirical demonstration. And rather than the prevarication of which he has been accused, some of his efforts to avoid overgeneralization can be read as a spirit of scientific caution. He is slow to draw, and quick to qualify, generalizations. Explaining the way the imagination "rages" in melancholy persons, for example, he remarks that they maintain

> the species of objects so long, mistaking, amplifying them by continual and strong meditation, until at length it produceth *in some parties* real effects. (I,2,3,2, emphasis added)

Only continual and strong meditation—obsessive rumination, we might say—will *in some, not all, people*, bring these results. Burton's suspicion of generalization, tendency toward qualification, and preparedness to acknowledge the telling exception, all favor an empirical over a dogmatic frame of mind. As a final example of these glimmers of what is recognizably scientific in the modern sense, we can return to Burton's example of the man and the plank. Exemplifying an approach that is experimental in spirit, he remarks that

> Let those who deride the effects of the imagination set to walke upon a planke on high, they would be giddie, upon which they dare securely walk upon the ground.

---

71. Thomas 1997:209–10.

Agrippa is quoted here ("strong hearted men otherwise, tremble at such sights, dazell, and are sicke, if they looke but downe from an high place"). "What moves them but conceit," he then asks? (I,2,3,2:253). This reasoning is not science in Babb's terms. Nor is it an appeal to book learning. Rather it is a *thought experiment*, applying an understanding of human behavior to counterfactual but grounded—and entirely persuasive—speculation.

THE SCIENCE OF EXPECTATION

All experience is mediated by expectations. But within the broader category lies a subgroup of effects variously known as context, psychosocial, positive care, placebo effects, or meaning responses.[72] As placebo effects, these form an integral part of experimental design in the study of treatment effectiveness. Even so, their status as genuine or "real" neurobiological phenomena has been questioned.[73] That certain changes might be receptive to influence through expectation in something like the ways Burton describes, is today more widely accepted, and effects like these have been demonstrated in at least four areas: analgesia, motor performance, mood, and brain responses in drug addiction.[74] For example, on a regimen of inert pills provided as placebos, those with mild to moderate depression show measurable improvement that almost matches the improvement shown by those receiving antidepressants.[75]

In addition to placebo effects, *nocebo* effects have been observed, occurring when expectations of sickness, disability, or deficiency, and the affective and imagined states associated with such expectations, actually induce or augment them. Following the second edition of his work and thus, we can suppose, reflecting the reception of the earlier one, Burton issues a warning about nocebo power: Reading

---

72. Nayak and Patel 2014, Kaptchuk and Miller 2015.
73. Finnis et al. 2010, Meissner et al. 2011.
74. Finnis et al. 2010.
75. Brown 1998, Kirsch 1999, Kirsch, Moore, Scoboria, and Nicholls 2002, Turner, Matthews, Linardatos, Tell, and Rosenthal 2008, Kirsch et al. 2008, Fournier et al. 2010.

about melancholy might invoke it.[76] Reading is both cause and cure in the *Anatomy*, it must be stressed. The imagination heals melancholy through reading when it serves to distract and soothe us, and dispel dark and troubling moods.[77] Reading and words will thus harm, or help, according to their context and semantic content; the imagination is in this respect Janus-faced, as Burton recognizes.

Ethical constraints must particularly prevent their full study, yet nocebo effects have also been observed by contemporary researchers.[78] In a typical example, subjects receiving placebo in an antidepressant drug trial experienced the typical and familiar side effects that would have been predicted to occur only in the recipients of the actual drug. Unaware whether their tablets were placebo or not, and knowing the actual treatment brought these minor effects (such as a dry mouth), the placebo takers responded accordingly, experiencing those effects even with inert substances.[79]

Several brain systems have been associated with outcomes such as these effects, moreover placebo mechanisms seem to occur in different systems in healthy and disordered people.[80] A recent summary notes that placebo responses are "complex, multiform, and multimodal. Their neural substrates are many interacting neuronal systems that orchestrate changes in pain ... motor control ... mood, anxiety, memory, motivation.... Both conscious expectations (augmented by desires, hope, and belief), and unconscious conditioning ("embodied experiences" or "remembered wellness") can move the molecules of change along the distributed biological systems, sub-serving cognition, emotions, pain control, reward, and learning" (Nayak and Patel 2014:74). In

---

76. Those who are "actually Melancholy" should avoid the "Symptoms or prognostickes in this following Tract" for fear that "he trouble or hurte himselfe" (I,24).
77. Indeed, it has been pointed out that the *Anatomy* itself can be viewed as a "reading" or "textual" cure (Lund 2010).
78. Hahn 1997, Kaptchuk and Miller 2015.
79. Mora et al. 2011.
80. Thus, in depression, neurobiological mechanisms including changes of electrical and metabolic activity in different brain regions such as the ventral striatum have been observed; in anxiety there are changes in activity of the anterior cingulate and orbitofrontal cortices, genetic variants of serotonin transporter, and tryptophan hydroxylase 2 (Finnis et al. 2010:688).

addition, seemingly related placebo and nocebo effects stem from different brain mechanisms, as indicated by neuroimaging.[81]

Researchers today have become wary of the kind of broad definition of placebo (and nocebo) effects relied on in earlier times, since the mechanisms by which these effects occur have proven to be various. So it is more accurate to speak of placebo effects in the plural, even in the limited instance of the kinds of symptoms Burton was concerned with. Moreover, claims about whether and how placebo effects occur remain somewhat contentious. In part this is because ethical considerations prevent their thorough study. It is also because of methodological impediments to that study. Three aspects of placebo effects have been subject to divergent interpretation. Although the evidence is compelling, the placebo-effect findings viewed as unequivocal and robust data are one of these.[82] The explanation of those findings is another. [83] And finally, as a consequence of unresolved questions in these two areas of focus, placebo effects still lack an agreed-on definition.[84]

The healing capabilities of the imagination applauded in the *Anatomy* are today associated with the work of the mid-twentieth-century physician Henry Beecher, whose influential paper declaimed the "power of the placebo" in medicine. Based on his observation of the effectiveness of inert (saline solution) injections for pain in injured soldiers during the World War II, Beecher measured the effectiveness of placebo over a range of conditions in a large sample of patients. From his meta-analysis, he concluded that placebo was pervasive, with "real," as distinct from merely psychological (or imaginary), effects.[85] Beecher's assertions as to their prevalence have since prompted a refinement of the concept of placebo effects. Certain confounding factors diminish his claim, as they must weaken Burton's account, as well. The natural course of a disease or symptom cluster is variable. Many depressions, particularly, seem to be episodic and thus self-limiting. The purely statistical phenomenon

---

81. The hippocampus and regions involving anticipatory anxiety have been said to be implicated in nocebo effects (Finnis et al. 2010, Kong et al. 2008).
82. See Jopling 2008:117–40.
83. See Harrington 1997.
84. See Jopling 2008, Moncrieff, Wessely, and Hardy 2004.
85. Beecher 1955.

of regression to the mean might further muddy the effects, as might response bias (in the patient who wants to please, for example) and the effects of concurrent treatments.[86] (Eliminating such confounding factors to establish the actual limits of the placebo effect, it has been pointed out, would at the least add a group of subjects receiving no intervention whatsoever to research protocols that presently comprise treatment and placebo groups—an arrangement incompatible with the current structure of research trials and likely impossible to achieve.[87])

The Declaration of Helsinki (World Medical Association 2001) prohibits as unethical placebo-controlled trials for life-threatening conditions, or when proven safe and effective treatments are available. Moreover, a strong ethical prohibition on deceiving patients complicates the design of placebo-controlled studies.[88] Because of ethical limitations like these, together with the methodological considerations noted above, efforts to understand, define, and explain expectation effects remain, today, without an authoritative formulation. In their general features, however, Burton's descriptions find affirmation. Placebo (and nocebo) effects are made possible by what has been described as a complex interplay between "belief, hope, expectation, and emotions" (Jopling 2008:146).[89] It is the same combination of feeling, thinking, and imagining that Burton claims can both incite and reduce the symptoms of melancholy. The *Anatomy* account of the influence of the imagination in lessening and also triggering disordered states, is incomplete. But it cannot be said to have been thoroughly overtaken or surpassed by settled scientific knowledge. To the contrary, the healing power of placebo effects is increasingly recognized within medicine. Empathic healthcare, it has been acknowledged, "creates cognitive-affective-sensory orientation, tapping into conscious and non-conscious mechanisms that can predispose patients toward reduced symptom severity and lessened reactivity to underlying pathophysiology ... healing

86. Finnis et al. 2010.
87. See Jopling 2009.
88. World Medical Association 2000.
89. A thorough review of recent efforts to define placebo effects, with a revised definition, is provided by David Jopling (2008:132–47).

interactions 'frame,' 'anchor,' or 'nudge' patients towards shifts in their perceptions of their symptoms and illness, making them less disturbed or perturbed" (Kaptchuk and Miller 2015:9).

In an endless exchange, the products of the imagination affect the feelings and inclinations making up the passions, and those feelings and inclinations in turn prompt further imaginative activity. This account of the normal imagination finds strong confirmation in some of the observations and theorizing of today's sciences involving the ubiquitous category of simulation. The conception of the activities making up imagination, which encompasses remembering, forming images, and dreams (both sleeping and waking), is one example of this; the importance, and properties, of the default attentional mode, with its associated mind-wandering states to which Burtonian descriptions apparently correspond, are another; and the power of expectation, particularly in relation to healing, is a third. Whether there is also support for the medieval idea that a disturbed or deficient imagination (or defective simulative capabilities) explains affective disorder is explored more fully in the chapters to come.

Chapter 3

symptom, disease, cause

What a Disease is, almost every Physitian defines. (I,1,1,2:129)
After offering a range of others' efforts to define disease that variously stress what is unhealthy, imbalanced, or dysfunctional, our author declines to select between them. So what conception of disease *does* underlie Burton's references to the "epidemicall disease" that is the subject of his book? And how does it match present-day conceptions? Today's philosophy of science and medicine employs a group of contrasts: reductive and nonreductive ontologies, signs and symptoms distinguished from their causes, etiological from symptom-focused classifications and analyses, and categorical from dimensional disorders. Although there are exceptions, biological medical psychiatry customarily takes a stand on each of them. It presupposes the elegance, measurability, and scientific uniformity of mind-body reductionism, adopting reductive over nonreductive ontologies.[1] Reflecting an etiological model of disease, it casts signs and symptoms as the causal products, to a greater or lesser extent, of an *underlying, endogenous factor,* variously depicted as a condition of dysfunction, imbalance, deficit, vulnerability, or disorder. (In the terminology of psychology and psychometrics, these factors are latent variables.) And finally, it favors classifications positing diseases as categorically distinct.

---

1. Empirical reductionism, it has been asserted, is merely methodological: a form of analysis into constituent parts to aid understanding. A more fundamental, metaphysical reductionism, by contrast, is "*ipso facto* a statement about the nature of the world: living systems (like all else) can be completely understood in terms of the properties of their constituent parts" (Woese 2004:174). Between these, the usually unthinking allegiance of biological psychiatry seems more often to the metaphysical form.

Although Burton does not always plump for one rather than another of these alternatives, they can be used to frame answers to the above questions about his conception of disease. The ontological matter has been addressed already: The *Anatomy*'s dualistic model avoids mind-to-body reductionism. Arguably, it does so while at the same time sidestepping some of the errors associated with other forms of substance dualism, as we saw earlier; but Burton never doubted that the rational soul was irreducibly distinct from its material container.

Considering Burton's conception of disease in relation to these other modern-day categories and contrasts, it will first be helpful to place the *Anatomy* account within the legacy of ideas inherited from classical works as well as those of his renaissance and early modern contemporaries. Aspects of the symptoms of melancholy identified this way include their role in definitions, their place within causal sequences, and their number, variety, and mutability. Later in this chapter we turn to present-day conceptions of disease shaped by advances in medicine since the nineteenth century, that emphasize the causes of disease as typically singular and uniform in their effects. By contrast with these conceptions, causes in the *Anatomy* are confusingly heterogeneous, and symptoms and natural history have relative prominence. In this difference, Burtonian Melancholy proves more consonant with present-day network models of depression, such as those put forward by Kenneth Kendler and colleagues, than with the models inherited from nineteenth-century medicine that have proven useful in understanding many other, nonpsychological diseases. The newer ideas seek to unseat those common-cause etiological disease models in application to mental disorder. Burton did not describe the symptom profile of the melancholic as an interactive network, yet his analysis suggests one.

SYMPTOM-BASED DEFINITIONS

There are many references to corporeal states and parts in the *Anatomy*, to the humors, animal spirits, and organs (particularly the heart, liver, and brain). But unlike its formal classification among other disorders, the definition of melancholy makes reference to symptoms. As we saw earlier, it is

> a kind of dotage without feaver, having his ordinary companions, feare, and sadnesse, without any apparent occasion. (I,1,3,1:163)

Dotage (also known as Fatuity or Folly), it is explained, occurs when one of the mental faculties, such as imagination, or reason, is "corrupted," or, we might say, impaired in its observable functioning.[2] The associated affections ("ordinary companions"), of melancholy are groundless fear and sadness or sorrow. Both the corruption of a faculty and these affective states are symptoms in the present-day, and everyday, sense. Similar appeal is made to observable symptoms where, in a loose separation, melancholy is distinguished from madness. (Within the ancient, three-part classification of *delirium*, each of Melancholy and Madness (or Mania), is divided from Phrenitis (or frenzy) in being unaccompanied by fever, and chronic rather than acute.[3]) Madness is defined by Burton as:

> a vehement Dotage, or raving without feavere, farre more violent than Melancholy. Full of anger and clamor, horrible lookes, actions, gestures troubling the patients with farre greater vehemency both of body and Mind, *without all feare and sorrow*, with such impetuous force and boldnesse, that sometimes three or foure men cannot hold them. (I,1,1,4:132)

---

2. *Dotage* is "some one principall facultie of the minde, as imagination, or reason, is corrupted" (I,1,3,2:163). Burton acknowledges the variations in terminology around the terms "Dotage," "Fatuity," "Folly," "Phrenitis," "Madnesse," "Phrenzie," and "Melancholy," noting that some authorities "make Madnesse and Melancholy but one Disease," yet explaining that he will follow Galen, Aretaeus, and "most of our neotericks [newer thinkers]" in handling Madness and Melancholy apart (I,1,1,4:132).
3. In so separating melancholy, Burton was aiming for an essentialist definition along Aristotelian or Galenic lines (Gowland 2006:59). His acknowledgment in later editions that while characteristic, fear and sadness were not unfailingly present as "inseparable companions," leaves the analysis short of that goal.

Both definitions are taken directly from Du Laurens, and echo other early modern medical works derived from Galen's definition of melancholy from *de locis affectis*. And, employing the same symptom-focused differentiation in characterizing madness, each notes the observable features of greater vehemence and violence, along with the absence of fear and sadness. In another allusion to the distinction between Melancholy and Madness, Burton elsewhere speaks of those men, far gone with melancholy "if not quite mad," who have "more need of Physicke ... more need of Hellebor," than those "that are in Bedlam" (III,4,1,3:388). Melancholy calls for *medicine*, this implies, madness, for *inpatient care*. But again, the distinction is symptom focused.

Definitions can be distinguished from classifications, though. In these same ancient traditions, diseases of the black bile *are classified* together by dint of their associations with imbalances of that substance. The eponymous Melancholy was one of the several diseases of the black bile (alongside dysentery, psoriasis-like skin conditions, hemorrhoids, and dyspepsia).[4]

In definitions like those above, the term "symptom" is employed in the way that is familiar from today's medicine: an observable, and often a subjectively voiced and psychological complaint.[5] However, the symptoms of melancholy as Burton understands them are distinguished by both a characteristic causal history and a characteristic mutability. Most importantly, they are not simply the more readily observable indications, and causal results, of an underlying bodily condition along the lines of many diseases familiar to us from today's medicine. Sometimes, changes in the black bile (in turn resulting from an internal

---

4. At least in some of his writing (the *Methodus Medendi*), Galen was emphatic that diseases must be precisely defined in terms of body parts and the causal effects of physical remedies, and these ideas were closely followed by the neo-Galenic Montanus, a sixteenth century physician whose work Burton often cites. In each patient, individualized remedies grew out of carefully observed symptoms. On the Galenic revival during the sixteenth century, and the influence of Montanus on Burton, see Tilmouth 2005:531–2.

5. Signs are sometimes differentiated from symptoms today, in not requiring the patient's awareness or acknowledgment, but Burton uses these terms interchangeably: Signs and symptoms are equally indicators of disorder. Placed in contrast to disease (Latin *morbus*) Burton uses "symptom" and "sign," while medical writing of that time also used "affection" (from the Latin *affectus*).

or environmental source) are indeed a cause of melancholy. But more commonly, melancholy is attributed to the imagination. While it will *result in* a changed humoral temperature in the body, the faculty of imagination, and thus the soul or psyche, is in this case the precipitating cause. In addition, the interactions within the embodied mind are rarely (if ever) unidirectional, as we saw. Imaginings affect bodily states and feelings, but bodily states similarly affect psychic functioning. Mental and bodily are endlessly linked through feedback loops: the humoral temperature, affected by all manner of internal and external effects (digestion, bad air, exercise, and sleep, to name a few), in turn alters the mind. Within the mind, perceptions, thoughts, and imaginings lead to feelings that then engender further humoral changes—and bring further thoughts, then giving rise to new feelings. From these incessant, looping combinations Burton stresses that the same attributes may be both the causes and symptoms of Melancholy. Hippocrates is quoted, naming Sadness or Sorrow "The mother and daughter of melancholy, her Epitome, Symptome, and chiefe cause":

> They beget one another, and tread in a ring, for Sorrow is both Cause and Symptome of this disease. (I,2,3,4:256)

Prompted by some external cause, this passage suggests, we experience passing melancholy in feelings of sorrow—an initial symptom that through repetitive thought patterns and its effect on the humoral temperature, yields further gloomy feelings engendered by disturbed bodily states. Thus "treading a ring," symptoms are at the same time further causes in the chain. Inclinations toward solitude, and other behavioral traits, are analyzed similarly: "too much solitariness, by the testimony of all Physicians, Cause & Symptome both" (I,2,2,6:242). We seek solitude out of, and as a symptom of, our melancholy, yet that solitude in turn produces further melancholy. (Research in social cognition seems to confirm this analysis: Increased social isolation, and the disregulated moods of depression, have been found to become mutually reinforcing.[6])

---

6. Hammen 2006.

The traditional Hippocratic and Galenic accounts can be read as assigning to humoral disturbances the role of *precipitating cause of all melancholy*, and Burton has often been taken to adhere to this view also.[7] Both his analysis of melancholy, and his own reflections on his position, suggest otherwise, however. To see why, it is first worth noting that these matters were not very settled in that day, at least by Burton's assessment:

> What this humour is, or whence it proceeds, *how it is engendered in the body*, neither Galen, nor any old Writer hath sufficiently discussed . . . : the Neoterics cannot agree. (I,1,3,3:166, emphasis added)

The new medical thinking (the Neoterics) was also unresolved over the issue of causation, this passage makes clear, and Burton does not take sides as, continuing, he describes the difference between the non-Galenists and Galenists on these points. In the causal language and conceptions of medieval and renaissance medicine more generally, humoral arrangements seem to be represented as both sole, idiopathic causes of melancholy and, perhaps more commonly, as diatheses or tendencies that combine with some experience or psychological state to bring about changes. (These were familiar from ancient medical lore about the humors and spirits being excited by an outside cause (*inaequalem et turbulentem et inordinatum*, in the Roman phrase)). The *Anatomy* accommodates both alternatives—and includes a third: working solely through their effect on the imagination, exclusively "adventitious," or external, causes can bring about melancholy symptoms (and subsequent humoral changes).[8] Thus, as the result of three different patterns of proximate causation, Burtonian Melancholy is initiated by

---

7. The Galenic account treated the sadness and unwarranted fear that constituted psychological symptoms of melancholy as the direct result of the black bile and its effects, and subsequent medical accounts almost always followed this analysis, according to Gowland (Gowland 2013).
8. See I,2,1,5:203, for example.

(i) humoral imbalances[9]; (ii) thoughts, feelings, and perceptions; and (iii) combinations of the two.[10]

Functions of the Imagination are the locus of disorder once melancholy has set in. But quite apart from that, an overactive imagination is the *commonest precipitating cause* of melancholy symptoms, by Burton's reckoning. As *"astrum hominis*, the rudder of this our ship" (I:2,3,2:254), it steers, and leads. The scant references to instances when bodily states initiate melancholy in the *Anatomy*, it has been pointed out, are considerably exceeded by instances of nonbodily initiating causes.[11] Moreover, the attitude adopted toward those whose melancholy was brought about by solely bodily states has been judged more sympathetic, because they are unavoidable:

> this Melancholy which shall be caused by such infirmities, deserves to be pittied of all men ... as comming from a more inevitable cause. (I,2,5,2:374)

The *Anatomy* account was not alone in its divergence from classical analyses. Galenic and humoral ideas may have predominated, but there was not uniformity in conceptions of disease causation during the centuries leading up to Burton's "anatomizing." Medieval and renaissance medical thinking exhibited variations, and differences between "Empiricists" and "Dogmatists" were recognized and remarked. The Empiricists limited their findings to what could be observed, whereas Dogmatists were closer to today's standard medical approaches, attributing underlying endogenous causes, albeit that these were mysterious and unobservable.[12] A further difference often characterized the Dogmatic position: humoral imbalances (the underlying causes to which diseases were attributed) were more holistic and systemwide, rather than localized, in

---

9. By comparison with astrological influences, humoral complexions can be robust causes. As "causes," the stars are said to "incline" but not "compel"—and that gently, allowing their influence to be resisted (I,2,1,4:199). But as causes of psychic changes, humoral states are offered as sometimes explanatorily sufficient.
10. Although unusual, and a break from Galenic orthodoxy, a similar acknowledgment of bidirectional causality is found in the work of Burton's near contemporary Ferrand. See Gowland 2013:78.
11. Tilmouth 2005:530.
12. Wear 1985:129.

their manifestations.[13] Disease was sometimes described as affecting one bodily part or system rather than another, it is true, and included those that were specific, local events or morbid states of particular bodily organs.[14] Nonetheless, humoral temperatures and constitutions usually identified whole-body states, affecting every organ and part uniformly.

Whether as observable or hidden, systemwide or localized, medieval and renaissance writers ranged over these differing conceptions of disease. And Burton shows himself quite aware of the implications of their varying accounts. It is vain to speak of cures, or think of remedies, he observes, quoting Galen:

> *untill such time as we have considered the Causes* ... those cures must be unperfect, lame and to no purpose, wherein the causes have not first beene searched ... Empericks may ease, and sometimes helpe, but not thoroughly roote out ... if the cause be removed, the effect is likewise vanquished.

Yet, in what seems a refutation of this reasoning, he immediately goes on:

> It is a most difficult thing (I confesse) to be able to discerne these causes whence they are, and in such variety to say what the beginning was. (I:1,3,4:171)

Entirely effective remedies depend on knowledge of causes, it is thus granted—and yet *the illimitable number and variety of causes must frustrate that inquiry*. This recognition that the ideal falls so short of the real seems to be closest to Burton's settled conclusion. It best explains the qualified and pessimistic attitude expressed toward the many remedial and preventive efforts enumerated in the Second Partition.

---

13. The variability over this point is evident in the *Anatomy*, where some forms of melancholy are assigned bodily locations in the head or hypochondries, while others are explicitly said to be bodywide in their effects. Remedies are similarly specified, in some instances, as "Cure[s] of Melancholy over all the Body" (II,5,2,1:259). But for the most part, the remedies Burton proposes are systemwide in their effects.
14. It has been pointed out that this variety contradicted the commonly accepted view that until the nineteenth century medicine was *entirely* holistic. See Wear 1985:130.

Regarding melancholy as solely caused by bodily humors is not an unreasonable expectation, since, as we saw in chapter 1, some of Burton's contemporaries (Bright and, arguably, Du Laurens) do seem to have followed classical medicine in accepting that, in Hippocrates's words, "All human diseases arise from bile and phlegm; the *bile and phlegm produce diseases* when, inside the body, one of them becomes too moist, too dry, too hot, or too cold" (Hippocrates 1988:7).[15] With its frequent references to the humoral state of any given person at a particular time, its attribution of some specific melancholy symptoms to changes originating within the body, and its acknowledgment of the inherent tendencies of those with naturally melancholic temperaments, the conception of disease in the *Anatomy* may at first appear to accept that symptoms inevitably result from endogenous, humoral states within the person, just as, in our contemporary etiological models, causes are endogenous organic states.

However, this superficial parallel is misleading, I will insist. For it leaves unexplained passages in the text that express important and repeated themes and form central aspects of Burtonian psychology. We explore these themes now, the first relating to anomalous features of symptoms, and the second to Burton's emphasis on melancholy habits.

SYMPTOMS AS NUMEROUS, VARIOUS AND MUTABLE

Aside from its account of "how [Melancholy] is engendered in the body," the *Anatomy* portrays the symptoms of melancholy as distinguished by their mutability from those of many, if not most, other diseases. Burton frequently stresses the individual variation in the observable manifestations of melancholy from one person to another ("so many men so many minds" [II,4,1,5:225]). Then, following the constantly fluctuating mixtures making up individual "temperatures," the indications of melancholy

---

15. Bright, we saw, offers what looks to be a solely etiological definition of melancholy with his reference to "a doting of reason through vayne feare . . . *procured by fault of the melancholie humour*" (Bright 1586:3).

are also depicted as varying incessantly within each person. This means the symptoms of melancholy are illimitable, even infinite. They are

> irregular, obscure, various, so infinite ... Proteus himself is not so diverse as the symptoms of melancholy [and] ... you may as well make the Moone a new coat, as a true character of a melancholy man. (I,3,1,4:407)

> The Tower of Babel never yeelded such confusion of tongues, as this Chaos of melancholy doth variety of Symptomes. (I:3,1,2:395)

Support here is provided through appeal to ancient and renaissance medical writing:

> *Arculanus in 9. Rhasis and Almansor, cap.16* will have these Symptomes to be infinite ... indeed they are, varying according to the parties, for *scarce is there one of a thousand that dotes alike.* (I,3,1,2:384)

This emphasis on the mutability of the symptoms of Melancholy has parallels in early modern claims about another mental disorder, hysteria, the manifestations of which were also said to vary radically between people and within the same person at different times. Indeed, the great seventeenth-century disease classifier Thomas Sydenham (1624–1689) saw little difference between hysteria, hypochondriasis, and melancholy, proposing that they be classified together on the basis of this similarity.[16] Of hysteria he observed that it was a disease "not more remarkable for its frequency, than for the numerous forms under which it appears" (Swan 1742:371).

Burton names as sources or causes of melancholy every possible factor of personal natural history—from inherited tendencies to the effects of life experience, to behavioral habits such as solitariness and idleness, to all manner of cognitive and affective processes—even climate, astrological arrangements, broadly social and political context, and, albeit

---

16. For a history of the diverse appearances of hysteria, see Scull 2009.

indirectly, demonic influences.[17] (Original sin is also included as a very significant cause, as are the factors addressed in the Third Partition, such as jealousy, and love.[18]) And matching the protean range of causes, is the range of symptoms. For symptoms and causes "tread a ring," in what we would call feedback loops, the diversity of causes bringing a diversity of effects:

> as the causes are diverse, so must the signes be, almost infinite. (I:3,1,1:381)

This dizzying range of cause and symptom has led some commentators to reject the very category of melancholy on grounds of its complete incoherence.[19] Burton seems to almost agree, but believes progress can be made by sorting out passing from habituated states, and normal from diseased ones.

The illimitable variety of causes and symptoms of melancholy explains some of its anomalous nature as disease. Burton may not have disagreed with traditional medical lore when it came to other diseases. But Melancholy was different. The frequent use of the nominative form of "disease" reveals no allegiance to a particular conception, it should be added. *Disease* was a broad term. Throughout medieval and early modern times, especially within religious discourse, it had traded on its power as what would today be regarded as metaphor. "Ills," "illnesses," "maladies," "sickness," "diseases," even "sores," were attributes of the soul as much as the body, often reflecting exclusively moral or spiritual deficiencies. So

---

17. The Devil is ready to try and torment, he points out, and "His ordinary engine by which he produceth this effect, is the melancholy humour it selfe, which is ... the Divels bath.... The body works upon the minde, by obfuscating the spirits and corrupted instruments" (III:4,2,3:412). By contrast, Burton notes the medical thinking of his contemporaries on the means through which this demonic influence occurs, with which he disagrees: "many Phisitians are of opinion, that the Divell can alter the minde, and produce this disease himself" (I:2,1,2:193).
18. Although not a topic for the present book, the tie to original sin, particularly, is an important and reoccurring theme in the *Anatomy*.
19. Before the Napoleonic wars, it has been asserted, melancholia was but a rag-bag of insanity states whose "*only* common denominator was the presence of a few (as opposed to many) delusions" (Berrios and Porter 1995:385, emphasis added).

allusions to melancholy as disease in the *Anatomy* might be seen to have referred equally to imbalanced or deficient psychic and spiritual states, as to imbalanced or deficient bodily ones—although, as we have seen, these were barely distinguishable in the embodied whole of Burton's kind of dualism. And even seemingly straightforward assertions about melancholy as disease must be approached with a recognition of the earlier usage, before such attributions had come to be construed in exclusively metaphorical terms. (We see closely related ambiguities to these, even today. Philosophical accounts of disease in our own time include those that are explicitly and entirely normative, those that aim for a solely naturalist account, and hybrids, such as the well-known definition of disorder as harmful (organic) dysfunction.[20] This last, composite account may be the one closest to Burton's conception, where both humoral *imbalance*, and implied moral deficiency, each attend states of habituated melancholy.)

Burton's complex and somewhat anomalous conception of melancholy as disease illustrates that several different etiological elements make up any such conception: its actual causal claims and emphases, and the basis of its definitions and taxonomic, or familial, background. Burton's conception of disease differs from the classical models of Hippocratic and Galenic medicine in only some of these features. Symptoms and symptom sequences, rather than causes, guide definitions and emphases with Burtonian Melancholy, but as one of the diseases of the black bile, it is fitted within the classical etiological taxonomy.

HABITUATION

Melancholy symptoms can be seen as mental and behavioral habits, on Burton's account. They come incrementally, often by stealth, as we'll see, to form repeated patterns of feeling and thought (and habituated behavioral responses). In this respect, we may describe the model of disease he employs as a cumulative one, based on *habituation*. The transformation

---

20. Schwartz 2007.

from brief and passing states into the intractable condition that resists all efforts at remedy takes time. It is through the repeated occurrence of thoughts and feelings that states that have gone unchecked bring about their unhappy result. Entrenched and more severe forms of the disorder result from repetition. Because of that, the notion of a temporally extended natural history of melancholy, involving a causal sequence through stretches of time, is not only characteristic but *constitutive* of the analysis. And in any given individual, the method by which more severe and intractable melancholy is distinguished from passing states rests on its particular natural history.[21] Severe melancholy, is identified with the "chronic," habituated condition.

> This Melancholy ... a Chronic or continuate disease, a settled humor ... not errant but fixed, and as it was long increasing, so now being (pleasant, or painful) *grown to an habit*. (I:1,1,5:136, emphasis added)

This emphasis on the natural history, or *course*, of the condition echoes the Hippocratic observation that "If fear and sadness *last for a long time* it is melancholia" (Hippocrates 1923–31:185, emphasis added). It would also reflect familiarity with the taxonomy of disease stages laid out by the Hellenistic philosophers, beginning with the predisposition, followed by the temporary affection or disorder (*pathos* Greek, *affectus* Latin); the *nosema*, or chronic illness, regarded as a stable condition; and finally an inveterate disease where no cure could be possible.[22] In

---

21. Case material scattered through the *Anatomy* often makes casual reference to this aspect of Burton's conception of disease. See for example, reference to an advanced stage of melancholy in "a Parish Priest at Prage in Bohemia," who "was *so farre gone with melancholy, that he doted*, and spake he knewe not what" (II:4,2,1:229, emphasis added).
22. Every habit and faculty is "preserved and increased by correspondent actions," as Epictetus explains, whether in relation to bodily movement in the habit of walking, or with regard to the operations of the soul. For "it is impossible, but that habits and faculties must either be first produced, or strengthened and increased, by corresponding actions. Hence the philosophers derive the growth of all maladies. When you once desire money, for example ... if you apply no remedy, it returns no more to its former state, but, being again similarly excited, it kindles at the desire more quickly than before; and by frequent repetitions, at last becomes ... fixed" (*Discourses* I: xviii, 118).

the same way, Burton allows for a range of stages: the first melancholy leanings, with the willful and self-indulgent daydreaming he names "melanchologising" (also spelled "melancholizing"), which are still amenable to intentional efforts aimed at self-care, are separated from the full-blown, often delusional, states of disorder that resist any treatment. Paraphrasing the philosopher Philo Judaeus, he notes, "*if they be reiterated,*" perturbations

> penetrate the mind and *produce an habit of Melancholy at the last* ... having gotten the mastery of our souls. (I:2,3,1:248, emphasis added)

The cumulative effect of repeated "Melancholy provocations" will vary with the individual: "that which is but a flea-biting to one, causeth insufferable torment to another." Yet,

> as it is with a man imprisoned for debt, if once in the goale, every Creditor will bring his action against him, and there likely hold him. If any discontent sease upon a patient, in an instant all other perturbations ... will set upon him, and then like a lame dogge or broken winged goose hee droopes and pines away, and is brought at last to that ill habit or malady of melancholy it selfe. (I,1,2,1:1389)

Other metaphors also illustrate the habitual quality of melancholy: As children are frightened in the dark, "so are melancholy men at all times," having

> the inward cause with them, & still carrying it about ... a perpetuall fume and darknesse, causing feare, griefe, suspition, which they carry with them, an object which cannot be removed; but sticks as close, and is as inseparable as a shadow to a body & who can expel, or over-run his shadow? (I,3,3,1:420)

Our habits are attached to us.

On this way of construing melancholy, Burton's attention and emphasis must be directed toward the natural history of the condition as it is observed through time. A snapshot assessment that captures a moment only will fail to reveal whether some melancholy mood or state is a passing one, or indication of chronic, habituated disorder. Observing a longitudinal course to establish diagnosis involves a distinguishable methodology from the more familiar ones of today's medicine. The scans, blood tests, and other technological aids of biological medicine allow the measurement of underlying disease states. And these procedures often obviate the cumulative, longitudinal approach, and history taking, required by a symptom-focused or syndromal perspective. (Although psychological medicine employs comparable techniques using standardized interview procedures and self-report questionnaires, the analogies, and their success, are more controversial.)

The habituation model of disease thus has considerable implications for the difference between those with healthy but melancholic constitutions, and those who are truly diseased. By contrast with Du Laurens, who upheld that distinction, Burton may be supposed guilty of blurring it. But this assessment fails to recognize the full import of Burton's description of melancholy as disease as a "Chronicke or continuate disease," and a *"setled* humour" (I,1,1,5:136). His primary criterion for melancholy as disease involves habituation, and a habituation analysis is of its nature graduated, or dimensional: it cannot recognize a categorical distinction between mild, natural states of melancholy and diseased states. With additional adventitious causes, and neglectful habits of self-care, the natural temperament or passing state of sorrow or fear may, through time, become the untreatably severe condition of disease. Indeed, it is more likely to do so in the melancholy temperament than in any other. On a habituation analysis, repetition accounts for severity.[23]

---

23. Gowland has pointed out that in theory, the complexion was innate whereas the disease was adventitious, and the two also differed in severity of affliction. But the "natural toxicity of the humour ... eroded the boundary between the theoretically healthy "stable imbalance" of a complexion, and the condition of disease" (Gowland 2007:70–71). Even in theory, however, a habituation model where repetition explains severity cannot accommodate categories that are hard and fast. So to the extent that Burton adopted a habituation model, his account diverges from this aspect of humoral theoretical orthodoxy.

DISEASE CONCEPTIONS IN MODERN TIMES

To place Burtonian disease within our contemporary mind science, we must turn to the history of medicine between his era and our own. The germ theory of disease, based on microbial causes, and developed during the nineteenth century, has been judged radically different from the humoral conception it replaced. Disease now ceased to be primarily identified in terms of imbalance, and became infection, according to historians of science and medicine.[24] Before this change, medicine paid more attention to symptoms, rather than underlying causes, it has been asserted. In our contemporary medical terminology a "syndrome," no more than a cluster of symptoms, is distinguished from a full disease with a known or hypothesized etiology. Thus, a "syndrome driven," or symptom-focused account has been attributed to the conceptions of disease prevailing until well after the early modern period of the *Anatomy*.[25] Except when disorder lay in a wound or a morbidly affected organ, remedies sought to achieve balance (or *krasis*), affecting the bodily system as a whole. And attention lay with the observable symptoms as they progressed through the disease course.

This sketch may oversimplify the matter.[26] And in the *Anatomy* at least, as we saw, the picture is certainly more complicated. Burton's emphasis on causal factors *in addition to those* originating with humoral disturbances, left his model of disease or disorder a mixed one, not antithetical to, but not entirely consistent with, those depicted above by historians of early medicine. Whatever may have been exhibited by other accounts, the incessant, bidirectional sequences of causes and symptoms indicate that Burton's account, at least, was focused on symptoms and natural history.

---

24. Thagard 1999.
25. Thagard 1999, Carter 2003.
26. Other evidence suggests that an earlier shift away from a symptomatic conception (associated with the Hippocratic texts) towards a more anatomical one (associated with Galenism) occurred, and that each conception could be found throughout the period leading up to the nineteenth century. See Wilson, A. 2000.

The broad contrasts drawn above between etiological and symptom-focused analyses permitted by the perspective across several centuries are only very loose and schematic generalizations, however; they can at best be understood in terms of prototypes. One such prototype, in early modern times, is the thoroughgoing syndrome-driven analysis associated with Sydenham, whose efforts, modeled on botanic taxonomies, resulted in a scheme also emphasizing the natural history of diseases. Sydenham's painstaking observational work is quite foreign to Burton's textual and quotational style. Shared between these two massive seventeenth-century endeavors, however, remains their emphasis on symptoms understood longitudinally, as individual natural history. A Symptom may come and go, and perhaps indicate some other disease, Burton observes, illustrating this emphasis on disease course, and the part played by habit. But

> *if it continue* [it is] a signe of Melancholy itself. (I,1,1,4:132, emphasis added)

Of the attention to symptoms, Sydenham points out that the causes of the majority of diseases are "inscrutable and inexplicable" (Sydenham 1979:20). *What short way*, he asks "—what way at all—is there towards either the detection of the morbific cause . . . or towards the indications of treatment which we must discover, except the sure and distinct perception of peculiar symptoms?" (Sydenham 1979:15). Indeed, the physician *should* confine his observations to the "outer husk of things," he opines in *Theologia Rationalis*, his reasoning that God had so shaped the faculties to "perceive only the superficies of bodies, and not the minute processes of Nature's 'abyss of causes.'"[27] The *Anatomy* shows no such religious qualms—but nor does it trace all melancholy to the underlying states of humoral imbalance described by Hippocrates.

Aside from theological reticence such as Sydenham's, medicine's emphasis on symptoms would have been dictated by the state of knowledge in those times. Inhibited by the authority and viability of humoral

---

27. This passage from Sydenham's *Theologia Rationalis* is reproduced by Arikha (2007:2000).

explanations, and without the means and technology to discover underlying causes of disease symptoms, medical practitioners were limited. Of physicians, Burton remarks:

> many diseases they cannot cure at all, as Apoplexy, Epilepsy, Stone, Strangury [incomplete urination], Gout ... quartan agues; a common ague sometimes stumbles them all, they cannot so much as ease, they know not how to judge of it. (II,4,1,1:211)

Historians confirm this assessment: The diagnosis and successful treatment of most contemporary illnesses in the early seventeenth century exceeded the capabilities of doctors.[28]

The shift away from largely syndrome-driven approaches has been dated to early nineteenth-century medical thinking and discoveries.[29] The germ theory postulated by Koch (1884) ushered in a new "aetiological standpoint" (Carter 2003), made possible only when diseases ceased to be conceived, and defined, in terms of symptoms.[30] Different lines of research on several key, bacterially caused diseases had culminated in the conclusion that only by discovering the universal and necessary causes of diseases could medical intervention be successful. (This interest in universal necessary causes is unique to, and a defining

---

28. Thomas 1997:9.
29. See Carter 2003, for example. The presumption that any single disease model prevailed throughout renaissance medicine has been subject to challenge (Wear 1985).
30. The contrast between, and respective advantages offered by, these two approaches are familiar from twentieth-century psychiatric classifications, particularly the decision to adopt a syndrome-based "descriptive" rather than an etiological nosology in the third edition of the *Diagnostic and Statistical Manual of Mental Disorders* (American Psychiatric Association 1980). The contrasting interpretations differ importantly in explanatory potential, favoring the model encompassing deficient underlying processes (Kendell 1990, Schaffner 2002, Radden 2003, Murphy 2006). Other limitations associated with contemporary symptom-based, descriptive approaches to classification include the feature of "hyponarrativity" (Sadler 2005). The self-related and context specific aspects of the person's life understood holistically are abstracted away, leaving an impoverished "hyponarrative" that arguably detracts from treatment (Sadler 2005, Tekin 2013). With its focus on symptoms, the natural history approach to disease associated with early modern medicine seems more likely to have avoided this danger, at least inasmuch as it incorporates a holistic longitudinal picture of the patient through time.

characteristic of, modern Western thinking about disease, it has been asserted.[31]) Thus:

> the same cause was common to every instance of a given disease, becoming its defining feature, so that without its cause, a disease of that kind was not judged to be present. By the second half of the nineteenth century, medicine was beginning to emphasize and value causes of a particular kind: "universal necessary causes that met recognized criteria, that explained disease phenomena and held out promise of control . . . [and] the greatest success of this effort was the bacterial theory of disease. (Carter 2003:143–4)

The etiological standpoint (or at least some versions of it) identified by Carter and other historians of medicine thus differs from the *Anatomy*'s not in its classificatory basis, but in several other ways. It differs (i) in its conception of causes as singular defining conditions that are both necessary and sufficient; (ii) in the orderly and consistent part played by one cause rather than many; (iii) in its emphasis on endogenous causes rather than mixtures of endogenous and exogenous ones; (iv) in its finite, coherent, and stable symptom profile; (v) in its depiction of causes as more often specific, local events or morbid states in the body than effects that are holistic and systemwide;[32] and finally, (vi) in that it affords atemporal analysis, allowing snapshot forms of observation and identification for diagnostic purposes.

CONTRASTING CAUSAL MODELS OF DEPRESSION

The *Anatomy*'s anomalous conception of disease has intriguing parallels in theorizing about today's depression. Within contemporary mind

---

31. Carter 2003:1.
32. Carter resists any reference to specificity in his account, complaining that the term is vague and ambiguous (Carter 2003:9). However, we can safely recognize the more specific and localized aspect of the causes described in the etiological standpoint *relative to* whole-body humoral complexions and temperatures.

science, we find the long-entrenched descendants of nineteenth-century disease models, but also, challenging them, newer ideas. These include several quite distinct ways of understanding the relation between symptoms and disorders, of which not all make any reference to causes.[33] The elements of Burton's conception of melancholy as disease that leaves it ill-suited to the etiological standpoint, we'll see, are particularly consonant with one of these alternatives: the conception that identifies depressive disorder as *a network of symptoms together with the direct causal relations between them.*

Before we turn to these comparisons, it must again be stressed that despite parallels between melancholy and today's depression, the two conditions cannot be equated. Granted, there are similarities. They include the shared emphasis on the affective states at the center of the clinical picture; the negative moods (of sadness, fear, dejection, hopelessness, and apprehension), predominating; the temperamental risk factors that are taken to partially explain some of these disordered moods, and also the recognition that individual differences and natural histories will account for why one person remains resilient in the face of life's inevitable setbacks, while another succumbs to illness. The relationship between melancholy and depression has sometimes been described as one of Wittgensteinian family resemblance, and that seems as far as we can safely go.[34] To equate present-day conditions with the disorder Burton describes would encourage us to accept an etiological disease model whereby its diverse symptoms, and changing symptom profile, are bound together by a single unifying cause.[35] That model is inimical to much that Burton says about the causes and symptoms of melancholy, and ill fits the account he provides, however. Moreover, whether or not such a model is assumed, equating conditions from two different eras incurs problems. German Berrios has

---

33. Constructivist accounts hold that disorders are sets of symptoms conveniently grouped for some practical purpose, for example, while dimensional perspectives view diseases or disorders as continua rather than discrete classes. For analysis of these alternatives, see Borsboom 2008.
34. See Gowland 2006:81; in particular, melancholy has been assigned the relationship of "distant cousin" (Kramer 2005:10).
35. See Radden 2003, 2013, Varga 2013.

spoken of the anachronistic reading of cultural categories as a "continuity mirage." The common (but unwarranted) belief that regardless of historical period, terms such as *hypochondria*, or *melancholia* "must refer to more or less the same 'clinical' phenomena is difficult to ... extirpate," he complains. No matter how often specific research shows that throughout history the same terms *have named different behavioral packages*, the mistaken "search for 'invariants' continues" (Berrios 2011:xv).[36] Evidence argues against continuity, not for it, he warns, and we should remain wary of the tendency to equate disorder categories from different eras.

The diverse causes of Burtonian melancholy would not seem entirely exceptional in contemporary psychiatry today: multicausal and also multilevel causal analyses are sometimes acknowledged.[37,38] They have been long recognized in "final common pathway" analysis of depression, whereby many different causal or risk factors are sufficient to produce similar symptomatic effects, for example.[39] And while still adopting a fairly conservative conception of mental disorders as distinct and discrete kinds, some theorists nonetheless acknowledge that particular disorders need not stem from a single cause. Rather, there are "multiple different systems interacting in different ways picked out by cognitive neuroscience and neurobiology, that produce the same or similar kinds of psychopathology" (Kincaid 2014:151). Nonetheless,

---

36. The dubious exercise of *retrospective diagnosis*, invited by the continuity mirage, it has been noted, "suppresses precisely ... the content of past descriptive and diagnostic categories," and this content is what determines what medical practitioners saw (Wilson 2000:304).
37. See Shaffner 1993.
38. Causes in psychiatry have been shown usefully construed as INUS conditions (Schaffner 2002). That is, they are insufficient (alone) but nonredundant (and thus necessary) subparts of an unnecessary but sufficient condition. Among a plurality of causes, several different assemblages of factors, say ABC as well as JKL and XYZ, might each be sufficient to bring about the same effect (any given letter in such a configuration is an INUS condition). Since some the possible INUS conditions will remain unknown, causal general. Although Burton provides us with too little to confidently identify the causes of melancholy as INUS conditions, this analysis at least emphasizes the illimitable diversity of causes he describes.
39. The classic work on the final common pathway is Akiskal and McKinney 1973. But see also Klein 1974, and more recently, Cramer et al. 2012.

according to the most commonly accepted and familiar model of depression, the major diagnostic category of unipolar depression, today known as depressive disorder, is assumed to involve a single, endogenous cause. This has been referred to by several names: as the "common cause" hypothesis, and as a "diagnostic" perspective.[40] Associated with the American Psychiatric Association's *Diagnostic and Statistical Manual of Mental Disorder* (DSM), the model holds that beneath the potentially misleading appearances of symptoms, real disorders involve objective dysfunctions that account for why the symptoms occur. All the causal work, on this model, is attributable to "a single, essential underlying pathological process," earning it the label *essentialist* (Zachar 2014). The "harmful dysfunction" definition of disorder forming the theoretical core of both the fourth and recent fifth editions of the DSM, illustrates this model. A mental disorder is defined as "a syndrome characterized by clinically significant disturbance in an individual's cognition, emotion regulation, or behavior that reflects *a dysfunction* in the psychological, biological, or developmental processes underlying mental functioning" (American Psychiatric Association 2013:20, emphasis added).[41] The application of such a model to the particular disorder of depression occurs in the following typical definition: "Depressive disorder is a long term, relapsing condition associated with high levels of disability and mortality. *It has a neurobiological basis* and is associated with *functional and structural brain abnormalities*" (Palazidou 2012:1, emphasis added). Presupposed here is that beneath the observable surface, depressive disorder involves brain dysfunction that accounts for why the symptoms occur, and occur together, to produce a characteristic symptom profile.

Depression symptoms include the behavioral, bodily, and mood features familiar from diagnostic psychiatry and epidemiological findings. Hypotheses and research projects abound, but the exact

---

40. Cramer et al. (2012) employ "common cause"; because it descends from the classical idea of diagnosis as it originated in medicine, Borsboom (2008) names it the "diagnostic view."
41. The theoretical origin of this harmful dysfunction definition is Jerome Wakefield (Wakefield 1992).

underlying cause or causes of depression symptoms remain, as yet, incompletely understood. The endogenous cause giving rise to depression, on this model, has been hypothesized as states of structural or neuronal dysfunction, chemical imbalance or abnormality, inflammation, or some combination of these—as well as traits, genetic or otherwise, that function as diatheses or risk factors predisposing the individual to disorder.[42] (There are parallels with these etiological models in Freud's metapsychology. Behavioral symptoms, conscious feelings, and intentions also emanate from a hidden, unconscious locale—although it is usually depicted as ideas and memories, not brain or bodily states.)

Clinically and from the experiential perspective, depressive disorder generally presents itself as a series of temporally separated episodes that, on the etiological model, are part of a single disease entity—not a series of separate disorders. The contrast between two medical conditions, herpes and the common cold, illustrates these presuppositions and the linguistic conventions around them. The reoccurrence of a cold at different times reflects separate illnesses, not the occasional reemergence of the same one. In his influential 1938 critique of the division between endogenous and reactive depression, this point was made by Aubrey Lewis. Of periodicity (being episodic) as a distinguishing feature of the former, he wrote that it may be no more indicative of an intrinsic rhythm, or a biological periodicity "than is a series of a colds in the head."[43] On the etiological disease model, depression is more analogous to herpes than to a common cold, a reoccurring series of symptoms stemming for a single underlying state of disease. (This counting system may have considerable implications for the individual diagnosed with depression, it should be added. Being the bearer of a single, persisting disease that is "in remission" or "nonsymptomatic" presents itself differently from having a disorder and knowing one might in time have

---

42. See, for example, Kramer 2005: "In the new model of depression, underlying physiological defects (like a deficit in resiliency factors or a small hippocampus) are made worse by stress . . . a host of injuries combine to cause a common downstream process that becomes self-sustaining" (Kramer 2005:122).
43. Quoted in Shorter 2007:8.

another. The effects of diagnosis on self-identity are profound, and will include attitudes affected by these differing ways we count diseases. Among their unintended consequences, it has been demonstrated, the sciences of mental disorder serve as epistemic sources for those who must create self-narratives encompassing their diagnosis, disorder, and treatment.[44] And data on the subjective effects of essentializing mental disorder confirms such differences.[45])

Common-cause, etiological models of disease appear to have many, appropriate applications throughout medicine.[46] Yet they may not be as fitting for depression as has been widely presupposed, and recently several alternatives have been proposed. One alternative account most closely seems to reflect Burton's conception of disease: On it depression symptoms are not the result of a single underlying disease process or dysfunction, but instead comprise a causally related cluster of features—a network—that may be attributable to a range of causes.[47,48] Within this network model, psychiatric disorders arise from causal interactions between their component symptoms. In network approaches to psychopathology, disorders or diseases result from the *causal interplay between symptoms* (such as insomnia, worry, fatigue, and the like), when this may involve feedback loops. The disorder is a symptom cluster, and through time, the totality of symptoms constituting it forms a circuitry of causal relationships. As the result of mutual reinforcement and feedback loops within these symptom clusters, particular features enter into a large number of mutual relationships with other symptoms in the network.

44. See Tekin 2010, 2011.
45. Adriaens and De Block 2013.
46. And for the greater part of the modern scientific history of clinical psychology, as it has been pointed out, the common-cause idea seemed the only analysis available (Borsboom and Cramer 2013:93).
47. The more general network hypothesis is that not only depression but also other psychiatric disorders all result from interactions between their component symptoms. See Kendler, Zachar, and Craver 2011, Borsboom et al. 2011, Wichers 2014, Zachar 2014, Cramer et al. 2012, Borsboom and Cramer 2013.
48. Empirical research on the networks model of depression is thus far limited. But one study of symptoms caused by stressful life events has shown the network model to have significant predictive advantages over common-cause hypotheses (Cramer et al. 2012).

Depressive disorder is characteristically episodic, but whether depression more closely resembles the common cold or herpes will on the network model be an empirical, not a conceptual question. It is hypothesized that, with additional episodes, what has been described as an inescapably vicious circle of experiences will likely result.[49] When a depression reoccurs, on this account, new precipitating causes enter, and are reinforced, within an already established causal network. These additional, reinforced interactions leave the person increasingly unable to escape, and less dependent on new triggers for subsequent episodes.[50] (The sensitization phenomena known as kindling, taken by some researchers to reinforce this process, is introduced in chapter 5.)

One persuasive aspect of a network model for mood disorders like depression is that typical depression symptoms such as fatigue and insomnia, or hopelessness and sadness, seem more likely correlated because of an immediate causal relationship between them than because of an underlying liability independently affecting each. It stands to reason that insomnia might directly cause fatigue, and that a pattern of symptoms might emerge proceeding from that fatigue to concentration problems, to self-reproach to depressed mood to insomnia, in a loop that, with repetition, and through time, brings about, and in part constitutes, a depressive episode.[51] Similarly, hopelessness can be expected to engender sadness, which will in turn bring inertia, followed by self-reproach. These symptoms will have partly distinct etiologies: the connection between tiredness and insomnia involving more physiological homeostatic mechanisms, and that between depressed mood and self-reproach, more cognitive ones. But separate symptoms are not each the direct result of a single underlying state of dysfunction.

Also favoring the application of the network model for depression is that it seems implausible to suggest that depression might be entirely asymptomatic, in the way true of diseases more obviously fitting the etiological model, such as some early-stage cancers.[52] With disorders

49. Wichers 2014:1353.
50. Zachar 2014:167.
51. See Cramer et al. 2012.
52. The "masked," "hidden," or "latent" depression associated with the psychodynamic psychiatry of the twentieth century, no longer supported within contemporary

apparently unable to occur in the absence of psychological symptoms, it has been charged, conceiving of underlying causes that exist independently of the symptoms used to identify them must involve an unwarranted reification.[53]

Several points of contrast between network and etiological conceptions have bearing on the *Anatomy* account. On a network model of depression (i) its causes may be many, and include stressful life events that, rather than weak, incomplete, or partial causal antecedents, are sufficient to bring about the disorder; (ii) the disorder may be a fuzzy-edged rather than a sharply delineated, discrete entity; (iii) observation of its disease course through stretches of time will be required to identify it and determine its severity; and (iv) while not essential to it, some symptoms will be more central, as the result of many incoming and outgoing relations from and to other symptoms in the cluster. We can take these four features in turn.

(i) Some etiological accounts accommodate multicausal explanations such as Burton's, as we saw.[54] Only the etiological account that emphasizes a single, *common* cause is applicable here, and it is the one against which network models have been juxtaposed. Within the kind of kinds identified by philosophers of science, this alternative network model has proposed that disorders like depression comprise the cluster of causally related properties known as mechanistic (or homeostatic) "property clusters."[55,56] Depression will vary in its individual instantiations. But due to shared causal mechanisms (albeit a multitude of them rather than a single one), such as the link between insomnia, tiredness

---

classifications or research, was understood in terms of a preponderance of somatic, behavioral, or affective symptoms that concealed, or indirectly expressed, the affective states typically characterizing depression. Most recent thinking accepts that no mental disorder *can be asymptomatic* this way. If there can be masked depression, it will perhaps be more easily accommodated on the etiological model. On a network view, with its fuzzy edges, masked depression might or might not correspond closely enough to the more customary symptoms to warrant diagnosis as depression.

53. See Borsboom and Cramer 2013.
54. One example is to be found in Kincaid 2014.
55. See Boyd 1991, Kendler et al. 2011.
56. Homeostatic property clusters denote the co-occurrence of properties in the cluster sustained by a similarity generating or homeostatic mechanism (Craver 2009:575).

and concentration problems, it will form a loose cluster, unified by the causal relationships between its properties. The property cluster view of kinds, some have supposed, has an advantage in the context of psychiatric diseases more generally *because* they seem to be brought about by such a range of different causes.[57]

Troubling life events as the causes of depression have received extensive empirical study.[58] In recent work on symptoms caused by stressful occupation, finances, relationships, and so on, the network hypothesis proved a better predictor of correlation patterns between depression symptoms than did the common-cause model. From this it has been concluded—as Burton never doubted—that stressful life events are strongly implicated as causes of depressive episodes. And further confirming this conclusion, it has been established that stressful precipitants bring about clusters of symptoms that differ distinguishably according to the particular stresses involved.[59]

(ii) On a network model, symptom clusters or syndromes will vary in their degree of coherence and in the fuzziness at their boundaries, the networks expanding and contracting, for example, with alterations in their constituent symptoms. This leaves them dissimilar to the categorical kinds associated with most etiological models.[60] Networks exhibit more and less prototypical cases, and even the status of the symptom clusters as distinguishable entities may shift with changes within the networks involved.

With multiple causes and only loosely similar symptoms, a network relies on the stability of its constituent symptoms to provide

---

57. Murphy 2014:109.
58. Long-established correlations have indicated that stressful life events are sufficient causes of depressive states (Kendler et al. 1999, Jacobs et al. 2006, Munafo et al. 2009, Cramer et al. 2012).
59. Sadness, loss of interest, and loss of appetite more commonly resulted from the death of loved ones or dissolution of an intimate relationship, it was shown, whereas other precipitants more often prompted fatigue (Keller, Neale, and Kendler 2007). See also Cramer et al. 2012.
60. Some theorists are liberal enough in their conception of mental disorder categories that, while adhering to a broadly etiological model, they also acknowledge such fuzzy sets, as we saw (Kincaid 2014:151). But again, this is not typical: Etiological models customarily presuppose discrete boundaries.

coherence sufficient for diagnosis. The network model thus presupposes the presence of a finite set of symptoms forming a cluster that is relatively cohesive and at least temporarily stable, even though each of these interrelated symptoms may not possess any commonality. (By contrast, a common-cause etiological model can accommodate an illimitably diverse range of symptoms, unified, and afforded coherence, by its hypothesized discrete underlying disease entity.) In this respect, network models reflect "imperfect communities" (Zachar 2014:238). Some symptoms and symptom clusters in the domain overlap with others in the domain, but no shared common feature may unite all of them. These are also features of melancholy as Burton characterizes it: an amorphous whole, unified only loosely through its tendency to exhibit unwarranted fear and sadness.

The person's repeated, pervasive moods and apprehensions are indications of depressive disorder on a network model when, because, and to the extent that the connected links and loops occur often enough to become entrenched and self-sustaining, even to the point of no longer requiring any triggers. Within the network model, internal (causal) relations between symptoms determine the profile of the disorder (as well as its severity in particular cases). In this sense, depressive disorder comprises a loosely bounded syndrome. The individual symptoms in a network "sustain the other symptoms characteristic of the illness. Illnesses will ... appear as more or less stable sets of traits, in part because the traits are mutually reinforcing" (Kendler, Zachar, and Craver 2011:1147). The network model thus presupposes that depression symptoms make up the loosely coherent and finite set established by correlations between symptoms, observed through empirical study. And taxometric studies of depression, as well as brain studies, have together been judged to confirm the stability and relative coherence of depressive disorder (as defined through the DSM diagnostic criteria).[61]

(iii) Another feature of the network model of depression with parallels in the *Anatomy* lies with its temporally extended, cumulative nature.

---

61. For a summary of these findings see Kincaid 2014:165–70.

The examples used earlier, where symptoms like insomnia, fatigue, concentration problems, and low self-esteem become in their turn the causes of further symptoms, illustrate a natural history, or sequence. At least in part, the model relies on a cumulative effect, where severity is a function of the extent of the network and the number of repeated feedback loops linking symptoms together.[62] A cumulative assessment will establish the severity and extent of the accurate—or better, plausible—diagnosis of depression. In another example, depression's low mood and social isolation enter into a large number of mutual relationships with other symptoms in the network. Because reduced social interaction would result in more negative moods, it has been explained, "*cumulatively* . . . this dynamic interplay would result . . . in the clinical expression of anhedonia and social isolation" (Wichers 2014:1353, emphasis added). Limiting assessment of a network to a time slice, it has been observed, would "diminish the base rates and reduce the plausibility of the disorder's attribution" (Zachar 2014:136).

Among chronic rather than acute diseases, some are assigned to the category of being *progressive*, they worsen through their course.[63] Some are also *episodic*, with symptoms declining and reappearing through stretches of time. Burtonian Melancholy is one of the former: With repeated melancholy states, it becomes progressively severe. (We find little evidence of the episodic feature in the *Anatomy* account, although Burton's brief and secondhand case descriptions are insufficient for us to entirely rule it out.) As a chronic but episodic condition, typical unipolar depression is both similar and different to Burtonian Melancholy in these respects. Depression has been observed to run an interrupted but often progressive course, increasing in severity and frequency through the sequence of repeated episodes.[64]

---

62. This is not to deny that severity will rest on other causal factors as well (temperamental tendencies and environmental triggers, for example).
63. In physical medicine, progressive conditions exhibit a course that worsens or spreads through time, to the point of organ failure, death, or extreme debility. With mental disorder, the first element may alone be applicable: The condition worsens through time in some qualitative or quantitative dimension.
64. Although this absence of an episodic nature separates melancholy from depictions of depression, the progression through ever-worsening episodes of depression is

Like melancholy, depression allows of milder and more severe, even delusional, states. Data about milder forms of depression is not always borne out in more severe cases. (The relationship between more and less severe forms is also disputed, as we'll see in chapter 4.) So, for example, antidepressant medicines have long been shown to outperform placebo more robustly with severe disorder.[65] While Burton's conclusions have bearing on milder states of disorder, it may be supposed, they are less applicable when it comes to debilitating and severe conditions. Such a suggestion disregards the *Anatomy*'s emphasis on the difference between passing and more habituated or chronic melancholy, however. Entrenched and relatively severe forms of the disorder are those resulting from repeated feedback loops linking symptoms and causes. Unchecked repetition is in this respect one significant mark of severity. On Burton's practical criterion, more severe and chronic forms of melancholy are distinguished by neglecting personal efforts at prevention. When we have indulged our imagination and passions to the point that we can no longer adhere to the required behavioral and cognitive regimen and need to seek outside help, *our Melancholy has become a recalcitrant and dangerous disease*.

(iv) The unwarranted fear and sadness that are associated with melancholy are *typical* symptoms, as depicted in the *Anatomy*. They are less than unfailingly present, Burton concludes by the 1624 edition—not, as he had earlier supposed, "inseparable companions" (I:163). But they are strongly characteristic, affecting "most Melancholy, not all."[66]

The fit with the *Anatomy*'s ideas about melancholy and network models of disorder is thus considerable. Burton throws up his hands over any hope of identifying and isolating the rapid and incessant shifts and changes

---

sometimes portrayed in terms very similar to Burton's. Thus Kramer speaks of the *career* of depression and of its "late stages" in depleted inpatients, on whose charts "you would see notations that stretched back over decades. Accounts of recurrent hospitalizations and incomplete recoveries" (Kramer 2005:20).

65. Many studies have since replicated the first observation of this effect by Donald Klein (1974).

66. The whole passage reads: "*Feare* and *Sorrow* are the true Characters, and inseparable companions of *most* Melancholy, *not all* . . . for some it is most pleasant, as to such as laugh most part; some are bolde againe, and free from all manner of feare and griefe" (I:1,3,2:163, emphasis added).

making up the particular course of the disorder. So the network model provides a conception of causation more accommodating of the chaotic plurality of multilevel, multicausal explanations for melancholy, including stressful experiences, as well as the incessant feedback loops, where elements are transformed from cause to symptom to cause and back, "treading a ring." Its diseases are fuzzy rather than sharply edged and discrete entities, exhibiting relative stability of symptoms across episodes, and between individuals, and requiring observation of each particular disease's course to identify and measure severity. The picture he presents diverges from the common-cause etiological, disease model of depression still guiding much psychiatric medicine. But, as in the network model, the *Anatomy* depicts reoccurring states and traits (particularly groundless fear and sadness) that, if not common to all melancholy, are at least common enough to form a characteristic and typical pattern. Melancholy is a loose syndrome, comparable to the network model's imperfect community comprising depression symptoms.

On a network model, symptoms do not *define* the disorder in an essentialist sense, as we have seen. They are only contingently related to diagnosis, a diagnosis that could alter, or even cease to apply. Adhering to a network model in the face of a radical transformation of the symptom picture, we might be tempted to say the disease category "depression" had disappeared. Its relative stability and cohesiveness thus play a different epistemic role with the network model than with the common cause one, which could better weather such a radical transformation. Extreme changes in the symptom profile may also present a diagnostic challenge, on the etiological model. But they do not require us to say one disease has disappeared or been replaced by an entirely different one.

This is a not an inconsiderable concern, for two reasons. The history of psychiatric disorders has included transformative symptom shifts of this type; and recent theorizing has also attributed such changes to depression. Hysterical paralyses, the once common symptoms of hysterical and neurasthenic conditions, illustrate the first of these.[67] So do the symptom clusters that are apparently made possible

---

67. On these symptoms, see also Shorter 1992, 2013.

by constellations of cultural and technological changes.[68] The sociologist Alain Ehrenberg argues that depression has seen a similar symptom transformation, altering the meaning of the disorder.[69] As well as, or even replacing sadness and anxiety, Ehrenberg asserts, the symptoms of what was once known as depression now present a different profile, characterized by feelings of exhaustion, impotence, inhibition, vulnerability, paralysis, dependency, lack of self-confidence, or inability to deal with frustration. "Depression" has expanded as a category, encompassing more ills than before. But it has also become unrecognizably changed from the earlier disorder known by that name, and should not be confused with it. Such extensive transformation may leave unaltered the core of the disease on a common-cause etiological model. But the content of its symptom clusters on a network model are only as valid as the strictly empirical observations confirming their presence.

COMMON CAUSES AND MAGIC BULLETS

Burton was not a scientist in the modern sense. Indeed, he was an unabashed moralist. But far from detrimental to his account, Melancholy's compatibility with a network disease model of depression leaves his mind science in good standing. Moreover, his conception of disease and causal explanation has far-reaching implications for his ideas about remedying and averting melancholy, as well. The great advantage of isolating the cause of a condition with precision lies in the power it should afford us to find an effective treatment (whether that cause is endogenous or environmental). With a sufficiently precise treatment, and a coherent disease entity whose causal properties are fully understood, a single, specific cause can be expected to only require a single remedy.[70] It has proven to do so in many of the triumphs of modern medicine over diseases. The emphasis in earlier times had been *strengthening*

---

68. See Hacking (1995, 1998) for examples.
69. Ehrenberg 2010.
70. See Thagard 1999, Carter 2003, Healy 1997.

the host, or what Burton describes as "mending the Temperament."[71] But in descriptions of these oft-cited, recent triumphs, more bellicose language abounds: Rather than strengthening the host, on this model, the goal is to attack the invader. Specific ("targeted") responses to particular diseases, identified by way of their causes, are magic bullets, as medicine battles to vanquish disease.[72]

These triumphalist metaphors and successes, however, were over the horizon, way beyond what Burton could have envisioned. Along with maintaining humoral balance and righting imbalance, his modest remedial goal was avoiding suffering and distress, and averting worse dysfunction.[73] More importantly, and even beyond these differences, it would not have occurred to Burton to adopt a magic-bullet model for remedying melancholy, nor would it have appealed to him. His conception of that condition is anomalous within these contemporary models. Its causes are illimitable, even infinite, in number: Its boundaries are loose and inexact, and it is far from a coherent and discrete disease entity along the lines of the bacteriological infections that gave rise to the common-cause etiological models. (To the extent that they also lack coherence and discreteness, indeed, any diseases understood as networks will be similarly unsuited to the magic-bullet reasoning.)

The idea of these specific responses draws strength from a conception of underlying dysfunction or deficit that is localized rather than more systemwide. Humoral temperatures and complexions were for the most part construed as a whole-body state, affecting every organ and function. By contrast, the twentieth-century conceptions usually

---

71. The temper "is to be altered and amended, with such things as fortify and strengthen the heart and braine, which are commonly both affected in this malady, and doe mutually misaffect one another" (II,5,1,5:246).
72. For an example of such reasoning, see: "The ability to identify small groups of patients who can benefit from targeted treatments is necessarily built upon two major factors. First, diagnostic tests are required to identify relevant genetic polymorphisms, biomarkers, and other specific aspects of disorders. Second, new interventions must be developed that are targeted directly to the disease mechanisms identified by the diagnostics" (Cuthbert and Insel 2013:1076).
73. As well as averting melancholy in this sense of avoiding or preventing its occurrence, Burton also speaks of enemas and suppositories as more literal "averters" due to their purgative function.

construe disease as localized within some particular organ or system. Again, we turn to the germ theory of the nineteenth century and particularly the work of Virchow (1821–1902), to find the origin of this assumption and its incumbent emphases. Virchow had instilled the idea that all diseases can be traced to causes that are localized.

CATEGORIES AND DIMENSIONS

Within medical psychiatry, both dimensional and categorical models are employed, and particular psychiatric disorders such as depression, as well as the overarching category of psychiatric disorder, have provoked debate about their status as dimensional or categorical.[74] Where Melancholy lies, according to this division, is surprisingly unclear. Both humoral medicine and network analyses are dimensional, allowing us to place melancholy on a continuum stretching between brief sad moods, through increasingly habituated and extreme gloominess, to delusional obsession. And in keeping with the legacy of renaissance humanism, this is for the most part the picture envisioned by Burton. A continuum is explicitly endorsed in one passage:

> as they write of heat and cold, we may say of this humour, one is *melancholicus ad octo*, a second two degrees lesse, a third halfe way. 'Tis super particular . . . all these Geomentricall proportions are too little to expresse it. (I,3,1,4:404–5)

Even habituated melancholy, the disease proper, when placed in contrast to more passing states, is construed as "super particular" and continuous with those states. Yet, references to melancholy that resists efforts of self-help, or reaches the point where the black bile is burnt or *adusted*, suggest a categorical difference. And a further categorical separation can be found where Burton speaks of the combination of a flawed imagination with a defect of reason that accounts for the delusional thought afflicting some, but not all, melancholy sufferers. (This is discussed in chapter 6.) Moreover, in a third

---

74. The status of disorders as natural kinds has been the locus of some of this debate. See Kincaid and Sullivan 2014.

differentiation, Burton briefly hints that a shift in the individual's usually stable humoral *complexion* occurs with the emergence of more serious disorder.[75] We are left with several criteria by which a discrete category might be delineated. This seeming confusion shows the *Anatomy*'s to be neither an exclusively dimensional nor a solely categorical account, however, and to rely instead on a breakdown orthogonal to that much-used binary. What is more significant for Burton, practical treatment issues are appealed to in dividing melancholy, and these are neither categorical nor dimensional in the sense usually intended. In one passage, the practical contrast is neatly reiterated and explicitly linked to incurability:

> this disease is either in habit or disposition, curable or incurable. (II,3,8,1:206)

At other times, emphasis is placed on the point where remedial self-help proves alone insufficient. Distinguishing disorder that is incurable, or has advanced beyond the point where self-help can provide a sufficient remedy, does introduce categories of a kind. But they are categories arising out of practical life, not biology.

This is an approach that has its defenders, it should be acknowledged. Some have argued that the idea of an unchanging general-purpose classification for psychiatry is mistaken, and any divisions ought to be guided by the pragmatic goals of practice and science (including reliable diagnosis, prediction, and identification of risk factors).[76] Other research has similarly emphasized that the binary distinction between categorical and dimensional conceptions of disorder conceals further separations, of which "practical" kinds (Zachar) is one.[77] (What counts as a good dividing line around mental disorders such as depression "depends on what we want/need the classification to do for us," it has been observed [Zachar 2014:177].) And from the perspective of such contemporary analyses, the forms of untreatably severe melancholy described by Burton constitute kinds (or a kind) unto themselves.

75. I,1,1,5:138.
76. Zachar 2000, 2003, 2014.
77. See Haslam 2002.

In relation to the present-day contrasts by which causes are distinguished from signs and symptoms, etiological accounts of disease from symptom-focused ones, and categorical from dimensional disorders, Burtonian Melancholy exhibits several anomalies. The signs, symptoms, and natural history of melancholy are its focus; in this respect, we can say, it is understood on a "syndromal model." This emphasis on symptoms and course is only in contrast to exclusively endogenous causes, however: Multiple causes are acknowledged (at least as many of them exogenous as endogenous), leaving the picture quite consonant with contemporary network models of depression. Finally, Burton's melancholy can be seen as a more dimensional than categorical condition. Yet his is also a pragmatic account: neither entirely dimensional nor entirely categorical, and orthogonal to that contrast. Melancholy itself, and also its subdivisions, are instead "practical" kinds of entity.

There is an important consequence of the analysis in this chapter: The analogies between melancholy and depressive disorder, in this and what follows, can be recognized to be at most analogies. To go further would be to risk Berrios's "continuity mirage." But in addition to Berrios's concerns, there are theoretical implications that are likely to be considerable, and may prove unwelcome. Any variation in the symptom pictures characterizing each of melancholy and depression can be accommodated if they are construed as anchored by an underlying, idiopathic state, and equating today's mood disorders with melancholy quite naturally invites an etiological model of disease. Yet that model fits little else that Burton says about the causes and symptoms of melancholy. In equating the two disorders through the embrace of an etiological disease model, we confront daunting disparities within the descriptions of each disorder. Stronger analogies actually unite Burtonian Melancholy with some aspects of today's depression if the latter condition is understood on a network model of disease. Networks do not support the idea of unchanging cross-cultural or cross-historical disease identities, however. In light of these tangles, and the epistemic hazards of the continuity mirage, *analogical* relations between these two conditions—*not identity*—will be presupposed in the rest of this book.

Chapter 4

between the confines of sense and reason

With its signature disturbances of fear and sadness, Melancholy is primarily a disorder of affect, and the evaluative, attenuated, and cognitively based Passions are as central to the *Anatomy* as the Imagination, that faculty unique in its tendency, and ability, to affect them. The Passions are endlessly troubled and troublesome at all times, but particularly so as,

> the fountain, the subject, the hinges whereupon [melancholy] turns (II:2,6,1:100)

This chapter explores the particular feelings of ungrounded and sometimes objectless sorrow, sadness, and fear that, as the prototypes of melancholy suffering, form the "hinges" on which melancholy turns. They are considered here in terms of the contemporary philosophical category of moods, in their relationship to one another (as "German cousins"), and as their status as Passions contrasts with the deracinated category of emotion employed in much affective science today. The distressing feelings assailing the melancholic bring us to some of the commonest symptoms, and most intransigent classificatory issues, confronting contemporary medical psychiatry. They prompt obvious parallels with today's states of depression and anxiety. But in addition, they seem to carry implications for the problem of "comorbidity" arising from the relationship between depressive and anxiety disorders inasmuch as they are interpreted on etiological disease models. Finally, this chapter requires us to enter the fraught arena of present-day psychiatric classification, for the canon on melancholy of which Burton's work forms a part has been explicitly invoked within depression classifications. Parallels are sometimes drawn between melancholy and depression, as we know, but in recent years they have also been drawn between melancholy and the particular category, or subcategory, of Melancholic Depression. Neither comparison can be entirely dismissed, it will be concluded here. Yet neither fits Burtonian Melancholy as readily as these casual comparisons would suggest.

The mid-seventeenth century saw philosophical interest in affective states and processes unmatched since Stoic times. Major works were devoted to their explication and classification, particularly Descartes's *Passions of the Soul* (first published in 1649), and Spinoza's *Ethics* (1677). The classical categories and conceptions largely accepted throughout medieval and renaissance eras were now subject to fresh, analytic attention and powerful systematic analysis. *The Anatomy of Melancholy* comes before these explorations, or at least before Burton could have known of them, and his approach is less original, systematic, and sophisticated. Yet, as we have seen, Burton has an advantage when it comes to the passions. His attention on the aberrant case of affective disorder, and respect for the long tradition that placed fear and sadness at the center of melancholy suffering combined with his embodied interactionism to leave him immune from the extremes of much dualistic modern psychology. (In analyzing the passions, Descartes himself accepts something close to the same notions as Burton's.[1])

The earlier centuries had also given rise to some works devoted to the passions. And one of these, *The Passions of the Mind in General* by

---

1. Traditional models had assumed a kind of transparency about the operation of the passions, Cottingham explains: We are aware of what we ought rationally to do, and we are also aware of emotions often pulling us in the opposite direction. But Descartes's insight is that "the causal genesis and subsequent occurrence of the passions is intimately linked to corporeal events in ways which often make the force of the resultant emotion *opaque to reason*" (Cottingham 1998:92, emphasis added).

Wright, introduced earlier, Burton read and seemingly knew well.[2,3] There is little mention of melancholy in Wright's work, which is on the passions more generally understood.[4] And other than borrowed phrases, Burton's debt to Wright is rather an *attitude* toward what Wright calls the "garboil of these tumultuous Passions." With his inimitable turn of phrase, Wright says of these Passions that they "toss and turmoil our miserable souls as Tempests and Waves the Ocean Sea, which never standeth quiet but either is ebbing or flowing—with winds that buzz about it, or rains alter it, or earthquakes shake it, or storms tyrannize over it" (T.Wright 1986:327). And Burton wholeheartedly accepts this kind of depiction.

The *Anatomy* employs unquestioningly the categories from the earlier, medieval era, with its rich inheritance of ideas about the passions from Greek, Roman, and Thomistic sources. These include some traceable through the sixteenth-century neo-Stoic revival associated with Justus Lipsius (1547–1606). As well as a broad classificatory scheme, such sources provide an enumeration of each particular one of the passions. Some of these are felt states (fear and sorrow, for example). Others, like emulation and mercy, seem more akin to what we might call settled attitudes, or motives; still others are desires and inclinations. Burton adopts a standard list, as we saw earlier, and in recounting the

---

2. There are two acknowledgments of Wright in the *Anatomy*, in each case identifying him as a Jesuit (at I,2,3,1 and I,3,3,3). In addition, one of Burton's most striking descriptions of the perturbations and passions echoes lines of Wright's. These feelings, the *Anatomy* reads, "dwell between the confines of Sense and Reason, yet . . . rather follow Sense than Reason, because they are drowned in corporeall organs of Sense" (I,2,3,3:255). The passage in Wright's *Passions* goes: "[these passions] inhabit the confines of both sense and reason. . . . For passions are drowned in corporeal organs and instruments . . . passions follow rather Sense than Reason" (Wright 1986:95).
3. Whether he also read the influential *A Table of Human Passions* by the French bishop Nicolas Coffeteau (1574–1623), which had been translated into English in the year that saw the first edition of *The Anatomy of Melancholy*, is not clear.
4. Offering examples of how the passions alter the body, Wright does speak of those who have permitted themselves to be "o'rruled with the melancholy Passion," explaining that "The cause why sadness doth so move the forces of the body . . . [is] the gathering together of much melancholy blood about the heart, which collection extinguisheth the good spirits" (Wright 1986:136).

different ways the passions have been divided he avoids taking sides. The language in the *Anatomy* is of "perturbations," "affections," "passions," and "inclinations." Each of these terms finds its source in Latin translations of the Greek *pathos* by Cicero and Seneca. (There are nuances of difference between them, however. The course, and cognitive complexity, of the states they name vary, as does their association with identifiable feelings and sensations.) "Emotion" comes in later, as we'll see, and brings new connotations more apposite for the part played by feelings as objects of scientific observation and study.

The passions and affections dwell, as (borrowing from Wright) Burton says, "between the confines of sense and reason," and are "drowned in corporeall organs of Sense," so that they are closer to sense than reason (I,2,3,3:255).[5] They include "lusts" and "appetites." Unfailing control of any of these states is rare. Only "a few discreet men" can curb their affections.[6] Most cannot, and instead

> precipitate and plunge themselves into a Labyrinth of cares; blinded with lust, blinded with ambition.

Giving way to violent passions, they "crucify their own souls" (I:2,3,4:256).

The most important passions are listed as love, joy, desire, hatred, sorrow, and fear, to which are added affections reducing to them (anger, envy, emulation, pride, jealousy, anxiety, mercy, shame, discontent, despaire, ambition, avarice, "&c.").[7] Any one of these passions, "if they be *immoderate*" can "macerate ... mindes" in such a way as to bring about, or exacerbate, melancholy (I,2,3,4:256, emphasis added). So, as well as being feelings whose object is unknown, or somehow illogically grounded or distortedly conceived, one way passions can make

---

5. This point is stressed in descriptions of emotions from the seventeenth century; for example: "as properties of the sensitive soul, the passions just are ... *simultaneously physical and psychological*. Bodily motions are shot through with feeling, and feeling is expressed in ... bodily manifestations" (James 1997:65, emphasis added).

6. I,2,3,3:255.

7. I,2,3,3,:255. Anxiety, along with a range of other feelings, was a "fearfull branch" derived from one of the two stems of feare and sorrow (I,2,3,5:260).

trouble is by their sheer *excess* or inappropriate persistence. Feeling too intensely, or too long, in relation to an object, even when that object is appropriate, will incite melancholy. (Illustrating the latter case, is the person who grieves overlong, a common matter in Burton's England noted by the practitioner Richard Napier in his case records.[8])

Like the later seventeenth-century philosophers, and the Stoics before him, Burton judges the passions to jeopardize and distort reasoning quite as much as they endanger a person's soul by inciting sinfulness and vice. Particularly influential is the idea that feelings lead us astray in our judgments. This view, associated with Stoic cognitivism, construes feelings as guided and partially constituted by beliefs. Thinkers from the preceding century had also emphasized this cognitivist analysis of the passions: Wright speaks of the way perturbations trouble the soul, blinding inclination toward virtue by "the corrupt judgement caused by inordinate Passions" (T.Wright 1986:133). So had Burton's closer contemporaries. About the idea that feelings must be controlled and trained, and that this "stubborn will of ours perverts *judgement*," Burton quotes approvingly from Luther's friend and contemporary Phillip Melancthon (1497–1560), for example:

> [judgment] sees and knows what should and ought to be done, and yet will not doe it. (I,2,3,3:256)

That perturbations and other affections had a special role in the presence and persistence of melancholy states is a central doctrine in the *Anatomy*. Quoting Philo Judaeus, who wrote in Alexandria during the first century CE, Burton notes (in his own translation) that

> Perturbations often offend the body, and are most frequent causes of Melancholy.

Moreover, repeated affective disturbances of these kinds explain the habituated states of melancholy that resist efforts of will. Again quoting

---

8. See Macdonald 1981a. Sorrowful occasions were so common in Napier's era, Macdonald points out, that excessive and prolonged grief was a preoccupation (Macdonald 1981a:158).

or paraphrasing from Philo Judaeus, Burton goes on to say that "if they be reiterated," perturbations

> penetrate the minde, and produce *an habit of Melancholy at the last* . . . having gotten the mastery in our soules. (I,2,3,1:248, emphasis added)

We saw in other passages that Imagination is named the most frequent cause of Melancholy, so this seeming assignment of the passions to that position must be explained by the interactive relationship between the two, with passions triggering imagination, and imagination in turn inciting passions. It is this iterative action that, with further repetition, brings about Melancholy. This imagination, Burton explains,

> is the *medium deferens* of passions, by whose meanes they worke and produce many time prodigious effects; and as the phantasie is more or lesse intended or remitted, and their humours disposed, so do perturbations move more or less, and take deeper impression. (I,2,3,3:255)

The broad links between affective and cognitive states posited by Burton find confirmation in aspects of today's neuroscience that are by now widely accepted. Just as the animal spirits transported messages (representations, we might say, or even tokens of propositions) to the heart, firing neurons send data to the brain's emotion centers, producing feelings and reactions experienced over or about the ideas and imaginings represented. The details of this process and the extent to which Burton anticipated its broad structure, were introduced in chapter 1.

SADNESS AND FEAR WITHOUT CAUSE

By Burton's time, renaissance humanism had challenged many of the tenets of ancient medicine, casting doubt on both practice and theory.[9] A little-altered aspect of that ancient medical lore, however, was the framing of melancholy as a condition of subjective distress—often depicted as mood states of apprehension and sadness without, or without sufficient, cause or warrant.[10] Bright is typical: The perturbations of melancholy, he notes, are for the most part "sadde and fearfull, and such as rise of them: as distrust, doubt, diffidence, or despair" (Bright 1586:59). The melancholike man properly so called, for Du Laurens, is "ordinarily out of heart, always fearfull and trembling, in such sort that he is afraid of every thing" (Du Laurens 1599:82). And, acknowledging Hippocratic and Galenic aphorisms, Burton names fear and sorrow Melancholy's " most assured signs, true characters and inseparable companions" and its "most grievous and common" symptoms (I,3,3,1:418).

> *Feare* and *Sorrow,* are the true Characters, and inseparable companions, and characters of most Melancholy. (I,1,3,1:163)

Burton appears to have puzzled over the relationship of these two to melancholy. By the 1624 edition of the *Anatomy* he has relinquished the claim that fear and sorrow are " *inseparable* companions" or, we might say, essential characteristics of melancholy. Instead, based on further reading of the classical canon on melancholy, he concludes that they are typical or characteristic aspects only (I,1,3,2:163).[11]

The striking persistence of these descriptions of sadness and fear without cause have been the grounds for claims about the presence of melancholia through the ages, the equation of melancholy and depression, and even the pancultural nature of these conditions.[12] Melancholia

---

9. See Babb 1959, Gowland 2006, Jackson 1986, Wear 1985, Kristellar 1988.
10. The continuity of these feelings through the premodern and modern era has been traced and confirmed. See Radden 2003, 2013, Varga 2013.
11. Rather than based on empirical observation, the qualification is attributed to reading Hercules de Saxonia's treatise about Melancholy.
12. For example, Andreason 1982, Jackson 1986. On the other hand, others have insisted that low affect was not part of the definition of melancholia until well after Burton's time (Berrios and Porter 1998). For a thorough and fair review of the force of the continuity between melancholy and today's affective disorders, see Varga 2013.

was "the term usually used to refer to the depressive syndrome," on one view.[13] We have seen already one reason why, despite notable similarities, any such inferences should be approached with caution. To judge these parallels to be identities would encourage us to embrace common-cause etiological models of disease, not easily accommodated by Burtonian Melancholy. Further reason for caution is that the medical descriptions echoing each other resoundingly through the ages are not empirical evidence in our modern-day sense. The continuity in symptom descriptions between past eras reflects adherence to medical and particularly Galenic lore as much as, or even more than, it does independent and corroborating clinical observation.[14]

Also, despite the centrality of the states of fear and sadness without cause as the inseparable companions of most melancholy, that condition is associated with other symptoms stemming from a disordered imagination as well. Thus while certain *symptoms* show continuity, full *syndromes* or symptom clusters cannot be assumed to do so. To illustrate: Burton's cases commonly indicate the presence of what we would today identify as other disorders. They include what we would call delusional ideas, usually depicted as unaccompanied by troubled feelings, as well as what resemble today's obsessions and compulsions, and the mistrustful attitudes that today betoken the separate disorder of paranoia. Grounds are there, then, for recognizing cross-historical continuity in the conjunction of sadness and fear depicted as emblematic of melancholy, but they are grounds not entirely apparent from these "case records." And certainly, the persisting symptom descriptions in the long medical canon about melancholy cannot be used in any unproblematic way to infer the presence of an unchanging disease entity.

The fear and sadness without cause that are the symptoms of melancholy are subjectively experienced complaints. Although, following ancient Hippocratic and Gallenic lore, melancholy is classified as one of the diseases of the black bile, the disease concept employed here is not quite that of today's medical orthodoxy, as we saw in chapter 3. This

13. Andreason 1982:24.
14. See Jackson 1986, Berrios and Porter 1995, Wear, French, and Lonie 1985.

leaves the expression *disease of the black bile* potentially misleading. Moreover, the status of chronic disease is accorded *only when melancholy becomes so habituated as to be beyond control through efforts of will*. (When, having "gotten the mastery in our soules," as it is put in the passage quoted above, melancholy the habit sets in, Burton says, it "may well be called disease[s].")

Not all melancholy is this severe, entrenched, and diseased kind. Melancholy distress may be brief and passing:

> these Melancholy fits . . . continue not; but *come & goe*. (I,1,2,1:138, emphasis added)

Such "dispositions" tend to become habituated, it is true. In any person, when passions and imagination are unchecked by reason, there is a risk that they can lead to ingrained, habitual, and eventually untreatable, melancholy.[15] Even for the "best and soundest of us all," this is a great danger.[16] Once ingrained, and a "Chronicke, or continuate disease," Melancholy is next to incurable:

> so now being . . . growne to an habit, it will hardly be removed. (I,1,2,1:139)

PHENOMENOLOGICAL EMPHASIS

If the most common and grievous symptoms are feelings and affections the subject stands in a privileged position to report and describe, then the personal sufferer can elucidate melancholy in ways not available to a more detached observer. This is not the incorrigibility associated with reports of feelings that became a feature of post-Cartesian

---

15. "it falleth out oftentimes that these Dispositions become *Habits*, and *many affects contemned*, (as *Seneca* notes) *make a disease. Even as one Distillation, not yet growne to custome, makes a cough; but continual; and inveterate causeth a consumption of the lungs*: so doe these our Melancholy provocations" (I,1,1,5:138).
16. I,3,2,1:408.

epistemology. We can misdescribe and misrepresent our feelings, inadvertently as well as willfully. Nonetheless, the Burtonian sufferer has a special relation to his feelings, and subjective experience is privileged.

This phenomenological emphasis alerts us to the significance of Burton's seeming hints that, like others, he writes of melancholy as a sufferer as well as an observer. Those others are of course legion, and famously include Ficino, Montaigne, and Luther. Also, there is Melancthon, whose *De Anima* (1540, revised 1553) Burton quotes with approval about the epistemic advantage firsthand experience provides. He was much troubled by melancholy, he says of Melancthon, and

> therefore could *speak out of experience*. (I,2,5,4:379, emphasis added)

Evidence that Burton himself suffered from melancholy comes from several passages, including "I write of Melancholy, by being busie to avoid Melancholy" (I,6), and "Concerning my selfe, I can peradventure affirme ... that which others heare or read of, I felt and practiced my selfe, they got their knowledge by Bookes, I mine by melancholizing" (I,8). Explaining why he writes about Melancholy, he observes that at one time he had been

> fatally driven upon this Rocke of Melancholy, and carried away by this by-streame, which as a Rillet, is deducted from the main Channell of my studies, in which I have pleased and busied my selfe at idle houres, as a subject most necessary and commodious. (I,20)

And he reports that he is "not a little offended with this maladie, shall I say my Mistris Melancholy" (I,7).

Such personal references may provide less than conclusive proof of Burton's own suffering. Each one is from the long, introductory letter added at the start of the second (1624) edition of the *Anatomy* (and subsequent ones), which has often been dismissed as exaggerated and unreliable.[17] Moreover, because Burton believes avoiding melancholy is possible—and advisable, his personal efforts to avoid it may have succeeded. And his "Rocke of Melancholy," at least, may have been little more than an obsessive scholarly interest in the topic. Regardless, the above remark about Melancthon, and his own that melancholy is "Something I can speake out of experience" (I,8) are sufficient to establish the general, epistemic point. Firsthand accounts of melancholy provide a valuable and perhaps indispensable addition to our understanding of it, reminding us of the virtues of what later came to be known as the phenomenological approach.

"SUCH A WANT-WIT SADNESS"

When he speaks of the unwarranted fears and strange ideas resulting from a disordered imagination unconstrained by reason, Burton often describes beliefs and feelings that are inappropriate to their objects, or causes.[18] He offers examples:

> Fear of Devils, death, that they shall be so sick, of some such or such disease, ready to tremble at every object. (I,3,1,2:385)

Unwarranted or ungrounded beliefs and speculations about the presence of demons, or sickness, or imminent death, produce *unwarranted* fearfulness in these examples, and not only apprehensive feelings, but their trembling bodily expression. In melancholy, fear and sadness are inappropriate—either in degree or kind—to the states of affairs toward

---

17. The Letter is apparently modeled on an earlier work from the sixteenth century: a widely circulated, anonymous, pseudo-Hippocratic *Letter to Damagetes*. See Gowland 2006:8–15. In the earlier document, the philosopher was writing a treatise on madness, it has been pointed out, while in retelling the tale of Democritus, Burton expands its subject matter to include melancholy as well as madness. By that means, the "psychologically disturbed and foolish melancholic was thereby presented as ... an incarnation of the necessary coincidence of misery, ignorance, and moral turpitude" (Gowland 2006:15).
18. "Object" and "cause" are each used to refer to what the feelings are about or directed toward.

which they are directed (their cause or object) or the context in which they occur. Extreme or prolonged distress over a trifling setback is an example of such "without cause"—or better, without sufficient cause. Or, Burton's more common example: excessive worry and concern over an imaginary illness or outcome. (Social norms of appropriateness are reflected in these judgments: what makes a setback trifling, a sadness undeserving of prolonged or intense grief, or a worry unwarranted, are to a great extent matters of cultural custom and agreement.[19])

However, this is only one reading of the phrase "without cause," which, taken more literally, can also denote an absence of recognized causes, and feelings that are less concise, more pervasive, even "objectless." Melancholic fear and sadness are sometimes not over or about anything in particular. Instead, they are ways of apprehending and experiencing the world as it presents itself in its entirety. The terms *mood* and *emotion* in recent philosophical writing mark the contrast between entirely without a subjectively recognized cause (a "mood") and without a cause that may or may not be fitting and appropriate to the occasion (an "emotion").[20] Moods are affections that color and frame experience in its moment-by-moment totality. If they are said to have objects at all, these have an elusive, indiscriminate generality that affects all experience. When a melancholy mood prevails, the whole world seems bleak, meaningless, and without consolation. (The German *Verstimmungen* is translated as the English "mood," and attunement metaphors capture some of this amorphous quality.[21])

Depressed moods have often been employed to illustrate these objectless, pre- or nonintentional states; anxiety that is "free floating" is also regularly described in our contemporary times. In moods of depression, everything appears gloomy or irritating; in apprehensive or fearful moods, everything takes on a threatening, unsafe, or ominous aspect. At times, Burton also points to such nebulous, apparently objectless

---

19. See Horwitz and Wakefield 2007, Horwitz 2014. Rashly, Horwitz equates "without cause" in this first sense with "endogenous," and we return to this equation later (Horwitz 2014:212).
20. For a summary of this distinction, see Radden 2013.
21. Heidegger 1996.

moods, at least of sadness. He speaks, for instance, of the sorrow afflicting melancholics as

> continual, and still without any evident cause ... grieving still, *but why, they cannot tell.* (I,3,1,2:388, emphasis added)

In another passage, referring to the melancholy symptoms in Maids, Nuns, and Widows, he describes how

> now this now that offendes, they are weary of all; and yet will not, *cannot again tell how, where or what offends them*, though they be in great paine, agony, and frequently complaine, grieving, sighing, weeping and discontented still. (I,3,2,4:416, emphasis added)

Some melancholic men, he explains, are "dejected, moped [mopish], in much agony, some by fits, others continuate, &c. (I,3,1,3:402). At least those who are "dejected" or mopish, not by fits but continually ("continuate"), apparently suffer moods rather than aberrant thoughts with more time-limited and precise objects. Moreover, the persistent presence of these objectless moods would appear to follow from the system linking imagination and the passions: with that interaction, every unwarranted and idle fear will in turn engender distressing moods—of apprehension, dread, and despair, as well as their "German cousins" of discouragement, dejection, and sadness.

Bright makes similar reference to these objectless states in his description of melancholy sadness and fear "whereof no occasion was at any time before, nor like to be given hearafter" (Bright 1589:99). Bright's emphasis in this discussion is on the internally caused or, as he says, "domestical" nature of these imaginings, unprompted by external perceptions. Recounting the effect of the heated vapors on the brain, he says they "counterfetteth terrible objects to the fantasie, and ... causeth it *without external occasion*, to forge monstrous fictions, and terrible to the conceate, which the judgement taking as they are presented by the disordered instrument" (Bright 1586:99, emphasis added). And later: "Thus the heart a while being acquainted with nothing else, but domestical terror, feareth every thing and the braine simpathetically partaking with the hartes fear, making doubt, distrusteth, & suspecteth *without cause*" (Bright 1586:103). This interpretation of "without cause" has been equated with internal, bodily, or "endogenous" causes. Edward Shorter goes so far as to say that endogenous depression "has traditionally served as a synonym for melancholia" (Shorter 2007:7).

Even if they remain unknown to the subject, however, causes can presumably be exogenous, and there is no suggestion in the *Anatomy* to the contrary. So Bright and Burton differ here. The purely domestic or internal fears, for Bright, were placed in contrast to those passions derived from objects in the external world acquired through perception and provided us through God's goodness. But Burton does not follow this reading of "without cause." As we have seen, the causes of melancholy are both internal and external, perceptible and imperceptible.

Although not a category expressly distinguished in the *Anatomy*, the idea of a prevailing mood that lasts through stretches of time is implied in Burton's emphasis on the habituated aspect of melancholy and the attenuated nature of all passions. Rather than momentary irruptions, these states are often trait-like in their duration, providing a prevailing, moody backdrop to other experiences. Moods such as these were recognizable in Elizabethan times and would have been as familiar to Burton as they are to us. "In sooth I know not why I am so sad," says the melancholy Antonio, in *The Merchant of Venice*:

> It wearies me: you say it wearies you;
> But how I caught it, found it, or came by it,
> What stuffe 'tis made of, whereof it is borne,
> I am to learne: and such a Want-wit sadness makes of mee
> That I have much ado to know myself. (Act I, Scene 1)

This "want-wit sadness" is not merely inappropriate to its object. Its source and object are unknown, and it clings and pervades tiresomely.

So "without cause" includes *without any* (apprehended) *cause*, as well as without appropriate cause. Burton separates fear and sadness, and we can discern something of a pattern in the case examples he provides. Fears are more often unwarranted (an inappropriate cause), whereas sadness and sorrow also seem to afflict their sufferers with a prevailing mood (*without* cause), as well as being inappropriate (in duration or intensity) for specific objects.

Both occasional and more prolonged and pervasive states seem to assail Burton's melancholic, and this is an observation confirmed in the notebooks of Burton's contemporary, the physician Napier. Patients with "baseless" sorrow are there, including those whose sadness was distinguished by its disproportion or duration as a response to actual and specific losses or setbacks. "Sorrow" and "sadness" are apparently synonymous in the *Anatomy* and used interchangeably. Less frequently employed today, "sorrow" is associated with a longer-term attitude, rather than a momentary feeling, however. Other forms of distress are described by Napier as well, some are states of such persistent "mopishness." And sorrow may suggest persistent, "mopish" suffering and low mood. From his case notes on this affliction, those who are mopish are said to be "despairing, heavy-hearted, exceeding sad" and "solitary and will do nothing."[22] These sorrowing, mopish habits appear to correspond to persisting, unspecific objectless moods – fitting within Burton's general category of sadnesses "without cause."

SORROW AND FEAR, GERMAN COUSINS, SISTERS

The relationship between sadness and fear (without cause) is a close one. They are related, Burton says, as cousins, even sisters, and as cause and symptom.

> Cosen german to *Sorrow*, is *Feare* or rather a sister, *fidus Achates*, and continuall companion, an assistant and a principall agent in procuring of this mischief; a cause and symptom as the other. (I,2,3,5:259)

---

22. See MacDonald, 1981a:158–61.

They can occur separately: Burton reports he is of the same mind as Hercules de Saxonia on this point:

> some feare and are not sad; some bee sad and feare not; some neither feare, nor grieve. (I,3,2,2:410)

While separable, however, they are more often found together and "continual companions." Despite these familial similes, the relationship between the feelings is potentially confusing. If fear is defined by objects that are fearsome, and sadness by objects or states of affairs that are construed as sad, such as losses, then in accord with the loosely cognitivist analysis Burton adopts of such feelings (where their objects are definitive, if not entirely constitutive, of them), these must be treated as separate affections. Something may be fearsome yet not sad—or sad without being frightening. Their relation is thus not conceptual, it is empirical, and Burton recognizes this. Fear and sadness occur together as a product of a causal sequence by which they follow one another, sadness succeeded by fearfulness, and fear in turn followed by sadness. Other possibilities might also explain this emphasis on the "continual companionship" of fear and sadness, and Burton may intend them as well. One is that the fear and sadness are experienced as two distinct feelings that occur simultaneously; another that they become blurred, phenomenological states of apprehensive sadness and dispirited anxiety that resist disambiguation, or are such mixed, subliminal forms of distress that fail to fully reach conscious awareness or attention.[23]

Even if related through nothing beyond causal propinquity, the feelings of fear and sadness are part of the way Burton distinguishes Melancholy from the allied condition of madness. The relation between melancholy and madness is complicated in the introductory Letter to the Reader, which conflates the two. (This conflation is discussed in chapter 7.) The rest of the *Anatomy*, however, adheres to the

---

23. In recent work on feelings that are inconspicuous and sometimes preconscious, Matthew Ratcliffe has described "existential feelings"; these are beneath reflective awareness and constitute a "space of possibilities within which we experience, think and act" presupposed by conceptual judgments (Ratcliffe 2008:368).

definition by which madness is more vehement, raving, and violent than Melancholy, and

> *without all feare and sorrow*, with such impetuous force and boldnesse, that sometimes three or foure men cannot hold [patients]. (I,1,1,4:133 emphasis added)

Feelings of fear and sorrow thus anchor Melancholy within Burton's loose taxonomy. At one extreme they mark the habituated form of suffering that can be neither controlled by its subject nor effectively treated. But they also comprise the passing melancholy states he believes can be dispelled or averted through activities such as the employment of imaginative and critical self-awareness and distraction.

In many instances described by Burton, melancholy is a condition where self-control is evidently retained, it should be noted, and this also is a consequence of the use of affective states to characterize melancholy. Some are "so gently melancholy," as he says, that

> in their carriage, and to the outward apprehension of others, it can hardly be discerned, yet to them an intolerable burden, and not to be endured. (I,3,1,4:404)

Outwardly, little may seem amiss, and cognition is also sufficiently intact for dissimulation and deception: melancholy states affect *feelings*, whose presence we can often choose not to show.[24] In this respect, the melancholic perhaps resembles those suffering the less severe forms of depression. Mood congruence combined with only very minimally impaired cognition allows a degree of self-presentation and -integration that serve to make the mildly depressed person intelligible to others.[25] The typical melancholic depicted in the *Anatomy* is similarly transparent to us.

---

24. Burton believes we should express them to those around us and not keep them to ourselves, it should be added. The best way for ease is "to impart our misery to some friend, *not smother it up in our owne breast* . . . for griefe concealed strangles the soule" (II,2,6,1:104).
25. See Radden 2013:90–91. Their mood-congruent nature is apparently the result of selective epistemic bias (hence the minimal cognitive dysfunction).

We cannot assume that feelings are unchanged when experienced by one person and another, let alone experienced in one era and another. Nonetheless, the *Anatomy*'s "fear without cause" does seem to have close parallels in the feelings of apprehension, dread, and anxiety we know today. (The German *Angst* translates into English as *fear* or *worry*, indeed.) The relationship between anxiety and depression thus warrants additional attention due to its seeming parallel with fear and sadness. As aberrant and pathological states, the relationship between the modern-day pair (anxiety and depression) has had its own complex, and partially separated, history.[26] It is a history frequently played out against a backdrop of classificatory decisions and assumptions rather than phenomenological analysis. Historians point to the emergence during the nineteenth century of nervous illness, and neurasthenia, existing alongside and arguably even occluding the diagnosis of melancholia. Nervous illness covered a broad group of traits including, but not limited to, mild depression or low mood: There was mild anxiety and somatic symptoms such as fatigue, chronic pain, and insomnia as well as mild obsessive thinking. Nervous illness also came in turn to be displaced by (or rather, subsumed within) depressive disorder. Mild depression or low mood acquired what one historian complains is a misleading prominence, since not all those diagnosed as depressed experience sad and despondent mood states.[27] And today, one trend in psychiatric classification would reinstate the nineteenth-century category of nervous disorder that encompasses anxiety and physical pain quite as much as sadness and despondency.[28]

At first glance, this expanded symptom profile for depression mirrors the illimitable symptoms of Melancholy recounted in the *Anatomy*. While something short of defining features however, sadness and ungrounded fear were aspects of melancholy too common, and too

26. These convergences and divergences are observable even by decade, it has been shown (Levine et al. 2001a). See also Berrios 1996.
27. Shorter 2013.
28. This brief description only points to a handful of the multitude of tributaries and streams into which depression and anxiety have been directed since the nineteenth century. For a thorough review, see Levine et al. 2001a, Berrios 1996, Shorter 2007, 2013, and Varga 2013.

important, to be displaced by other signs and symptoms such as fatigue. Added to that, as we'll see in chapter 7, sadness holds a special place in the *Anatomy* account, because of its relation to the universal sadness and unavoidable states of distress that are our human lot. So whatever may be the fate of the disorder of depression and its symptom of low mood and sadness, melancholy is linked to its fear and sadness without cause. They remain the continual companions, assistants, and principal agents, as Burton says, in "procuring of this mischief" of melancholy.

Just as Burton saw fear and sadness as continual companions, today's epidemiological data confirms that as symptoms and as forms of affective disorder, anxiety and depression occur together.[29] Disordered forms of anxiety and depression have been described as the most widely prevalent forms of mental suffering in the human species.[30] Indeed, a combination of anxiety disorder and depressive disorder, it has been established, is more common than either disorder considered alone, and results in more severe and lasting symptoms, as well as greater impairment and subjective distress.[31] There is not agreement over the explanation for this. Most contemporary psychiatry works with the assumption that felt symptoms are the causal outcome of a specific underlying disorder or dysfunction, as we saw in chapter 3. So the disease process is composed of such underlying states and processes together with these affective features (and other symptoms). Hence, we have the confounding, and unresolved "comorbidity problem," presented by anxiety and depression regarded as distinct, yet co-occurring, anxiety and depressive disorders. Anxiety and depression symptoms, respectively, each form part of separate disorders, on this model, yet they overlap in unaccountable ways.

The more symptom-focused network model better fitting the *Anatomy* account avoids such a conundrum. It allows that states of sorrow and anxiety act as mutual causes, just as Burton describes the

---

29. Kessler et al. 2005. The history of this relationship is given in Levine et al. 2001. Because somatoform symptoms are also strongly evident in these clusters, some researchers have titled them emotional, rather than affective, disorders. See Goldberg et al. 2009.
30. Roth and Mountjoy 1982:90. (These authors use the expression "morbid forms.")
31. See, for example, Maser and Cloninger, 1990, Angst, 1997, and Baldwin et al. 2002, Tsuang and Marneros, 1986.

actions of fear and sadness in melancholy, "treading a ring." Their co-occurrence can be explained by nothing beyond their tendency to trigger one another. From nearer our own time, one way the interactive effect might work is described by Darwin's writing in *The Expressions of the Emotions in Man and Animals* (1872). After the mind suffers from a paroxysm of grief and the cause still continues, he explains, "we will likely experience a state of low spirits or become dejected. Prolonged pain generally leads to the same state of mind. If we expect to suffer, we are anxious, if we have no hope of relief, we despair" (Darwin 2007:175). In this example fear is the object of distress; distress the object of fear. Yet in other cases, such as the instances of distress over one's health Burton often cites, both fear and sadness apparently share a third object not itself a feeling: The same source (my perceived illness) is at once the target of worry and subject of my sorrow. Either way, the network model can accommodate these relationships.

If we consider comorbidity from the perspective of a network model, it has been observed, then the term "comorbidity" also acquires a different meaning. The causal relations between symptoms constitute pathways that can connect different disorders by way of "bridging" or shared symptoms common to both disorders. A consequence of this formulation is that the boundaries between different disorders will be intrinsically fuzzy: "one may still define disorders as sets of more densely connected symptoms that show synchronized behavior (like a school of fish or a flock of birds) . . . [they are] literally intertwined with one another and cannot be neatly separated" (Borsboom and Cramer 2013:97).

Whether based on common-cause etiological model assumptions, and so viewed as a classificatory problem, or simply treated as a striking coincidence of causally interconnected symptoms, the anxiety–depression relationship has been the subject of many different classificatory revisions and proposals. Several of these echo— sometimes explicitly—the co-occurrence of apprehensive, fearful, and anxious states with sad and dejected ones found throughout the canon of writing on melancholy from Hippocrates and Galen, proposing that these states be classified as a unitary cluster. On one such revision, the disorder category of "mixed anxiety-depressive disorder" was advocated for a large group of patients with the combination of depression and anxiety symptoms that are insufficiently severe as to warrant a diagnosis of depressive or anxiety disorder.[32] The impairment exhibited by these patients has been hypothesized to be a shared diathesis, and best described by "the construct of *nonspecific negative affect*" (Barlow and Campbell 2000:1).[33] Because those with anxiety disorder and depression respond similarly to certain psychopharmacological interventions, it has been asserted that both states are better classified together for certain research purposes.[34] A further refinement allows that a measure of anxiety severity be assessed as a *dimension* of depressive disorder.[35] Each of these attempts to combine depression and anxiety described here has been strongly endorsed during the years leading up to the revised *Diagnostic and Statistical Manual of Mental Disorders* (American Psychiatric Association [APA] 2013). Nonetheless, present-day classifications (including the revised version) continue to present depressive and anxiety symptoms as manifestations of the respective disorders known as depressive disorder and anxiety disorder, and so to incur the comorbidity "problem" network models of disease can avoid.[36,37]

PASSIONS TO EMOTIONS

Burton's symptoms little resemble the isolated elements of affective upheaval that emotions increasingly came to be as modern psychology took hold. Nor do his passions readily reduce to a handful of basic states

---

32. See Boulenger et al. 1997. The category is found in DSM-IV, and omitted from DSM-5 without explanation (APA 1994:724–5, APA 2013). It is also in the current World Health Organization *International Classification of Diseases* (ICD-10); WHO 1992, due to be revised by 2018.
33. See also Goldberg et al. 2009.
34. See First 2011. Also, Stahl, 1997, Salin-Pascual 2002, and Levine, Cole, et al. 2001a.
35. First 2011.
36. See WHO 1992, APA 2013.
37. These different "emotional clusters" around depression and anxiety, it has been observed, ought not be allowed to obscure the similarities between all members of the cluster and "should not necessitate putting these disorders into separate chapters of the DSM and ICD classifications" (Goldberg et al. 2009:2054).

disconnected from higher cognitive influence, and closer to reflex-like physiological and behavioral responses, on the model of some contemporary emotions research.[38] The feelings of sadness and fear that so dominate the symptom picture of Burtonian Melancholy are part of an interactive whole uniting more and less sensory, and more and less purely cognitive, elements with bodily states, as we saw. They are also anchored by their natural history: Their meanings are tied to their past, so that they reflect the endpoints of sequences of interconnected loopings and interactions. Burton's passions are both like and unlike Freudian ones in this respect. Freud's symptoms emanated from deeper psychic states buried below immediate awareness. Burton, although indifferent to the divide between consciousness and unconsciousness, did not recognize this notion of burial, or repression, but he seems to presuppose, with Freud, that to understand a feeling is often to identify its causal antecedents in further psychic elements of imagining, memory, and feeling.

The affective states known as the passions underwent changes between the seventeenth and nineteenth centuries, scholars have asserted.[39] The ancient "Passions" came to be usurped by conceptions more consonant with modern scientific approaches. And just as Descartes' *Meditations* are often seen as influencing modern epistemology, his *Passions of the Soul* (1649) has been implicated in this severance of the passions of old from the more modern, and more scientific ideas that still dominate today's affective science.[40,41] To avoid connotations of passivity and aspects of the soul incompatible with naturalistic approaches, Descartes renamed the passions as, and conflating them with, emotions, it has been asserted. (Descartes's change of emphasis, he makes clear himself: "émotion" captured the way these thoughts (*pensées*) agitate and disturb the mind, and so are active in motivating us, disposing the soul "to want the things which nature deems useful to us."[42])

38. Such basic emotions are analyzed by Griffiths 1997.
39. These claims may be exaggerated. For a more nuanced account of the transition from the early modern to the modern periods, see James 1997.
40. Rorty 1982, Dixon 2003, Charland 2010.
41. This newfound attention to affective states and processes is a burgeoning research area: We are in the "age of emotion" (Charland 2010:239).
42. Descartes 1961:117–8.

The evaluative, attenuated, intentional responses, organized around a particular idea, that had been the passions, came to be marginalized, stripped of their ethical and spiritual associations, and replaced by "a crude, secular, amoral substitute" (Charland 2010:238). Characterized as occasional states, emotions were more momentary and sudden affections of short duration and extinction.[43] Affording easier scientific observation and method, these irruptions of feeling were eventually to become the exclusive subject of scientific investigation.[44] Descartes is depicted as having eschewed the passions construed as the enemy of reason and virtue in classical and Christian traditions—although whether he succeeded in replacing the old passions with emotions is debated.[45,46] And recognizing the loss entailed in these changes, some contemporary philosophers have attempted to revive the passions—or reassign to emotions some of the features associated with them.[47]

Descartes' role, and success, in this transformation from passions to emotions may be unresolved. But the extent to which the presuppositions of today's affective sciences diverge from the earlier conception put forward in the *Anatomy* by Descartes' near-contemporary in England is evident. Burtonian passions are far from the affective irruptions, and momentary and sudden states of limited duration and extinction, that the emotions have become. Despite these differences, we must not forget that Burton's passions share important features with the contemporary conceptions of emotion that today dominate emotions research in the mind sciences. Their effects on and close links with cognition, which have been shown to affect higher reasoning (the activities of Burton's

---

43. Charland 2010:249.
44. One example of such emotions would be those associated with contemporary affect programs. See Griffiths 1997.
45. As Noga Arikha has observed, moreover, Descartes' treatise on the passions remained as devoted to the causes of ethics and virtues as its predecessors had been (Arikha 2007:221); see also John Cottingham, who points out that with his work on the passions, Descartes reintroduced many of the moral categories and concerns that had been omitted from his earlier epistemological writing (Cottingham 1998:61–103).
46. Recent analyses suggest that he could not so readily dispense with the moral and spiritual elements of previous analyses (Charland 2000, 2004, 2006, Arikha 2007).
47. With his conception of emotional episodes, for example, Peter Goldie allows for the duration and temporal career associated with accounts of the passions (Goldie, 2000:12–16.)

faculty of Reason), are obvious illustrations of this. Reasoning, working memory, attention, and judgment are each intrinsically shaped by emotional elements. This way, contemporary models remain compatible with the Stoic-inspired, and broadly cognitivist account of the passions depicted in the *Anatomy*, wherein passions comprise representations (or we could say, data) that are conveyed to regions of the body through the vehicle of the animal spirits.[48,49]

Thoroughgoing cognitivist theories of emotion are overly intellectualistic, disregarding the sensory aspect of feelings. For this reason, they have been criticized within contemporary feeling theories of emotion.[50] The role played by the passions is a mixed one in the *Anatomy*, however, allowing it to avoid this critique. Sensory and bodily as well as more narrowly cognitive elements are encompassed within the incessant mind–body exchanges, so that Burton's passions are firmly embodied. And contemporary parallels to Burton's hybrid account in our own time are also found (in the research of Jesse Prinz, for example).[51] So, again, Burton's passions are far from today's emotions, but they are not entirely incompatible with some of today's emotion models. With his hybrid, embodied interactionism, which accommodates the sensory and intellectualistic aspects of passions, he would find much that was familiar in some contemporary theorizing and research.

TRUE MELANCHOLIA, TWO DEPRESSIONS

A perceived continuity linking melancholy and depression, and the reasons to resist such analysis, have been noted already. A more refined

---

48. For a review of much of this contemporary research see Oatley, Keltner, and Jenkins 2006.
49. Purely cognitivist accounts invite philosophical criticism because they ignore the physiological aspect of all emotions and the reflexive and involuntary quality of some (such as disgust), and cannot explain moods, which seem without apparent intentional objects or sometimes linger after cognitive correction has occurred (Griffiths 1997, 1998).
50. These feeling theories derive from William James' notion that emotions are, or are caused by, awareness of bodily changes. (Indeed, James' ["James-Lange"] theory of emotion is the influential expression of the accounts of emotion judged to have replaced earlier ideas about the passions.)
51. See Prinz 2004.

version of that illusory continuity demands attention, however, because of the claim that the subtype of melancholia or melancholic depression corresponds to melancholy in past times.

Attempts to divide depression by medical psychiatry have been legion. A confusion of pairings proposed throughout the twentieth century, has included that between endogenous and neurotic or reactive depression (famously, and effectively, challenged as unsustainable by Aubrey Lewis in 1938), and the separation of bipolar from unipolar conditions.[52] In some divisions these are separations within a single disorder category. Others are more radical. Our particular focus here is the contrast between melancholic depression and nonmelancholic depression, and these have been described—radically—in terms of diseases "as distinct as mumps and measles" (Shorter 2007:7).

The separation between endogenous and exogenous sources of depression is acknowledged in the *Anatomy*, although it is not the basis of further differentiations with regard to severity, course, or response to treatment. Similarly, the *Anatomy* offers occasional hints of mood swings suggesting bipolarity, but today's sharp separation between bipolar and unipolar conditions is not consistently discernable.[53] As we saw, not only these but also a range of other disorder types seem to be accommodated under the broad umbrella of Burtonian Melancholy. However, one among the many diagnostic kinds into which affective disorder has been divided deserves special attention. As a subtype of depression, melancholic depression had been acknowledged before, but since the last decades of the twentieth century it has become more clearly delineated, emphasized, and often accorded categorical status.[54] Contemporary

---

52. Lewis 1938. A discussion of the disagreements surrounding these proposals is to be found in Shorter 2007.
53. A hint of bipolarity lies in the passage quoted earlier, where Burton points out that most but not all Melancholy involves states of fear and sorrow, explaining that "to some [Melancholy] is most pleasant, as to such as laugh most part; some are bold againe, and free from all manner of feare and griefe" (I,1,3,2:163). Not merely the pleasant moods described and the absence of fear and grief, but that *"some are bold againe,"* suggests periodic or cyclical disorder.
54. DSM-5 (APA 2013), it should be noted, merely acknowledges melancholic features as one variant within the category of unspecified depressive disorders (those where symptoms fail to meet the criteria for any of the disorders in the depressive diagnostic class).

researchers claim this form bears little relation to the clumsy and inexact characterizations of depression more broadly understood. Obscured within a plethora of other complaints, and by the misleading diagnostic categories of major depression, and depressive disorder, associated with influential recent psychiatric classifications, the condition truly entitled to the name melancholic depression or melancholia reflects a distinct disorder that is sui generis, it has been conjectured.[55] According to these recent analyses, melancholic depression can be identified by appeal to four criteria: biologically; in its response to treatment; phenomenologically, and behaviorally. Evidence from these four sources is regarded by some as sufficient for clinical definition, validation, and treatment differentiation, inviting the conclusion that "melancholia is likely to be a categorical entity capable of being circumscribed" (Parker 2007:28).

The category of melancholic depression deserves particular attention here for several reasons. It is depicted in terms of the same unrelieved sadness so emphasized by Burton. (A typical definition makes reference to "an episode of persistent unremitting mood of apprehension and gloom that compromises normal daily activities," for example [Taylor and Fink 2008:82–3]). In addition, contemporary researchers have repeatedly appealed to characterizations of Melancholy, including Burton's own, in claiming its ancient lineage.

Biologically, melancholic depression exhibits its primary marker in dysfunctionally elevated cortisol levels within the endocrine system, identifiable through a dexamethasone suppression test (DST).[56] Electroencephalographs show distinctive sleep abnormalities, in

---

Melancholic features include loss of pleasure in all, or almost all, activities and lack of reactivity to usually pleasurable stimuli, together with three or more of six features including depressed mood, worsening morning mood, early morning awakening, psychomotor agitation or retardation, significant weight loss, and excessive or inappropriate guilt (APA 2013:184–5).

55. Just as Michelangelo could "see" the *Pietà* already formed in a block of marble and merely had to "set it free," says Gordon Parker, "we conceptualize melancholia as a categorical entity residing within a potpourri of depressive diseases, disorders and syndromes, and more, awaiting definition and measurement" (Parker 2007:21).

56. Carroll 1981. See also Parker and Hadzi-Pavlovic 1996, Shorter and Fink 2010, Day et al. 2015.

addition.[57] Then, in terms of treatment, melancholic depression has been found less responsive to placebo, unaffected by the newer antidepressant drugs, and most effectively treated by electroconvulsive therapy or by the earlier antidepressants.[58] Phenomenologically, as primary symptoms the patient experiences unrelieved, distressing sadness and or the unresponsiveness of anhedonia, with frequent psychotic dimensions that are absent from more ordinary depression.[59] And behaviorally, there is a stronger link to suicide and psychomotor disturbance. Of these features, the latter two might be discerned in the *Anatomy*, although the breadth and scope of Burtonian Melancholy must leave it even more likely to conceal a specific subtype than is the portmanteau category of depressive disorder. The moods of unrelenting sadness sound familiar from the *Anatomy*, yet Burton provides little evidence of anhedonia. (The concept of anhedonia itself lacks specificity, clarity, and empirical grounding, it has been pointed out, leaving it difficult to apply here.[60]) Psychomotor disturbance is not noted, but Burton acknowledges suicide a "common calamity" for those suffering melancholy.[61] We are given such limited case material and brief descriptions in the *Anatomy*, however, that the absence of some of these features cannot be entirely eliminated on the basis of his clinical tales.

57. Reduced REM latency, increased REM time, and reduced deep sleep have all been observed (Armitage 2007). See also Taylor and Fink 2008, Parker et al. 2010.
58. It responds to tricyclic antidepressants and lithium better than to newer agents. Parker and Hadzi-Pavlic 1996, Shorter 2007, Horwitz 2014.
59. Parker and colleagues describe "disturbances of affect disproportionate to stressors" as including unremitting apprehension and morbid statements, blunted emotional response, nonreactive mood, and pervasive anhedonia, with "such features continuing autonomously despite any improved circumstances" (Parker et al. 2010:745). See also Shorter 2007, 2011, Shorter and Fink 2010.
60. See Berrios 1995.
61. "'Tis *a common calamity*, a fatall end to this disease, they are condemned to a violent death ... furiously disposed, carried headlong by their tyrannizing wils, enforced by miseries, and there remains no more to such persons, if ... [God] doe not prevent (for no humane perswasion, or art can helpe) but to be their owne butchers, & execute themselves" (I,4,1,1:432, emphasis added). As a Christian, Burton frowns on suicide, it should be added, despite the respectful attitude toward it adopted by Seneca and other admired thinkers.

The difficulty distinguishing melancholic depression from the broader diagnostic categories of depressive disorder (and the major depression that preceded it) is widely attributed to the insufficiency and vagueness of the latter, broader categories.[62] In contrast to their unworkable flabbiness, the narrower melancholic depression is a more manageable and precise research topic.

Because Burtonian Melancholy is also a loose and capacious category, it might be doubted whether melancholic depression could have any parallels with Burtonian Melancholy. Yet it has been melancholic depression about which researchers have recently invoked the canon of writing on melancholy beginning with Hippocrates, of which the *Anatomy* forms part. Melancholic depression, not depressive disorder, has been identified with the allegedly unchanging condition referred to in that writing. Allusion has been made to "the *centuries old tradition* that associated melancholic depression with a disproportionate response to its context" and to melancholic depression as *"one of a small number of mental disorders with a claim to reflect a natural kind"* (Horwitz 2014:212, emphasis added). The image of melancholic depression has been said to be *"consistent with centuries* of observation" (Fink and Taylor 2008, emphasis added). Melancholia is described as "a heritage label for *an age-old concept"* (Shorter 2007:11, emphasis added). We have already seen the dangers of equating today's affective conditions with melancholy of the past, and the presuppositions entailed in such equations. Nonetheless, this is a widely repeated theme.[63]

---

62. Of the diagnosis of major depression associated with the third edition of the DSM (1980) it has been said, "it included a wide range of conditions within a single representation of a presumed natural kind. Conditions that had been distinct for thousands of years of psychiatric history became indistinguishable: the capacious major depression criteria encompassed conditions that were mild and severe, transitory and long-standing, and proportionate and disproportionate to their contexts" (Horwitz 2014:215).

63. By Melancholic Depression, it has been said, "we understand *classical melancholia* and its cousin psychotic depression. . . . The argument for preferring melancholia to endogenous depression is simply that of *historical steadfastness. Melancholia has borne well the vicissitudes of time and continues to delineate a homogenous population that responds more or less uniformly to certain treatments*" (Shorter 2007:7, emphasis added).

Some of these appeals to the ancient canon may be oversimplified, judging from what we know of the Hippocratic and Galenic texts.[64] But more immediately troubling, these equations demonstrate a misreading of Burton's own descriptions. Three features attributed to the canon on melancholy are noted in these accounts of melancholic depression: (i) a trend toward psychosis, (ii) being an endogenous rather than an exogenous condition, (iii) and relative severity. To highlight the disparities between melancholic depression and Burtonian Melancholy, we can take these by turn.

(i) Psychosis is said to be a common feature of melancholic depression, although not unfailingly present. Turning to the *Anatomy*, we must first identify what might correspond to today's conception of psychosis (a term that came into use only after the seventeenth century). By virtue of its severity, this will be Burtonian Melancholy properly so called, the habituated, chronic condition that is next to untreatable. In addition, since many cases described in the *Anatomy* involve delusional ideas (as well as some hallucinations), it may be safe to say that those, at least, are an indication of what would today be known as psychosis. The tales and case records Burton provides do not entirely mirror those associated with psychotic depression in their *content*. Psychotic depression is typically mood-congruent, and focused around guilt, dire and deserved punishment, and catastrophic and mournful states of affairs. But structural parallels are evident. (We return to these parallels and such extreme states of melancholy in chapter 6.)

---

64. Thus, extracting parts of a passage from the historical writing of Berrios, it is asserted that "in classical antiquity 'melancholia was defined in terms of overt behavioral features . . . states of reduced behavioral output . . . (and) . . . *symptoms reflecting pathological affect . . . were not part of the concept*'" (Parker 2007:22, emphasis added). There may be evidence of psychomotor disturbance in melancholic depression that has hitherto been underrecognized. And certainly emphasis on its affective symptoms varies with text and era, both before and after the seventeenth century. (See Varga 2013.) But since an association between melancholia and an uncommon degree of fear and sadness are to be found in Hippocratic and Gallenic works, this claim remains misleading. Fear and sadness that are prolonged indicate melancholy, according to the Hippocratic writing; and all melancholic patients demonstrate fear and despondency, says Galen. The formulation of fear and sadness without cause may be more closely associated with the early modern period. But uncommonly prolonged or intense fear and sadness had long been, and remained then, one form taken by the melancholic's disordered affect.

(ii) Psychotic depression has long been identified as endogenous within the influential, twentieth-century etiological division between depressions that are either endogenous or "reactive" (exogenous). And melancholic depression is consistently described as endogenous.[65] This association linking melancholy to endogenous causes seems incompatible with the range of causes and triggers for Burtonian Melancholy, even in its severest form (as Habit), however. There is no suggestion in the *Anatomy* that the severest, habituated Melancholy with delusional symptoms is limited to endogenous or inborn forms of disorder (in those with the melancholy temperament). Nor is Burton's conception unorthodox on this point, as we've seen.[66]

(iii) As to the question of severity, it is widely agreed that a feature of melancholic depression is its relative severity, in contrast with the milder states of distress and anxiety suffered by many of those diagnosed with the capacious major depression, or depressive disorder. (The current research is less clear on the relationship between this "new" category of melancholic depression and bipolar disorder, presumably since the relationship between bipolarity and unipolar depressions is somewhat contested.[67]) Severity is an inescapably practical criterion, of course, and one as useful for Burton as for these present-day researchers, as we saw. But beyond its interpretation in strictly practical terms, severity is vaguely represented in the *Anatomy*. According to the metrics in contemporary descriptions of melancholic depression, Burtonian Melancholy would be difficult to rank as to relative severity.

Some parallels with Burtonian Melancholy are suggested by the link between melancholic depression and suicide, since the suicide risk attached to the severest forms of entrenched melancholy is noted from time to time throughout the *Anatomy*. Similarly, the distinctive phenomenology of melancholic depression, with its unremitting sadness, also evokes many of Burton's descriptions. Based on melancholic

---

65. We saw earlier that Shorter bases this reading on Bright's analysis, from which Burton's departs.
66. The same appeal to a range of exogenous causes for all types of melancholy can be found in Weyer and Platter, for example.
67. See Leonhard 1959, McGuffin et al. 2003, Goodwin and Jamison 2007.

depression's unresponsiveness to treatment, Burton's depiction of severe, entrenched, and *incurable* Melancholy may be what we should expect. Yet, if anything, the *Anatomy* descriptions of melancholy seem to better fit the loose and inexact diagnostic classifications of depressive disorder, rather than anything more precise. And since the few treatments found effective for today's disorder of melancholic depression had not been dreamed of in the early seventeenth century, it seems unlikely the *Anatomy* could guide us as to this differentiation, even if it existed.

More generally, then, as long as some version of an etiological, common-cause disease model underlies these claimed parallels, they cannot be excluded. But to suppose on the basis of symptom descriptions alone that today's melancholic depression corresponds in any but the loosest way to Burtonian Melancholy, or to the melancholy of Hippocrates and Galen, is a misreading of the record. And attempts to establish a straightforward continuity between the melancholy of old and melancholic depression are as incomplete as we found were those equating melancholy with depression more broadly understood.

Although they also include such affections, passions in the *Anatomy* are more than the type of passing feeling states of short duration and extinction that are the primary subject of study within the affective mind sciences today. This leaves much research on the emotions incompatible with Burton's conception. Yet, we saw, fear and sadness without cause seem to accommodate contemporary philosophical analysis separating moods from emotions. And their relationship has considerable bearing on psychiatry's concern over the relationship between anxiety and depression expressed as the problem of comorbidity—a problem allied to its acceptance of an etiological model of disease.

Moreover, while the similarities claimed between melancholic depression and Burton's Melancholy cannot be entirely dismissed, there are limitations to this comparative endeavor. If any descriptive syndrome corresponds to Burtonian Melancholy, the unrelenting sadness of melancholic depression perhaps renders it eligible; but so, it might be said, is the disease entity of depressive disorder, although for different reasons. No matter how viable the separation between the two forms of depression, or what validity is granted to refined contemporary subtypes, attempts to link contemporary mood disorder with melancholy of old must remain fraught with epistemic peril. Intriguing similarities there certainly are, sufficient to direct an interest in the remedies Burton recommends for the disordered moods he describes. But such practical ideas will be the most important, and certainly the safest, outcomes of these cross-historical forays.

Chapter 5

the akratic melancholic

For the urgent matter of curbing the aberrant feelings and tendencies that beset the melancholic, Burton often turns to the Stoics. That Stoic legacies as they concern the passions, self-control, and the phenomenon, and phenomenology, of weakness of will were important for understanding melancholy, he is not in doubt, although he approaches these classical ideas critically and selectively. Regulating passions lay at the heart of preventing melancholy, and along with the Epicurians, the Stoics had paid unparalleled attention to the matter of regulating the passions.[1] In addition, the Stoic conception of philosophy was essentially practical, focused on the "therapeutics of the passions" (Hadot 1995:82). And with his great book also directed toward the prevention and care of melancholy, Burton's interest in these questions is similarly practical.

At the center of the problem, as he sees it, is the sheer sensory, or even sensual, appeal of melancholy habits—especially idle and solitary speculation, musing, and reverie. These temptations are risks for all of us. In a tendency that can be likened to moral weakness, we are endlessly drawn to these charms, at first bewitched, and later inured in dangerous habits of thought difficult, or impossible, to break. Contemporary research on mind wandering seems to confirm some of these ideas, emphasizing the compulsive aspect of such default system states of

---

1. The importance of the Stoics on these matters, remains unchallenged today. In the detail and power of their analyses of the relationship between emotion and belief, their emphasis on the evaluative element in emotion, their suggestions about the interrelationships among the emotions, and recognition of the significance of the emotional life, their work has been judged to exceed even Aristotle's (Nussbaum 1994:507).

mind. The exercise of the imagination Burton names "melancholising," particularly, bears a strong resemblance to the unproductive "depressive rumination" that has been associated with mood disorder in our own times. Other than because it is unproductive, why is melancholising such an abhorrent and feared activity? New work on rumination; correlations between rumination, mind wandering, and depression; and hypotheses about habituation may illuminate Burton's contrast between dangerous and valuable uses of the imagination, letting us better see why he might have described melancholising as he does, in terms that invite parallels with the classical philosophical notion of *akrasia*. Moreover, the akratic melancholics' repetitive habit seems to be evidence of the distorting function of availability heuristics today associated with mood disorder.

Burton's religious and ethical understanding of melancholy forms a seamless whole embodying a classical and medieval Christian alignment between psychology and the ethics of how to live well. For example, original sin represents the ultimate source of melancholy suffering, with repentance a "soveraigne remedy for all sinnes" *but also* "a charme for our miseries, a protecting Amulet" (III:4,2,6:428). Although they have little place in modern science, the *Anatomy* is threaded through with these religious and theological ideas, important recent scholarship has illustrated. Moreover, even Burton's practical emphasis on healthy habits of mind is part of a tradition of Christian spiritual exercises.[2,3] The tenet that moral as well as bodily health lies in the achievement of emotional tranquility is much older, coming to medieval Christianity through classical philosophical sources. Burton's conviction that the melancholic can work on his own mind, adjusting beliefs, attitudes, and imaginings, and thereby curbing the passions, most closely reflects the distinctive ideas about the passions, the self and its powers, values, and ends, associated with the Stoicism of Chrysippus, Seneca, Epictetus, and Marcus Aurelius.

These classical sources were available in two forms for seventeenth-century scholars such as Burton. There were not only the classical

2. See Gowland 2006, Schmidt 2007, Lund 2010.
3. See Hadot 1995.

Greek and Latin texts themselves but also later interpretations and translations from the renaissance. Quite apart from Burton's own reading, translation, and paraphrase of the original works, the *Anatomy* is a reflection of Hellenistic writing as it emerged through the neo-Stoic revival that, closer to his own time, was undertaken by the renaissance humanists. Erasmus (1457–1536) and Lipsius appear frequently in these pages (although usually in little more than footnote citations), to support and confirm Burton's own interpretations of passages from the ancients. In addition, of the several lenses through which the *Anatomy* can be viewed, we'll see, one is as homage to the "divine" and "wise" Seneca.[4]

EXPUNGING THE PASSIONS

Stoic writing emphasizes that affective states such as fear, anger, and passionate love are tied to erroneous judgments. The analysis of the passions was thus a cognitivist one, closely related to today's theories of emotion in which beliefs and belief-like states are essential, and identifying, features.[5] Thoughts and beliefs are open to adjustment through our own efforts, and will in turn alter the passions that contain, and are a consequence, of them. Although these relationships had been portrayed in different ways in Stoic thought, it was agreed that he who had attained moral and intellectual perfection would be blessedly free of such feelings, as of all misfortune.[6] The state of tranquility (*ataraxia*) is held to be one "without all manner of passions and perturbations whatsoever" (I:2,3,1:247).

---

4. Burton was not alone in his admiration for Seneca, whose work also formed the point of departure for Montaigne, and who has been described as the favorite pagan of the Latin church (Haddad 1958). Twenty-first-century judgments are more guarded. See Romm 2014, Wilson 2014, Beard 2014.
5. These accounts vary; in some their intentional objects comprise, and define, affective states; while in others they are regular accompaniments. See Solomon 1976, Nussbaum 1994, Deigh 2010.
6. For an account of these relationships, see Sorabji 2002.

A wise man's minde, as Seneca holds, is like the state of the World above the moone, ever serene. Come then what can come, befall what may befall. (II:3,3,1:169)

On Burton's reading, the Stoic's goal—with which he took issue—was that of extirpating all feelings, and there is support for his interpretation. But Stoic ideas on the role of the passions divided philosophers even in Roman days. Scholars still remain somewhat divided over this question of whether the passions were to be entirely expunged, although there is agreement that the Stoic sage aimed to expel all immediate, intense, and harmful reactions and feelings like anger, anxiety, jealousy, and dread. Stoicism involved a set of ideas that flourished for several centuries (roughly between the fourth century BCE and the second century CE), however, encompassing two distinct historical eras and languages.[7] It is not surprising that accounts of the desirability of entirely extirpating the passions show some variation. The issue also depends on how the passions are understood, moreover. In some writing at least, Seneca seems to be in agreement with Chrysippus in presupposing that, while the initial reactions or feelings, sometimes known as proto-passions, must be expunged, passions proper are appropriate and acceptably rational as the outcome of acts of assent when reason "commands," rendering them voluntary (*voluntas*). (Stoic epistemology was similarly bound up with the power of assent, it should be added. As imprints or alterations of the soul, every impression may be assented to or not—leaving it within our human power to be wise.[8]) Examples of rational feelings of this kind include innocuous and "calm" attitudes such as wishing others well, rejoicing in virtuous actions, and the felt satisfactions of a good conscience.[9] Moreover, among the Roman philosophers, the Epicurians

---

7. The first Stoics (Old Stoa) were Zeno (344–262 BCE), Cleanthes (died 232 BCE), and Chrysippus (died 206 BCE), only fragments of whose writing remain. From Imperial Roman times are Epictetus (c. 55–135 CE) and Emperor Marcus Aurelius (121–180 CE), writing in Greek, and Seneca (4 BCE–65 CE), whose work is in Latin.
8. Katja 2011.
9. These examples are Seneca's. The sage would experience feelings when they were attuned to reason, *eupatheiai*—literally, good emotions or feelings. So the joy or satisfaction felt over his virtue, was not *pleasure*—a mistaken feeling in that it treats the actual possession of an indifferent as a good (Parry 2009).

do not want to repudiate quite all feelings; nor did Burton's admired Cicero. But in the *Anatomy* the particular focus remains the Stoics. And, along with much of the neo-Stoic writing of the renaissance, Burton accepts the simplified interpretation. For him, the entirely apathetic state is depicted by Stoicism as a desirable one, where, "befall what may befall," a person is untroubled by feelings of any kind. And this simplified interpretation is the one with which he takes issue.[10]

In contrast, the approach and methods proposed by Stoicism for curbing the passions, including regular, careful critical analysis of one's cognitive states of belief and imagination, are entirely accepted, as we will see. Burton's primary divergence from the Stoics comes with the ends sought. The wise person should not aim to be "without all manner of passions and perturbations whatsoever." This attitude is more than a blind embrace of Aristotelian moderation, although in some ways Burton's view of the passions more nearly fits the Aristotelian one.[11] Arguments are introduced: The state of tranquility sought by the Stoics was neither possible to achieve, nor desirable. No mortal man is free from these perturbations, Burton insists,

> or if he be so, sure he is either a God or a blocke. They are borne and bred with us, we have them from our parents by inheritance. (I:2,3,1:248)

But nor was a state of apathetic tranquility desirable. Because of their close relation to the faculty of the Imagination, which can work on them for good as much as for ill, the passions are necessary and valuable ingredients in the mental economy. Just as the Imagination causes such passions as fear and grief, it is explained in another passage,

---

10. The Stoic sage "is not insensitive to painful or pleasurable sensations . . . he is impassive towards them. But he is not entirely impassive, contrary to the *popular conception of a Stoic*" (Long 1986, 206–7, emphasis added). It was a popular misconception even in their own time, when the Stoics were ridiculed for their views on the passions (Baltzly 2014).
11. These differences between the Aristotelian and Stoic positions had long been noted: even Cicero makes the above contrast, in *Tusculan Disputations* Bks III and IV.

so *conceipts alone*, rectified by good hope, counsel &c. are *able again to helpe*: and 'tis incredible how much they can do in such a case. (II:2,6,2:110, emphasis added)

Rather than seeking to entirely expunge all passions through a reconsideration of the mistaken ideas and imaginings that are engendered by them, then, Burton wants to control, tame, regulate, and change those feelings through habits of self-analysis (together with other efforts at self-care, including distraction, seeking the company of others, and a host of other pursuits). These exercises aim for a balance (or *krasia*) between the passions, imagination, and reason—a goal again placing Burton closer to Aristotle than to the Stoic ideas.[12] The moderate, rather than extreme, passions, achieved through their careful, habituated regulation, were central to the moral life and the achievement of *eudemonia* for Aristotle and Aristotelianism. But they must be of the right kind: at the right time, about the right things, toward the right people, for the right end, and experienced in the right way.[13] (In his own comparison between Aristotle and Seneca on this point, Burton explicitly sides with Seneca, confusingly blurring the contrast: "Though Aristotle deny any part of intemperance to be conversant about sorrow, I am of *Seneca's* minde, he that is wise is temperate, and *he that is temperate is constant, free from passion, and he that is such a one, is without sorrow*: as all wise men should be" [II:3,5,1:185]. But his more consistent opinion favors temperate passions over none.)

The emphasis on temperance reflects as much humoral balance as balance within these facultative functions. But this would follow naturally from the *Anatomy* account: A balanced complexion corresponds to one in which the passions are tempered by reason and imagination, not expunged entirely. (Burton is repeatedly drawn to balance and moderation; their appeal for him is evident in some of his broadest admonitions: "Nothing so good, but it may be abused," he remarks, illustrating this paean to moderation with the case of physical exercise: "nothing better than Exercise (if opportunely used) for the preservation of the

---

12. See Lund 2011:169.
13. Aristotle, 1985. *Nicomachean Ethics* Book II.

Body: nothing so bad, if it be unseasonable, violent, or overmuch" [I,2,2,6:238].)

Efforts to achieve balance by taming the passions parallel the balance of humors sought through other self-care measures. In this difference between Burton and the Stoics, we may see reflected Burton's point of departure in writing the *Anatomy*. Aberrant mood states and affections must be averted, and regulated, with the aim of achieving normal moods and more everyday miseries. This rather Aristotelian recognition of the worth of normal passions occurs only sporadically in the *Anatomy*, however. It is recognized, then lost, then recovered, as Burton seems to slip back into the Stoic and Christian attitudes of disparagement, where all feelings and passions are judged wrongful, unhealthy, and disordered.

THE AKRATIC MELANCHOLIC

Added to his admiration for the faculty of imagination, and emphasis on its power to adjust and expunge excessive and inappropriate feelings, this attitude toward moderation suggests a more nuanced view of the picture whereby Reason provides the only force against unruly and dangerous feelings. Guided by reason, the imagination also helps curb, deflect, and alter those states. Yet, as a compelling, and partially sensory inclination, imagination, too, is unruly. By injecting the imagination into the center of things, Burton complicates the relation between reason and the passions suggested by the traditional metaphor of Reason as charioteer. Despite being a sensory inclination, imagining is not a blind impulse; rather, it is a mindful and purposive activity. Like the passions with which it is so intimately entwined, it is rebellious and difficult to govern, yet unlike them, it is directly responsive to will.

Passions (*pathê*), were literally things undergone or suffered, as we saw. They were the appetites and fears associated with pleasure and distress, respectively.[14] On this matter, Burton seems to assume the Stoic

---

14. See Cooper 2012:449.

taxonomy, comprising four basic affective states: pleasure or delight (*hedone*), longing or appetition (*epithumia*), distress or pain (*lupe*), and fear (*phobos*). Conative contraries in this way distribute the passions into two broad categories, inclinations and aversions. (The inclusion of desire with other perturbations in such a taxonomy is an arrangement that may seem somewhat anomalous in our contemporary times. But it was standard in Burton's era, and recognized by other early modern thinkers as well. The role played by desire in reasoning and action differs from that played by more typical passions like sadness or fear. Yet the similarities linking desire to such states were nonetheless regarded as more significant than the differences.[15])We are so drawn to imagining and so enjoy our imaginary conceits, that the Imagination is for Reason an unreliable, if powerful, ally.

The uneasy, even warring relationship between Reason and the passions within Western philosophical traditions has been judged to have been nowhere played out more fiercely than in the sixteenth-century England that was the immediate setting of Burton's intellectual development.[16] And moral struggle and weakness are familiar themes in the *Anatomy*. Incumbent in the simile of Reason as the charioteer, always striving to curb his horses' headstrong careening, are instances when control is ceded to the passions and, while it judges rightly, Reason is temporarily powerless. These are occasions of what Aristotle knew as *akrasia* (incontinence) and we commonly refer to as weakness of will. *Akrasia* is a deficiency in the normal degree of self-control (*enkrateia*); thus incontinent or *akratic* action is in today's discussions said to be intentional action contrary to the person's better (and rational) judgment.[17]Although customarily described in moral language, the states of mind captured in the notion of *akrasia*, and the characteristic phenomenology associated with them, call for psychological analysis as much as any other aspect

15. James 1997:7.
16. Tillyard 1963.
17. Mele 1987:4. Not all cases of conflicted thinking reduce to *akrasia*, it should be added. There is also ambivalence. (See Rorty 2010.) Moreover, although Burton would not have countenanced any such dethroning of the rational soul, cases of "inverse akrasia" contradict this formulation, where sentiments or passions such as sympathy bring about right action by sidestepping rationality.

of mental life. Thus, while closely entwined with Burton's religious and philosophical preoccupations, his moral psychology is a critical aspect of the Burtonian conception of the mind and mental processes.

Burton is acutely aware of the ever-present challenge of *akrasia*, and in discussing the will, he offers his own account of such moments of weakness. Some actions of the Will are performed by "inferior powers" he explains, "which obey ... [it] as the Sensitive and moving Appetite." His examples are when we open our eyes, move about ("goe hither and thither"), refrain from touching something, or choose to "speake faire or foule." But such obedience is not consistent:

> this Appetite is many times rebellious in us, and will not be contained within the lists of sobriety and temperance. It was ... once well agreeing with reason, and there was an excellent concent and harmony betwixt them, but that is now dissolved, they often jarred, *Reason* is over borne by *Passion*[18] ... as so many wild horses runne away with a chariot, and will not be curbed.

He quotes Medea in Ovid[19]

> We know many times what is good, but will not doe it, as she said ... Lust counsels one thing, reason another, there is a new reluctancy in men ... We cannot resist.... So David knew the filthinesse of his fact, what a loathsome, foule, crying sinne Adultery was, yet notwithstanding he would commit murther, and take away another mans wife, enforced against Reason, Religion, to follow his Appetite.

Those "*Naturall* and *Vegetall*" powers bring

> head-strong Passions ... violent perturbations of the Minde ... vitious [vicious] Habits, customs, ferall Diseases; because we give

---

18. The harmonious earlier time referred to was before the Fall.
19. *Trahit invitam nova vis, aliudque cupido, Mens aliud saudet.* (We see the better and approve it, but follow the worse.)

so much way to our *Appetite*, and follow our inclination, like so many beasts. (I,1,2,11:161)

Along with any classically educated scholar of his day, Burton would have been familiar with the accounts offered to explain *akrasia* by Aristotle, the Stoics, and the medieval church. How to account for these moments of moral weakness has been a philosophical preoccupation ever since, with his insistence that we cannot knowingly do wrong, Plato had infamously seemed to deny the very phenomenon.[20] Aristotle's idea was that *akrasia* must be fought against with habituated virtues, and could only come about when knowledge was somehow obscured by the appetite at the very moment of choice. The Stoics had tried out different explanations, some denying, others acknowledging, the phenomenon of *akrasia*. In the seemingly *akratic* moment, according to Chrysippus, reason oscillates at imperceptibly rapid speed between the two incompatible evaluations.[21] Others emphasized that *akrasia* could be avoided, but only by achieving the state of tranquility (*ataraxia*) when all passions were expunged—an unlikely, and perhaps unreachable, position even for the sage. Later, in the writing of Church fathers Origen and Augustine, the conception of diminished will was ascribed to the akratic moment. Of these several accounts, Burton's reference to the danger of vicious habits in the above passage, suggests agreement with Aristotle's. The good habits of a regulated life must provide the best bulwark we could have against weakness of will. But that such *akratic* moments occur, Burton never doubts.

Regardless of whether the Stoic goal of apathy could, or should, be achieved, the role played by imagination in Burton's cognitive architecture seems to prevent his entirely settling for any of the classical accounts. The models of *akrasia* offered by Plato, Aristotle, and the Stoics each pit reason against the passions, and leave no room for the hybrid activity of imagining that partakes of the intellectual as well as

---

20. Plato also resorted to other unsatisfactory explanations, appealing to discord, lack of control, intemperance, and cowardice. See Sorabji 2002.
21. For an analysis and explication of this view, see Sorabji 2000:305–15. See also Gill, 2010.

the sensory and desiring. The inadequacy of classical accounts has been attributed to its "ratiocentric" focus on pure intellect that invites only two outcomes: rationality or aimless chaos. On this compartmentalized picture, "reason either remains firmly in charge, or else is taken over and dragged around by irrational forces." Such models, John Cottingham complains, betray the anxious fear that "unless reason remains fussily and firmly at the helm, our lives will lose direction" (Cottingham 1998:163–4).[22] Rather than these rational functions, what actually gives our lives direction are elements beyond reason's power to control and regulate; they provide "the springs of human creativity, inventiveness and imagination" (Cottingham 1998:164).

In the imagination's disorderly nature lies its power and value, on Cottingham's analysis. It will not always do Reason's bidding. And with this, at least, Burton would have agreed. The *Anatomy* picture is akin to Cottingham's in relying on the capacity of the imagination to curb, balance, and adjust the passions. We can regulate unwanted and dangerous responses and moods through the inventive freedom of imaginative creativity. Such inventiveness is at most guided by Reason, but brings its own direction and meaning to our lives. We are able to thus evoke, dampen, and redirect feelings in ways that far exceed what can be achieved through reasoning alone. This way, as Cottingham says, we use the capabilities of imagination to elicit feelings that enrich and shape us. Reason also had a role in the *Anatomy*, but the imaginative capabilities, which are as much assets and gifts as liabilities, provide a complex, interactive link between inclinations, reasoning, and willing, the intellectual and sensory. It is a scheme not easily allowed within traditional depictions, whether Aristotelian, Stoic, or Christian.

That the imagination and feelings actually dictate the direction of our lives more importantly than any of the classical, ratiocentric models

---

22. Whether this accusation is equally true for the Stoics may be questioned. Christopher Gill points out that the materialist and cognitivist features of passions they adhered to, combined with the psychological pull of the passions, allowed the Stoics to avoid dividing the psyche into rational and nonrational parts in explaining the internal conflict leading to *akratic* action. Gill 2010:151–2.

can allow has become a commonplace of our contemporary mind sciences. And Burton saw it only incompletely. When he did, moreover, it was perhaps more due as much to historical luck than reasoned argument. His focus was feelings, since the Melancholy he "anatomized" involved disordered moods. And he inherited a faculty psychology, together with attitudes toward, and medical lore about, the imagination, that assigned the relationship between the imagination and passions to a position at the center of his inquiries. Today, however, these tenets have the force of established fact. Findings from neuroscience such as Damasio's, about the complex interaction between cognition and affection, and LeDoux's account of the roles played by the amygdala and the cortex, strongly support Burton's tenets, and affirm the picture Cottingham develops—as do observations about the role played by the default system, and recent emphasis on emotions and the imagination in philosophical writing.[23]

The source of passions was willful impulses of all kinds. And Burton accommodates the focus on carnal sins and bodily appetites associated with notions of *akrasia* from Greek and particularly Christian traditions, as we saw above. Aside from the familiar bodily appetites, however, much attention in the *Anatomy* is directed toward inclinations that are, by contrast, more broadly sensory. Where the naturalness of carnal appetites egging us on by natural concupiscence is explained, Burton also acknowledges weakness over appetites more generally understood:

> Sensuall appetite seeing an object, if it be a convenient good, cannot but desire it . . . we are egged on by our natural concupiscence, and there is . . . a confusion in our powers, our whole Will is averse from God and his Law, not in natural things only, as to eat & drinke, lust, to which we are led headlong by our temperature and inordinate Appetite . . . we cannot resist . . . the seat of our affections, captivates and enforceth our will. So that in voluntary things we are averse from God and goodnesse, bad by nature,

---

23. See Moran 1994, essays in Goldie 2010, Lennon 2015.

by ignorance worse, by Art, Discipline, Custome, we get many bad Habits, suffering them to domineere and tyrannize over us. (I,1,2,11:160)

"The seat of our affections captivates and enforces our will." One reading of this passage it has been pointed out, leaves us all in a state of perpetual *akrasia*: Man, "knowing in his reason what he should do, yet doing instead what concupiscent appetite calls him to" (Tilmouth 2005:527). That Burton also alludes to the Fall here is not in doubt. But by remembering his emphasis on the lure of imagining, we can recognize a narrower, and more specific, reference in the bad habits that "domineer and tyrannize over us."

Imagining is a function of the sensitive or sensible soul, in the *Anatomy*'s faculty psychology. It partakes of the bodily and finds a place between the body and the pure intellect of the rational soul. Because of this, it seems to force a realignment of the customary oppositions: imagining can be pleasurable as well as intellectual. Inclinations can be partly bodily and partly intellectual. The imaginative play and fanciful speculation described in the *Anatomy* are (initially) intensely appealing and exciting, in the manner of bodily and localized pleasures—indeed, they do not seem sharply differentiated from these more familiar temptations. And the pleasures of "melancholising" are as much of a temptation, and as dangerous, as lust and gluttony.

MELANCHOLISING

Our struggles with these particular inclinations, and the hazards they represent (falling into severe, intractable melancholia), are repeatedly emphasized. And Burton's contribution to philosophical ideas about *akrasia* is found here, with pleasures provided by the imagination alone.

In the *Anatomy* the imagination is described in several ways: as *raging* excessively, as *crased*, as particularly *strong* and *apprehensive*, and as *restless, operative*, and *quick*. A similar range of adjectives conveys the normative element: The imagination is "unapt," "hindred" [hindered], "hurt," "corrupt," "injured," "false" and "violent." Characterizations of the unhealthy and dangerous aspects of the imagination are vague, despite this collection. They seem to want for features that would conclusively distinguish the unhealthy from the prodigious imagining Burton recognizes to be so unsurpassingly valuable in scientific, scholarly, and artistic efforts, and the useful imagination that can be employed to balance and regulate our passions.

That such descriptors, normative and neutral alike, sometimes indicate what would today be distinguished as hallucinatory and delusional states is evident from cases introduced by way of illustration. Citing Weyer, Burton notes that melancholy and sick men

> conceave so many phantastical visions ... and have such absurd apparitions, as that they are Kings, Lords, Cocks, Beares, Apes, Owls. (1,2,3,2:252)

But melancholy is also associated with tendencies less extreme than these. Sometimes it is a passing, pleasurable wool-gathering or reflection. At other times, while still recognized by its subject to be mere fantasizing, it is "melancholising" (or melancholizing)—the mental habit of the melancholic.[24] Rehearsing an idea over and over, elaborating, embroidering, worrying at, obsessing, ruminating—these are all ways we might capture the idle, repetitive, tenacious ideas and feelings described as melancholising. As depicted by Burton, some of these tendencies and habits call for effortful imagination, while others seem to be unbidden states and thought patterns. The language and categories are vague here (but so are our own, today). As it plays a part in engendering melancholy, two processes and experiences can be distinguished, although in some cases, they will later prove to have been merely different phases of a continuous sequence. The first stage involves the "fond conceits" entertained in solitary and idle moments that often lead to a habit of melancholising. At this point in the progression, it is suggested, we remain in control of ourselves. But the activity of melancholising

---

24. I,2,2,6:243.

can induce the more severe states of disorder over which the person is powerless. By then, the Imagination, and sometimes Reason itself have become corrupted. The first of these stages, and the psychology around the activity of melancholising are our subject here; in chapter 6, we turn to the more advanced condition.

Melancholising describes repetitive thought patterns—or, when the subject matter is negatively toned, a kind of gloomy ruminating. Yet the term is also used to describe positive and enchanting ideas:

> A most incomparable delight, it is so to melancholize, to build castles in the ayre . . . [But] Feare, sorrow, supsition [suspicion] . . . discontent, cares, and weariness of life, surprise them in a moment, and they can thinke of nothing else, continually suspecting, no sooner are their eyes open, but this infernal plague of Melancholy seazeth on them, and terrifies their soules, representing some dismall object to their mindes, which now by no meanes, no labour, no perswasions they can avoide. (I,2,2,6:243)

Burton establishes compelling parallels between sensual appetites and the way those who suffer or are prone to melancholy find themselves powerless to resist certain thoughts and fears, drawn on by such exaggerated and profligate imaginings, while at the same time knowing full well that they should dispel, or deflate, them, or use other means to distract, and redirect, their own attention. Although it is not a term Burton uses in this context, so comparable is this depiction of the pleasures of unfettered imagining to the more traditional passions and appetites that the notion of *akrasia* seems applicable. Like the more familiar *akratic*, who knows what he must do but is lured by bodily appetites, the melancholic is similarly, and equally, a victim of temptation:

> let him by all meanes avoide it, 'tis a bosome enemy, this delightsome melancholy, a friend in shew, but a secret divell, a secret poyson, it will in the end be his undoing . . . If he proceede, as a Gnat flies about a candle, so long till at length he burne his body so in the end he will undoe himself. (II,2,6,1:102)

The attitude toward those who succumb to melancholy conveyed in this passage has been identified as an anxious one. And Burton's apparently overblown fears perhaps illustrate this.[25] But it is not merely the attendant risks that are captured here: Also described are the comfort, enjoyment, and delight produced by engaging in these flights of fancy. The charms of imagining and melancholising lauded by the Elizabethan poets are familiar, and very real for him. The gnat flying into the candle is the ambivalent Burton himself.

While exaggerated in its language, the poem added to the third edition of the *Anatomy* most clearly conveys the intense tension set up by these contrasting attitudes of attraction and fear. Using rhyming couplets, Burton lays out in the Author's Abstract the matched joys and horrors brought by melancholy: "Naught so sweet as melancholy" yet also "A thousand miseries at once, Mine heavy hearte and soule esconce" (I,xix). The woes and distresses enumerated include solitary wakefulness, remembering past ill deeds; thoughts that tyrannize in their insistence; ugly images, fearful sights; bitterness, torments over love, and so on. It is widely held that Burton suffered from melancholy himself, and these lines capture the phenomenological frame so well, they might well be taken to bespeak personal acquaintance. Drawn to such deceptive and false pleasures (secret devils masquerading as friends) Burton writes vividly of the lure and pleasures of melancholising. Again in the Author's Abstract, he speaks of musing all alone; thinking of "divers things fore-knowne"; building castles in the air; pleasing oneself with charming fantasies; entertaining pleasing thoughts; thinking one hears sweet music, sees towns, palaces, and fine cities, rare beauties, gallant ladies, "what e're is lovely or divine," and imagining oneself in the embrace of a mistress—and all these solitary imaginings beguile most pleasurably. Yet, as the structure of the poem emphasizes, there is

---

25. Tilmouth points out that the incessant repetitions, and "self-propagating" nature, of the loops between feeling and imagination makes Burtonian Melancholy a condition that is "terrifyingly tenacious"—so much so that a recurrent fear must be attributed to Burton that melancholy "may not be suppressible; that man's descent into the disease may be unavoidable." The copiousness of his style is thus explained as "a nervous response to his sense of the overwhelming, ever-burgeoning and ungovernable scope of melancholy" (Tilmouth 2005:526).

endless danger to such fantasy and melancholising. As often as pleasure, the imagination brings suffering and distress. The scene is turned, the joys gone, as he says, and "Feare discontent and sorrowes come." This solitary pleasure is the route to melancholy, to "paines past cure," even despair, and thoughts of suicide ("Now desperate I hate my life, Lend me an halter or a knife").

The struggle described here shows the melancholic as an *akratic*— he knows he should not, yet gives in to the lure of these inclinations that bring so much effortless satisfaction and pleasure. Its language is exaggerated and jesting, yet the Abstract artfully illustrates the central, complex role of imagining in these inner sequences. The Imagination invokes images and thoughts that are both distressing and pleasing, fearsome and delightful. *And imagining of each sort comes with a powerful, repetitive, insistence*:

> still, still, still thinking of it ... still that toy runnes in their minde, that fear, that superstition ... that agony, that crotchet. (I,3,1,2:393)

With the inclination toward the pleasures of fantasy and imagination, the phenomenon of *akrasia* becomes more complex than in traditional analyses, where, as Burton puts it, "we are led headlong by our temperature and inordinate Appetite." This noncarnal kind of inclination is different, yet easily recognizable. To those given to Melancholy,

> most pleasant it is at first ... to ly in bed whole daies, and keep their chambers, to walke alone in some solitary grove, betwixt wood and water ... to meditate upon some delightsome and pleasant subject, which shall affect them most ... to goe smiling to themselves, acting an infinite variety of parts, which they suppose, and strongly imagine they represent, or that they see acted or done ... to conceave and meditate of such pleasant things, sometimes present, past, or to come, as Rhasis speakes. (I:2,2,6:243)

Just as solitude itself is pleasurable, so is the idle, isolated reasoning that, in producing fantasies and conceits, strays from consensual realities and the rub of interpersonal exchange. Bypassing the often unsettling processes of confirmation and disconfirmation, it can be a comforting and easeful experience. And so is pretending, adopting roles, imagining oneself to be other than what, or how, one is, this passage points out.

Frequent references to these distinctive pleasures associated with the initial activity suggest the source of its irresistible appeal. It is an appeal to our inherent laziness: It is easier to let our speculations, assumptions, and fantasies run free than to curb and critically evaluate them. It nourishes our self-loving, egocentric grandiosity. But it is also a feeling of exuberance: part curiosity-satisfied, part aesthetic appreciation, and part a sense of creative achievement. Later, this melancholising will sour and become unpleasant. But these initial pleasures and tendencies combine to yield, as Burton says, a most incomparable delight: They "bewitch" us.

The poem illustrates a second element important to understanding melancholising: It is a process. The compelling lure remains, whether its objects are pleasurable or painful; we resist each with difficulty. But this is a sequential analysis. First come the pleasures, then, once we have habituated ourselves to enjoying them, they are followed by suffering. The scene is turned, he says. Then "joys are gone," and "Feare discontent and sorrowes come."

"BE NOT SOLITARY, BE NOT IDLE"

Melancholising is an inner exercise, engaged in alone. And it is the inclination to fantasize *alone*, that puts us at extra risk—not fantasizing as such, but fantasizing and ruminating without the steadying balance provided by others' perspectives. In the engraved frontispiece from the third edition, solitariness is accorded a separate image, showing a lone figure in a landscape devoid of other people.[26] The yearning for solitude, the dangerous way solitude engenders melancholy states, and the further

---

26. It is richly peopled with animals, on the other hand—as he describes in the accompanying guide: "sleeping dog, cat: Bucke and Doe, Hares, Conies [rabbits] cuniculus and Owles."

isolating effects of those states, had all been part of the long tradition of writing about melancholy since Hippocratic times. The solitary life can be hazardous to one's health, as Seneca is enlisted to confirm. We are led to degenerate from sociable creatures to become "beasts, monsters, inhumane, ugly to behold" (I,2,2,7:245). And these outcomes are the worse for being self-imposed:

> *Thou hast lost they selfe willfully,* cast away thy selfe, though thy selfe art the efficient cause of thine owne misery, by not resisting such vaine cogitations, but giving way unto them. (I,2,2,7:245, emphasis added)

"Be not solitary, be not idle" is the succinct prescription that ends the entire book.[27] And the part of solitariness and its linked idleness in bringing about and fostering melancholy is important enough to be given its own subsection. Burton first explores the dangers of the solitary life (or at least that which is entered voluntarily). Voluntary solitariness, as he says, "gently brings on like a Siren" the horrors of melancholy, although "most pleasant at first." Those lured by it,

> could spend whole daies and nights without sleepe, even whole yeares alone in such contemplations, and phantasticall meditations, which are like unto dreames, and they will hardly be drawne from them, or willingly interrupt, so pleasant their vaine conceipts are, that they hinder their ordinary taskes and necessary business ... untill at last the Sceane is turned upon a sudden, by some bad object, and they being now habituated to such vaine meditations and solitary places, can endure no company, can ruminate of nothing but harsh and distastefull subjects. (I,2,2,6:243)

---

27. The full passage runs, "Onely take this for a corollary and conclusion, as thou tenderest thine owne welfare in this and all other melancholy, thy good health of body and minde, observe this short precept, give not way to solitarinesse and idlelesse. *Be not solitary, be not idle*" (III,4,2,6:445). Samuel Johnson's nice elaboration was, "if you are solitary, do not be idle; if you are idle, do not be alone" (Johnson 1893:293).

Remembering the valuable solitariness of the religious in their cells, and of philosophers sequestered from the tumultuous world, Burton hastens to qualify. There is some "profitable Meditation, Contemplation and kind of solitarinesse." Seneca's refinement is employed: It is only a "destructive solitariness" that thus "undoeth us." This last contrast seems to rest with the link between solitariness and idleness, "German cousins" that, as he says, go hand in hand:

> Nothing begets [melancholy] sooner, encreaseth and continueth it oftner then idleness. (I,2,2,6:239)

Idleness may be of body or mind, moreover. The idleness of the mind is much worse than that effecting the body, for "witte without employment is a disease" (I,2,2,6). Those who are idle are never well, in body or minde, but

> weary still, weeping, sighing, grieving, suspecting, offended with the world, with every object, wishing themselves gone or dead, or else carried away with some foolish Phantasie or other. (I,2,2,6:240)

Monks' and philosophers' contemplations are exempt. Although solitary, they are quite unlike these idle thoughts that, without order, discipline, or purpose, charm with foolish phantasies. Recent research on rumination has employed a contrast similar to the one Burton draws here, interestingly. Recognizing innocuous and even productive forms of mind wandering, it contrasts *rumination*, which is apparently maladaptive in allowing the person to disengage from activities and commitments, with *reflection*,[28] or *reflective pondering*.[29] Similarly, *brooding* and *obsessive* or *depressive* rumination are identified as the dangerous kind correlated with depressed mood or depressive disorder.[30]

---

28. Trapnell and Campbell 1999, Takano and Tanno 2009.
29. Treynor et al. 2003.
30. Kuyken et al. 2006, American Psychiatric Association (APA) 2013. On the tendency toward depressive rumination and negative thoughts, see Spasojevic and Alloy 2001, Watkins, E. and Teasdale 2001.

"BEWITCHING THOUGHTS"

In the *Anatomy*, the process by which these temptations incite idle, dangerous, and compulsive melancholising receives copious and careful phenomenological description. Of these "phantastical and bewitching thoughts," it is said,

> [they] so covertly, so feelingly so urgently, so continually set upon, creepe in, insinuate, possesse, overcome, distract and detaine them ... [the melancholic sufferers] cannot ... extricate themselves, but are ever musing, melancholizing, and carried along. (I,2,2,6:243)

While elsewhere sometimes distracting, Burton's prolix style works to unparalleled effect here in explaining the several ingredients constituting these irresistible thoughts. It is a complex gestalt; nonetheless, the compelling force of such ruminative activities remains clear. We cannot extricate ourselves; they carry us along in this "labarinth of anxious and solicitous melancholy meditations" (I,2,2,6:243).

Research on the mind-wandering states introduced in chapter 2 seems to confirm that similar experiences affect a subset of people in the irresistible way depicted in such passages. Even "normal" mind wanderers, studies have indicated, include a group who engage in excessive fantasizing, and for them, fantasizing is a barely controllable preoccupation.[31] Of this "compulsive fantasy," it has been observed that, "while they are fully aware that these fantasies are not real and are generally able to refrain from engaging [in them] ... during work or school, they find the compulsion to engage these fantasies uncontrollable *when they are alone*." The lack of control over their fantasy "not only differentiates them from 'healthy' individuals, but also contributes to their distress over issues of time diverted from social activity and important relationships" (Kam and Handy 2013:11, emphasis added) That distress sounds

---

[31]. Schupak and Rosenthal 2009, Bigelsen and Schupak 2011.

like the lament of the *akratic* melancholic: He knows he should be otherwise engaged, yet feels powerless to resist.

DEPRESSIVE RUMINATION AND AVAILABILITY HEURISTICS

Affective states have long been associated with ruminative symptoms. And clinical descriptions from today of the ruminating, negative, idle, repetitive ideas associated with depressive states depict very similar patterns of thought to those Burton describes as melancholising.[32] Contemporary research has also linked default system mind-wandering with depression.[33] If melancholising can be analogized to the ruminating that is a typical default system thought pattern, then here may lie a way to explicate Burton's references to melancholising and its dangers.

Such research concludes that, "depressed individuals are more likely to be in the default state and once engaged, are more likely to stay there" (Kamm and Handy 2013:12).[34] That "more likely to stay there," particularly, invokes the tendency toward a habituated condition stressed throughout the *Anatomy*. And it suggests another of Burton's themes. Studies of otherwise "normal" mind wanderers have identified some who engage in excessive and even compulsive, solitary fantasizing, for whom fantasizing is a preoccupation.[35] These current demonstrations of the addictive and compulsive qualities of mind wandering seem to capture some of Burton's observations about habituated, solitary musing.

The passages of the *Anatomy* cited earlier also anticipate recent research about the kind of "depressive" rumination, or "brooding" associated with mood disorder. (This association has been noted in anxiety disorders as well, but is most commonly introduced in relation to depression[36]). Rumination is variously defined and characterized in these

---

32. On the tendency toward depressive rumination in negative thoughts, see Spasojevic and Alloy 2001, Watkins and Teasdale 2001.
33. Killingsworth and Gilbert 2010. These links are explored more fully in a later chapter.
34. See also Spasojevic and Alloy 2001, Watkins and Teasdale 2001, Disner et al. 2011, Smallwood and O'Connor 2011, Marchetti et al. 2012, Marchetti et al. 2014.
35. Schupak and Rosenthal 2009.
36. Harrington and Blankenship 2002.

contemporary studies. It is self-focused thoughts;[37] a repetitive preoccupation with negative emotions;[38] brooding over the person's "symptoms of distress, and their possible causes and consequences";[39] and recyclic negative thinking resistant to distraction.[40] Rumination need not involve negative thoughts, these variations suggest. Nonetheless it is often so defined (or "depressive rumination" is introduced as a subtype of rumination more generally understood). Without yet fully identifying the mechanisms involved, research has shown consistent correlations between ruminative response style and depression.

According to one review of these findings, the habit of rumination exacerbates depression, enhances negative thinking, impairs problem solving, interferes with instrumental behavior, and erodes social support.[41] Speculations as to the exact relationship between rumination and depression have included the notion that common depression symptoms such as lethargy and decreased inclination toward engagement with the external environment, themselves due to impairment of effortful task-related processing, may be induced by rumination.[42] Ruminating has been shown to prolong and exacerbate depressed moods in experimental studies with dysphoric and depressed individuals.[43] Longitudinal studies have revealed that trait rumination predicts higher future depressive symptom levels, particularly in nonclinical samples.[44] And rumination on negative thoughts engenders negative moods, the interaction between the thoughts and moods creating, it has been hypothesized, a vicious cycle.[45]

Depressive rumination has also received particular attention among conjectures put forward to explain the persistence of depression symptoms.[46] While seemingly valueless, even depressive rumination may be,

37. Nolen-Hoeksema and Morrow 1993.
38. Nolen-Hoeksema 1991, 2000.
39. Nolen-Hoeksema, Wisco, and Lyubomirsky 2008.
40. Treynor et al. 2003.
41. Nolen-Hoeksema, Wisco, and Lyubomirsky 2008.
42. Watkins, E. and Brown 2002.
43. Kuehner et al. 2007; Kuehner et al. 2009.
44. Huffziger et al. 2009; Nolen-Hoeksema, 2000.
45. Disner et al. 2011.
46. For a review of these efforts, see Varga 2012b.

or may have once been, adaptive. Together with the set of depression symptoms with which it is associated (pessimism, despondency and low mood, diminished responsiveness, and lack of motivation), this habit has been hypothesized to conserve resources in the face of unachievable challenges or problems, for example. Thus, in the "analytic rumination hypothesis," the obvious costs of depressive rumination are assessed as outweighed by its role as a stress-response mechanism. Triggered by analytically difficult and materially significant problems (those with "fitness-related goals"), it is hypothesized to promote sustained analysis, and the generation and evaluation, of solutions to those challenges.[47] Quite contrary to such recent adaptationist hypotheses, however, are findings accumulated within many years of past depression research. Depressive rumination may have once served an evolutionary purpose, but instead of helping to provide solutions, these activities today seem to maintain and exacerbate affective disorder, as well as impairing cognitive capacities and hindering instrumental behavior—consequences plausibly interpreted as among the dire and deleterious effects that ensue from the dangerous habit of melancholising.

Much is yet to be learned about rumination. For example, some recent studies indicate that both the content and the context of ruminating alter its value. One form of problem-solving, social in focus, has shown itself to be enhanced, not diminished, in depressed patients when rumination is concrete, as distinct from abstract.[48] A different study suggests that the ruminative style inviting depression is particularly that involving thoughts focused on past events.[49] In other research, findings indicate that with normal subjects, only rumination following stressful events ("stress reactive rumination"), not rumination over other matters, predicts the onset, number, and duration of major depressive and hopelessness depressive episodes.[50] Burton's vague remarks about melancholising are of little help here, but nor has present-day science entirely established what makes some ruminating bad for our health.

47. Andrews and Thompson 2009.
48. Watkins, E. and Moulds 2005.
49. Smallwood and O'Connor 2011.
50. Robinson and Alloy 2003.

The negatively toned, repetitive objects of rumination have been the particular focus of cognitive therapy in its application to depression. Reoccurring, negative, often self-referential thoughts have been shown to spring to mind with the occurrence of triggers. (Such thoughts form part of the person's "schema," or conceptual scheme by which he or she habitually and automatically responds to, and interprets, experience.) In order to avert or lift the unwelcome moods, the goal of cognitive therapy is to disabuse the patient of negative, pessimistic, and repetitious ideas (or "negative automatic thoughts"). This is done indirectly, through a didactic process of correcting and challenging inference patterns and conclusions, as well as more directly, by efforts of self-control, such as the employment of distraction.[51]

There is considerable evidence that biased "mood-congruent" thought processing and focus of attention in depressed subjects allow easier recall of information and memories with negative content.[52] Thus, appeal is made to the "availability heuristics" (Tversky and Kahneman) employed for decision-making under conditions of uncertainty: the biased reasoning patterns that serve to skew judgements about predicted or hypothetical outcomes. (For further discussion of these biased reasoning patterns, see chapters 6 and 7.)

It has been shown that laboratory-induced sad and negative moods resulted in both easier recall of negative events and exaggerated predictions over the likelihood that negative events would occur.[53] And because the function of the Burtonian Imagination includes recall and remembering as well as what we would usually intend by imagining, these findings appear to apply to melancholising: Gloomy memories will be more readily recalled. (Since they are in apparent tension with the evidence supporting the "Sadder but Wiser" studies about what is known as "depressive realism," these conclusions are not uncontroversial. Those studies suggest that inaccuracy and bias over some matters, including past events, are actually greater with normal subjects than those who are depressed, and we return to this issue in chapter 7.)

---

51. Beck et al. 1979, Clark et al. 1999.
52. See also Matthews and MacLeod 2005, Watkins, P.C. et al. 1996, Biegler 2011.
53. MacLeod et al.1997b.

Also closely related to the centrality of the imagination and imagining in the *Anatomy* are studies using a form of the availability heuristic known as the "simulation heuristic" (Kahneman and Tversky).[54] Predictions about the likelihood of eventualities have been shown to be dependent on the *ease* with which those eventualities can be imagined, constructed, or simulated. A number of judgments we make under conditions of uncertainty involve this activity: predictions about future circumstances; assessments of conditional probabilities, and assessments of causality, for example. The elaboration of a plausible imaginary scenario that leads from realistic initial conditions to a specified end state is often used to support the judgment that the probability of the end state is high, these researchers remind us. The simulation heuristic, associated with a risk of large and systematic errors, constitutes a persistent and serious form of cognitive bias found in normal reasoners, it has been concluded.[55]

Employing the conception of a simulation heuristic and its accompanying biases, subsequent researchers have hypothesized that the pessimism allied to depression is due to the exaggerated predictions that come from a greater ease explaining and imagining (or simulating) negative scenarios.[56] This would assign a role for imagining alongside recalling and remembering. As we saw above, these functions have been correlated with a similar bias favoring mood-congruent subject matter. In comparison with a control group without depression, those in the depressed group exaggerated the likelihood of negative events and the unlikelihood of positive ones; they were also more readily able to construct (envision, or imagine) explanations for the negative outcomes.[57]

These findings have been replicated in research that has described an "ease of recall paradigm." By measuring and controlling for that ease,

---

54. The term "simulation" is chosen here because "questions about events are answered by an operation that resembles the running of a simulation model" (Kahneman and Tversky 1982:201).
55. Kahneman and Tversky 1982:207–8.
56. These hypotheses found confirmation in parallel studies establishing that those prone to *optimism* are able to readily form mental images of positive outcomes. See Blackwell et al. 2013.
57. MacLeod et al. 1997b.

it is possible to determine the extent to which it affects other observed correlations (those between pessimism, depression, and judgments as to the likelihood of negative outcomes).[58] Designed to explain the positive correlation between depressive symptoms and pessimism using the ease of recall paradigm, one research study yielded evidence that the greater pessimism among individuals with dysphoria and depression is at least partially accounted for by "how easy it felt to imagine reasons why negative events would happen" (Vaughn and Weary 2002:700).

The focus on easefulness is particularly telling when considered in relation to melancholising. This is not an absolute inability to imagine positive as distinct from negative outcomes, but rather a relative difficulty in doing so. It is thus compatible with Burton's suggestion that with extra effort and self-control, imagining positive outcomes may often remain within our grasp. The finding that recall and remembering are limited by a bias governing mood-congruent content, may not in this way be quite as compatible with the *Anatomy* analysis. Inability to recall suggests something closer to complete incapacity. Emphasis on ease of imagining or simulating, by contrast, acknowledges the possibility of a capacity that is merely diminished—flawed, but not entirely broken.

In describing how the imagination explains the endless lure and dangerous persistence of melancholy, Burton speaks of an imagination that is hurt or damaged in being prodigious: too strong, too vivid, too "restless, operative and quick." This presents a puzzle in his account, as we saw, since the same adjectives are applicable to the exercise and products of the imagination that are lauded as creative and admirable. Contemporary research about mind wandering, rumination, and the cognitive bias resulting from these availability heuristics affecting recall and simulation may point to part of the answer to that puzzle. Three different traits seem to mark the troubling imagination and imagining to which Burton refers. As the above studies of mind wandering indicate and seem to confirm, it is idle, in the sense of unproductive and aimless. It is also appealing, at times almost irresistibly so—a consequence of which is that it is repetitive, with ideas played out over and over, ruminatively. Finally, when its

---

58. Vaughn and Weary 2002.

subject matter is related to uncertainties and hypotheticals, it seems likely (at least if negative outcomes are involved) to reflect bias brought about by availability heuristics of this kind. In contrast to the ease with which the person recalls and imagines negative consequences, recalling and simulating positive outcomes and scenarios is hampered, and relatively difficult.

Using the assorted findings from psychology cited above, we begin to see more clearly the meaning and importance Burton assigns to melancholising—once it has soured and become unpleasant. Melancholising is a form of imagining, or an exercise of the Imagination, that is idle and unproductive, initially difficult to resist and thus repetitive, and is marked by content that, due to the relative ease with which negative events are recalled and gloomy scenarios imagined (or simulated), tends eventually to depict negative and dire outcomes. To see the force of this final criterion, we must remember the sequential nature of Burton's account and his reliance on the effect of habit. The pleasures of melancholising are at first alluring and enjoyable. Then they turn, unexpectedly, bringing fear, sorrow, suspicion, discontent, cares, and weariness of life—these "surprise them in a moment," as he puts it. Suddenly

> the Sceane is turned . . . by some bad object, and they *being now habituated to such vaine meditations* . . . can ruminate of nothing but harsh and distasteful objects. (I,2,2,6:243, emphasis added)

"Some bad object'" is the telling phrase here. We cannot know what it might be, or when it will enter our thoughts. It may be of little consequence in itself, a small setback, or gloomy idea. But having allowed ourselves to be habituated to such vain meditations, as he says, we are somehow sensitized to respond negatively. Any small trigger might find us unable to resist the sequence of "harsh and distasteful" thoughts that follow. As this sequence makes clear, the power of melancholising comes with repetition and duration. It creeps up on us, at first pleasing, and only later, dangerously and inextricably painful. Melancholising is understood to be an activity of some duration, a process made up of a sequence of separate parts, rather than an activity that can be captured in a time-limited snapshot analysis. As long as it is thus construed, the final stages of melancholising can be seen to correspond quite closely to what today's researchers know as depressive rumination.

Contemporary studies, we have seen, offer some confirmation of the presence, and dangers, surrounding the activities at least similar to those Burton calls melancholising. Arguably, his account yet wants for a full explanation of how, through nothing beyond repetition, melancholy becomes so severe as to be next to incurably entrenched. Among contemporary hypotheses, those involving "kindling" and sensitization have been particularly identified in application to progressive forms of depression.[59] Sensitization to stimulants and stressors is said to involve "increasing reactivity to repetition of the same dose (or intensity) of the stimulus over time" (Post et al. 1999: 282). In earlier animal studies, motor seizures had been induced using repeated electrical stimulation, progressing from minor to major seizures, and finally to spontaneous ones. Later, it was hypothesized that sensitization to stimulants and stressors led to an increasing frequency, severity, and or spontaneity, of depression episodes.[60] And studies have confirmed that recurrent psychosocial stressors enhance the number and severity of further disorder to the point where depressive episodes emerge spontaneously. As an implication of these processes, early prevention is stressed, just as it is throughout the *Anatomy*.[61] Sensitization and kindling arguably themselves want for a more complete explanation. Yet they at least further illustrate and support, even if they do not explain, the nature of the habituation on which the concept of melancholising rests.

Influenced by classical and Christian sources alike, Burton is acutely aware of the danger inherent in the passions, as he is of the means of curbing them. We cannot control our feelings directly, the way we can

---

59. They have been applied to other disorders as well, including epilepsy and drug tolerance. See Post and Weiss 1998a, Post et al. 1992.
60. Post and Weiss 1998b.
61. "Early intervention before multiple episodes accumulate should help prevent aggressive episode sensitization ... from developing, and the earlier that this is instituted, the more likely it is to be successful. Each episode carries with it the risk for increasing pathological processes in kindling evolution" (Post 2009:363).

activities of the imagination; moreover, in the imagination we possess a special power to alter and regulate these passions. With that same power, our imaginings can also lead the passions astray, however, luring us toward habituated states where we eventually become powerless to control either feelings or thoughts. These states are a central focus in the *Anatomy*. Support for how that happens, we have seen, may be found within contemporary psychology, where correlations and particular reasoning patterns have apparent bearing on the activity Burton knows as melancholising.

If the analogies between these reasoning patterns are warranted, then the *Anatomy* account may contain ideas useful to contemporary science. Its recognition of the need for a longitudinal analysis of these thought patterns based on a progressive, or habituation model, is one of these ideas, seemingly confirmed by contemporary kindling and sensitization models in application to progressive depressive disorder. Another is the range of ways such thought patterns can be averted and avoided by their subject's own efforts. In the terms familiar from the phenomenology of classical *akrasia* where self control and creative uses of the imagination are called for, the lure of melancholising is an unavoidable feature of our nature, as inevitable as lust or gluttony. But it is not one we are entirely powerless to resist, any more than are lust and gluttony.

The inclination toward melancholising, and the form of weakness so closely modeled on classical *akrasia*, will be more likely to occur in those with inherently melancholy tendencies, Burton concedes. Nonetheless, it is a general danger that is described in the passages cited here, not limited to those temperamentally inclined toward melancholy, nor to those so afflicted that they suffer Melancholy the Habit, the chronic, next to incurable, disease. Potentially, the *akratic* melancholic is any one of us, and these warnings are issued in the spirit of general measures for mood-regulation. Melancholy understood as disease properly so called is the subject of the next chapter, where, we will see, findings from contemporary cognitivist psychology can again be appealed to in confirmation of Burton's claims.

Chapter 6

when Reason is also corrupted

Careless and self-indulgent uses of the imagination place anyone at risk of succumbing to habitual Melancholy; we are all in that respect potentially *akratic* melancholics. But the *Anatomy* loosely separates the less advanced states and tendencies that are within our power to avert and control, from the habituated, chronic condition. And the latter is the subject of the present chapter. Melancholic men, Burton says, sometimes see and hear phantasms, chimeras, noises, and visions. Their "corrupt phantasie makes them see and heare that which indeed is neither heard nor seene" (I,3,3,1:424).

> Some have a corrupt eare, they thinke they heare musicke, or some hideous noise as their phantasie conceaves, corrupt eyes, some smelling: some one sense, some another. (I,3,1,3:402)[1]

In addition to these cases of what we would suppose hallucinations, the *Anatomy* is filled with (and enlivened by), tales of those who have fallen prey to misapprehensions of delusional proportions. There are the woman said to have thought she swallowed a serpent; the gentleman who was "afraid to pisse, least all the towne should be drowned;" the man who supposed his nose so big that he should "dash it against the wall if he stirred"; and one who believed he was dead (II,2,6,3:112).

---

[1]. These perceptual errors are explicitly juxtaposed to what we would call mere *illusions*; one example given is when an oar in water "makes a refraction, and seems bigger, bended double, &c." In the case of the distortions afflicting the melancholic, it is "the braine that deceives them" (I,3,3,1:426).

WHEN REASON IS ALSO CORRUPTED

In this chapter we look at what Burton says about these extreme states of melancholy. If reason cannot be exerted the way it should, then in cases like these not merely imagination, but reason itself, has become corrupted.

This is melancholy the Habit, which is well beyond self-help. Our judgment has become

> so depraved, our reason over-ruled, Will precipitated, that we *cannot seeke our owne good, or moderate our selves.* (II,2,6,1:104, emphasis added)

Indeed, it may be beyond all help:

> you may as well bid him that is diseased not to feel pain, as a melancholy man not to fear, not to be sad: 'tis within his blood, his brains, his whole temperature, it *cannot be removed.* (II,2,6,1:103)

Burton mostly suggests that these cases of delusional and hallucinatory experience involve melancholy, rather than outright madness. Although many writers "make *Madnesse* and *Melancholy* but one Disease," we saw, he will follow the newer thinkers ("our neotericks") who "handle them apart" (I,1,1,4:132). In light of this resolve, the passage asserting that some melancholic men are mad is best understood to imply that severe cases of melancholy *can become madness,* which he readily admits.[2] Where these states would be assigned according to today's disorder categories is also a matter of potential confusion. Melancholy is distinguished from madness by Burton in terms of its predominant moods of sadness and fear and its relative lack of vehemence and violence. Today, by contrast, more severe states of disorder are often distinguished clinically by the

---

2. "Some laughe, weepe, some are mad, some dejected" (I,3,1,3:402). The confusion engendered by calling everything Melancholy (normal passing sadnesses and worries, the entrenched, habituated condition, and delusional forms) explains Burton's apparent inconsistencies. But we remember that it is a consequence of his habituation model, where repetition can transform each of those three states to the next: passing sadnesses and worries to the habituated condition, and the habituated condition in turn to the delusional one.

presence of psychosis (along with indications of social and behavioral dysfunction), identified through evidence of delusions and hallucinations. And although they occur in what is known today as psychotic depression, delusions and hallucinations are less commonly associated with mood disorder than with schizophrenia and related conditions, categories not in use until after the early modern period.[3] Burton's admission that some melancholic men might be mad seems to better fit this contemporary rubric (where, indeed, psychosis is aligned in common parlance with the less polite "madness.") However, historians assure us that in seventeenth-century England, these delusional states would not have been judged that way.[4] Madness might be the eventual outcome of severe Melancholy. As defined in the *Anatomy*, madness had a violence and vehemence not present even in cases of severe melancholy. If delusions were not madness in seventeenth-century England, however, they were very close to it. And, rather than any consistent linguistic practice, Burton's practical contrast (the melancholic should have physic and

---

3. The term "psychosis" was not coined until 1845 (Beer 1996).
4. None of the English delusions were thought of as madness, it has been asserted, and the addition of delusions and hallucinations to the signs of acute insanity (together with the spread of the idea that suicide was a symbol of disorder, rather than a sin and crime) date to the seventeenth and eighteenth centuries: Until then, delusions and hallucinations were thought of as *aspects of melancholy rather than madness*. These changed conceptions have been attributed to a long antagonism to religious enthusiasm. (See MacDonald 1981a:155–7, and 1981b.) Yet in a passage from the fifteenth-century *Breviarie of Health*, quoted earlier, we find melancholy and madness equated, or even conjoined: "This sicknes is named the melancholy madness which is a sicknes full of fantasies, thinking to here or to see that thing that is not heard nor seene, and a man hauing this madness, shal thinke in himself that thing that can never be, for some bee so fantasticall that they will thinke themselfe God or as good, on such lyke things pertaining to presumption or to desperation to be dampned, the one hauing this sicknes doth not go so farre the one way, but the other doth dispayre as much the other way" (Boorde 1547: fol 78r). And only a few short years after Burton, Descartes was writing the *Meditations*, where, beset by bilious vapors, his madman entertains all manner of distorted and mistaken, and what we would count delusional, misapprehensions. Although commonly rendered "madness" or "insanity" in English translation, Descartes' original Latin uses *insanis* and *amentis*. This blending within the same passage may suggest that the English differentiation was at most specific to that language. If delusions were not madness in seventeenth-century England, they were very close to it. (On claimed regional and national differences in how melancholy was understood during the early modern period, see Bell 2014, chapter 4.)

hellebore, the madman Bedlam, as he puts it), seems likely to ground the attribution of melancholy to these delusional, yet outwardly calm, cases.

That said, retrospective diagnosis holds many dangers, fostered by the lure of the "continuity mirage" (Berrios 2011). To avoid those dangers, it is sufficient to conclude here that many of Burton's tales depict symptoms *delusional enough that today they would be classed as indicative of severe disorder.*

MELANCHOLY IN HABIT

The all-encompassing and flexible humoral system allows Burton to identify as Melancholy states of disorder according to four different dimensions. They are more and less permanent, more and less severe and dysfunctional, more and less intractable, and more and less temperamentally engendered. This is useful for his account, but invites confusion. At the beginning of the *Anatomy*, he takes some care with distinctions:

> Melancholy . . . is either in Disposition, or Habit. In Disposition, is that transitory Melancholy, which goes & comes upon every small occasion of sorrow, need, sickness, trouble, fear, grief, passion, or perturbation of the Mind . . . from these Melancholy Dispositions, no man living is free. . . . This Melancholy of which we are to treat, as in Habit . . . a Chronic or continuate disease, a settled humor . . . not errant but fixed, and as it was long increasing, so now being (pleasant, or painful) grown to an habit, it will hardly be removed.

While acknowledging that the one can lead to the other, Burton here promises that his work will be limited to melancholy properly so called, that is, understood as disease (Melancholy the Habit). He falls short in this resolve, and the book is unwieldy, but more interesting and valuable, as a result. As is implied in much of the *Anatomy*, however, melancholy properly so called (the habit) is, in some sense, disease and aberration— in contrast to the many normal passing states that, while resembling it, result from life's vicissitudes. Several pairs of contrasts thus occur in this dense passage, corresponding to the dimensions noted above. The general contrast between states that are passing and those that are more chronic is the broadest one, with application to both normal and abnormal states. A normal, passing or "errant" state may grow into a habit, as he puts it. Through our own doing, when we indulge melancholising tendencies and allow them to go unchecked, it might become an abnormal, intractable condition. At other times, and in other people, these states will be passing and insignificant in their effects, never becoming more chronic diseases. In addition, both passing and longer-term feelings of melancholy may reflect nothing more than normal responses to the inevitable occasions of, as he says, sorrow, need, sickness, trouble, fear, grief, passion, or perturbation of the mind.

There are also those with inherited melancholy temperament. Reviewing ancient medical authorities on the contribution of parents as the cause of melancholy, Burton concludes: "I need not therefore make any doubt of Melancholy, but that it is an hereditary disease" (I,2,1,6:206). The melancholy temperament of the seventeenth century—described as sober, contemplative, and timorous—was thought to stem from an abundance of the "natural" form of the melancholy humor, rather than its corrupted, adust form.[5] In addition to the temperament we receive from our parents, Burton acknowledges a host of causes of melancholy that we are powerless to avoid, those from angels, devils, God, and witches, as well as old age.

Like the separation between habit and disposition, the one between temperament and more occasional states can be expressed without reference to humoral language, and exhibits obvious parallels with today's talk about genetic and other endogenous risk factors for mood disorders such as depression. There is one difference: Humoral temperaments were not in themselves abnormalities. By contrast, even the dysthymic

---

5. Bright makes a clear separation between natural and unnatural forms of the humor. Unnatural sorts of humor, on his account, have been "wholly changed into another nature by an unkindly heat" (Bright 1995:2). Thus, any of the four humors might become unnatural due to overheating or excess, differing as Burton says, "according to the mixture of those natural humours amongst themselves, or foure unnaturall adust humours, as they are diversly tempered and mingled" (I,1,3,3:166–7).

temperament is often regarded as pathology within medical psychiatry today. Peter Kramer, for example, insists that because the number, severity, and duration of depressive episodes "sit on a continuum of risk," they all form, as he says, part of "a single picture," and we should understand their manifestations "*as pathology all along the spectrum*" (2005:166, 170). Kramer's reasoning here is based on research showing that early depression is, as he says, both a disease and a risk factor: a predictor of future and worsening episodes.[6] Illustrating such reasoning, the trait-based disposition toward pessimism and sadness, formerly known as dysthymia, has been merged with chronic major disorder in the most recent psychiatric classification (DSM-5). This yielded the composite persistent depressive disorder: a chronic form of depression whose diagnostic feature is "depressed mood for most of the day, for more days than not," for at least two years in adults, and one in children (American Psychiatric Association [APA] 2013:168).

The passage from the *Anatomy* quoted earlier, where Burton lays out these different ways Melancholy is to be understood, goes on to explain that the term melancholy has looser and more precise uses:

> In which *Equivocal and improper* sense, we call him Melancholy, that is dull, sad, sowre, lumpish, ill disposed, solitary, any way moved, or displeased. . . . Melancholy in this sence is the Character of Mortalitie. (emphasis added)

This loose, equivocal, and improper sense, affecting all of us with melancholy, is the subject of the chapter following this one (chapter 7).

DELUSIONAL FEAR AND SADNESS

Moods of nebulous, seemingly objectless apprehension known as free-floating anxiety are familiar today, yet they are barely recognizable among Burton's examples. Cases of fear in the *Anatomy* have precise,

---

6. Kramer 2005:158–71.

and usually fanciful, objects. Today, we would count them delusional or the creatures of delusional thought processes. Their themes run along familiar lines: guilt, impending disasters stemming from personal attributes (the nose) or unavoidable circumstances, and excessive responses, mountains made of molehills—misapprehensions that provide reasons, albeit bad ones, for the states of distress that accompany them. These, as we saw earlier, are fears "without cause." They are without sufficient cause, in excess of, or inappropriate to, their cause.

Burton was a storyteller. So little of importance about the symptom picture of melancholy, let alone about seventeenth-century epidemiology, can perhaps be drawn from these examples.[7] In particular, they cannot reliably guide us as to the frequency of delusionally based fears and worries in contrast to the presence of dejection and sadness—or (the more literal interpretation of "without cause") to the prevalence of nebulous moods without any apparent or recognizable object. The strange and wonderful fears that resulted from bizarre delusional beliefs make for more lively reading than accounts of the mopish moods of downhearted melancholics. Viewed as epidemiological data, the apparent prevalence of single-themed delusions, observed by some commentators, seems likely to be similarly wanting. Citing the man who supposes himself made of butter and fears he will melt in the sun,[8] the one frightened that he will "speak aloud . . . something indecent" during a sermon,[9] or he who fears he is suspected of imaginary crimes,[10]

---

7. Themes involving sex, jealousy, and religion each play a prominent role in the content of delusions observed in the clinic today. Yet despite the Third Partition, devoted to melancholy as it involves these themes, and Burton's seeming recognition that these particular ideas are regular incitements to, and components of, psychic distress and imbalance, the analysis of these particular forms of melancholy fails to improve on or alter those offered in the first two Partitions. Establishing that these aspects of our lives make us vulnerable to disorder is the limit of Burton's interest. For example, of the religious "prophets and dreamers amongst us," he remarks, "whom we persecute with fire and fagot, I thinke the most compendious cure for some of them at least, had beene in Bedlam" (III,4,1,5:395). The satirical thrust of such passages about religious melancholy, whereby superstition and zealotry are a form of illness, it has been noted, anticipates the later critique of nonconformist religious experience as dangerous *enthusiasm* (Lund 2015:88).
8. I,3,1,3:402.
9. I,3,1,2:385.
10. I,3,1,2:386.

Tilmouth concludes that a single obsession "dogs the imagination" (Tilmouth 2005:529). Certainly, as we have seen, the habit of melancholising will ensure that these distorted ideas are dwelt on repetitively. Moreover, some habitual melancholy is in one passage described as having lucid intervals, "(*lucida intervalla*), sometimes ill, sometimes well" (II:3,8,1:206). And in another, Burton describes some sufferers who are "like Comets, round in all places, but onely *where they blaze*." Though otherwise with "impregnable wits ... and discreet," in their particular idea or obsession, "their madnesse and folly breakes out beyond measure" (III,4,1,3:388, emphasis added). But again, we are not told enough to assess the extent of the delusional thought patterns that might have been associated with these cases. And whether they more closely correspond to what are today often distinguished as limited *monothematic* delusions, or to more elaborated *polythematic* ones, remains unclear.[11]

When delusions have become entrenched (our judgment depraved, as Burton says, our reason overruled), and self-control is temporarily lost ("the Will precipitated"), efforts at self-help must prove fruitless. His cases include milder melancholic states as well, but Burton frequently describes obsessions and bizarre ideas that would today be deemed evidence of psychosis. And he joins other thinkers from before and since his time in identifying a disordered imagination, rather than disordered reason, as the unfailing source of the aberrant thinking we associate with delusion. In all melancholy men, Burton says, referring to their natural temperament, the faculty of imagination is "most Powerful and strong." But in melancholy as disease, it is excessively so, producing "strange conceptions and absurd shapes." The misapprehensions that arise this way are bizarre and extreme, about people who

> suppose they have no heads, flye, sinke, they are pots, glasses, &c. is wind in their heads. (I,3,3,1:420)

The imagination produces not only these delusional ideas but also sensory-based hallucinations. Some melancholy men

---

11. On the distinction between monothematic and polythematic delusions, see Davies and Coltheart 2000.

have a corrupt eare—they think they hear musicke, or some hideous noise as their phantasie conceaves, corrupt eyes, some smelling: some one sense, some another. *Lewis* the Eleventh had a conceat everything did stinke about him; all the odiferous perfumes they could get would not ease him, but still he smelled a filthy stinke. (I,3,1,3:402)

An overactive imagination explains all melancholy tendencies, even milder ones, however. And it is equally the source of valuable forms of creativity and self-healing. So how is this point to be identified at which all self-control is lost? Burton gives two kinds of answer to that question. One resorts to the criterion of self-care or self-governance. Those with such extreme misapprehensions are at least temporarily beyond helping themselves, and must turn to others. A second, seemingly more precise account, suggests that the point of separation involves the parts played by imagination and reason, respectively. Once reason has become corrupted, then the creations of the imagination cannot be corrected—by ourselves or our friends. Arguably, these two approaches reflect degrees of disease severity. When the imagination alone is disturbed, friends can sometimes help, as we'll see below. But when reason is itself corrupted, even friends will be powerless.

WHAT FRIENDS CAN DO

The role of friends in averting and expunging the apprehensions of the melancholic, carefully explained in the *Anatomy*, takes us some way in understanding the kind of entrenched and habituated melancholy that is beyond any help we can undertake *on our own*, cases where

> the heart will not lay aside these vicious motions, and the phantasy those fond imaginings.

In that circumstance, we have "another form of government to enforce and refrain our outward members, that they be not led by our passions." At such times, our judgement be so depraved, our reason over-ruled, Will precipitated, that we cannot *seek our owne good*, or moderate our selves ... the best way for ease is to impart our misery to some friend, not smother it up in our owne breast ... for griefe concealed strangles the soule; but when as we shall but import it to some discreet, trusty, loving friend, it is instantly removed, by his counsel haply, wisdom, persuasion, advice, his good means, which we could not otherwise apply unto ourselves. (II,2,6,1:104, emphasis added)

The effects of friendship on the imagination explain how this works:

Friends confabulations are comfortable at all times ... the simplest narration many times easeth our distressed minde, and ... *a faithfull friend* ... *sees that which we cannot see for passion and discontent*, he pacifies our mindes, he will ease our paine, assuage our anger. (II,2,6,1:105, emphasis added)

The friend offers us a clearer view, he or she sees what we are temporarily blinded to: Feelings of friendship embody expectations and attitudes that are hopeful and reassuring. Only when the person is not able to resist or overcome these heart-eating passions, Burton goes on, "his friends *or physician* must be ready to supply that which is wanting" (emphasis added). Although physicians are included, what follows makes it clear that Burton supposes friends of equal or greater value here. He quotes Hippocrates: Physicians alone cannot effect a cure ("They must all joyne,") and explains that melancholy discontented persons must

not bee left unto themselves, but with some company or other, least by that meanes they aggravate and increase their disease. (II,2,6,2:106)

The more obvious duties of friendship in such a situation are enumerated: Friends and companions must be especially aware of the discontented person, not leave him with strangers, alone, or idle, and divert his thoughts with "some businesse, exercise or recreation" (II,2,6,2:107). More precise recommendations then follow: These deal with the distorted beliefs and misapprehensions that come with severe melancholy when the sufferer's weakness "be such that he cannot discern what is amiss, correct, or satisfy." In that circumstance, it behooves friends,

> by counsell, comfort, or perswasion, by faire or foule meanes, to alienate his minde, by some artificiall invention, or some contrary perswasion, to remove all objects, causes, companies, occasions, as may any waies molest him, to humour him, please him, divert him, and if it be possible, by altering his course of life, to give him security and satisfaction. (II,2,6,2:107)

The obligations of friends can thus be quite considerable, even burdensome. They will take time and attentive, thoughtful effort. They may also be disagreeable, testing the friendship in other ways, the reference to "fair means or foul," indicates. Burton countenances the deceptions commonly employed in his times, as we saw earlier. "Sometimes . . . by some feigned lie, strange news, witty device, artificial invention, it is not amiss to deceive them," he expands (II,2,6,2:111). Approvingly, he offers examples: there was the woman who thought she had swallowed a serpent, was made to vomit, and given to believe that she succeeded in expelling the creature, after which she was cured. In our later, more modern times, such subterfuge on the part of anyone would be unacceptable. Apparently ready to ignore the dubious aspect of the practice in dire circumstances, Burton applauds it as a demonstration of the power of imagination and expectation. With this and several other examples, he is unabashedly intent to show such deceptions work.[12] This not only elevates the duties of friendship well beyond where we would today assign them. It also seems to show a premodern disregard for the demands of what we would today recognize as the moral integrity of the friend and the dignity of the melancholic sufferer.

When self-care fails ("we cannot seek our owne good, moderate our selves"), there are always friends, then. And friends play a number of roles, not all of which we would endorse for the treatment of any

---

12. See Macdonald 1981a:153–4.

disorder today. Beyond that, some disorder, when it is "within his blood, his brains, his whole temperature" may be without remedy. Then, it "cannot be removed."

IMAGINATION OR REASON, ALONE, OR BOTH

There is also a more technical answer to the question of when severe and likely incurable disorder sets in. That the imagination is somehow deficient is not doubted. Because such extreme imaginings would usually be kept in check by reason, however, not merely a runaway imagination but also a failure or lapse of reason must be invoked for a complete explanation of these errors, Burton explains. Learned debates over whether delusion ("the affection") "be imagination or reason alone, or both," are reviewed. Galen's view is that melancholy primarily affects the imagination, while others are named as believing that the understanding is the damaged faculty. In Burton's words,

> reason was in fault as well as Imagination, which did not correct this error.... Why doth not reason detect the fallacy, settle and persuade, if she be free? Avicenna therefore holds both corrupt, to whom most Arabians subscribe . . . no man doubts of Imagination, but that it is hurt and misaffected here. (I,1,3,2:164–5)

Appealing to the authority of Avicenna and the other scholars in his tradition, Burton here postulates that reason, on particular occasions, has lost control of the melancholic's wild imaginings. Here, reason itself is somehow more deeply compromised, so it not only fails to, but *cannot*, engage in its usual function of curbing and correcting. The exact deficiencies attributed to reason and the imagination in these passages are not entirely clear. And Burton's elaboration about those occasions when the humor has become heated (*adusted*), so that smoky vapors obscure our reasoning, does not substantially advance our understanding. Quoting again from Wright, he explains that the mind is in these cases confined "within a perpetuall dungeon," and oppressed with "continuall feares, anxieties, sorrowes, &c." which have become entrenched. Such melancholy men have not a true object of fear, but an "inward cause" within themselves (I,3,3,1:419-420).

Even today, delusional thinking lacks a clear-cut and agreed-on definition, and is incompletely understood.[13] However, present-day psychiatry regularly identifies several parts that go wrong in sustained delusions. A collection of problems attaches to the initial, delusional idea: its often implausible content and the means of its acquisition through evidently flawed reasoning and ungrounded flashes of intuition. Then there is the unaccountable tenacity with which the notion often continues to be embraced despite the disconfirming evidence provided by the epistemic community, common sense, or past experience.[14]

This second defect allows delusions to become entrenched beliefs, or belief-like (the matter of how to describe them is contested), rather than being dismissed as passing fancies and illusions. It is a failure to "detect the fallacy, settle and persuade," as Burton puts it. That the implausibility and tenacity exhibited when there is sustained delusional thought somehow correspond to these separate functions of imagining and reasoning identified by Burton seems beyond doubt. The imagination is responsible for conjuring up the original, strange ideas, whereas the process by which they are maintained in the face of countervailing evidence reflects a malfunction of reasoning. Reason, as Burton says, should have corrected the error. Alone, the products of the imagination are innocuous. It is by assenting and blindly clinging to them that we fall into states of error that indicate disease. So Burton's account differs little from contemporary analyses employing these broad categories.

Also important in the *Anatomy* account is that the separated failures of reasoning and imagining are *initiated* by a flawed imagination. About the causal relation between and direction of their respective deficiencies, Burton quotes "a learned doctor of Padua," concluding that if the disease be chronic (" inveterate, or . . . more or less of continuance"),

---

13. See Bayne and Pacherie 2005, Radden 2011.
14. These characteristics of delusional thought are described by Karl Jaspers (Jaspers 1963), but see also Davies and Coltheart 2000.

I determine . . . that it is first in Imagination, and afterwards in reason.

This analysis is repeated in the Third Partition, and employed to confirm that love melancholy is appropriately so called. In its sufferer, "both imagination and reason are misaffected, *first one, then the other*" (III,2,1,2:58, emphasis added).

Any later effects, including those on reason, are thus secondary ("accidental"). Appealing to another authority (Hercules de Saxonia), Burton concludes that the imagination is the source of all the errors that follow:

> Faith, opinion, discourse, ratiocination, are all accidentally depraved by the default of imagination. (I,1,3,2:165)

In this determination that both imagination and reason are responsible for delusions, Burton aligned himself with Du Laurens, as well as the majority of thinkers in his day.[15] (Such an assignment of function reflects the faculty psychology associated with the era and with the emergence of modern psychology. The separate modules of imagination and reason could each become independently impaired.[16]) There remains some unclarity in the roles assigned to reason and imagination, nonetheless.[17]

The man who supposes he has no head has a flawed idea, attributed to his imagination, which will in turn affect what else he can believe, for example, whether he needs to wear a hat. This second idea (no hat necessary) will indeed be "depraved," but merely "accidentally" so. If some idea is adopted on the basis of hallucination, subsequent beliefs will similarly be accidentally inaccurate. This is "perceptual delusion,"

---

15. Jackson 1986:90.
16. See Varga 2013:147–8.
17. Burton introduces and seems to endorse a three-part division derived from Rhases, distinguishing cases where delusional thoughts are acted on (they "put in practice that which they think or speak" [I,3,1,4:406]). But this is in a context where the sheer variety of melancholy effects is emphasized, and is a merely functional distinction. There is no reference to changes in the black bile, or adustion, nor anything implying a uniform pattern of progression.

when mistaken beliefs result from the sensory or phenomenal experience prompted by mistaken perception.[18] Whether or not such "accidental" inferences are to be called delusions, rather than illusions, they do seem different from cases where the delusion derives from reasoning that is itself amiss. Some contemporary theorists have defended the rationality of such perceptual delusions, and even analogized every case to these accidental ones. On such a theory, all delusions represent efforts to make sense of anomalous perceptual experiences.[19]

THE MIND SCIENCE OF DELUSIONAL THOUGHT

Pathologies of belief, or delusions, have been the subject of much research since the last decade of the twentieth century. Contributors have been philosophers of mind, experimental and cognitive psychologists, and many whose work straddles, and blurs, such disciplinary divisions and boundaries.[20] The question of how to explain and classify such delusional states, and account for puzzling features like their resistance to evidence, has given rise to extensive theorizing and empirical study. While multifactorial explanatory hypotheses have been increasingly proposed since then, much of this attention initially resembled Burton's two-stage, or two-part process of delusion formation. Delusions occur

---

18. See Bayne and Pacherie 2005, also Radden 2011:26–7. Delusional perception, by contrast, occurs when an apparently normal perceptual experience triggers a delusional idea.
19. This is the one-factor account of Brendan Maher. On it, delusion is a hypothesis designed to explain unusual perceptual phenomena and developed through the operation of normal cognitive processes (Maher 1999:18). The misapprehensions that result from hallucination only differ from delusions proper in that the former stem from experiences that are more accessible to conscious awareness and are identified as perceptual experiences. Or, as it has been put, "there is nothing irrational about forming false beliefs on the basis of illusions and hallucinations" (McGinn 2004:115).
20. See Berrios 1991, Garety and Hemsley 1994, Davies and Davies 2009, Bayne and Pacherie 2005, Davies et al. 2001, Broome and Bortolotti 2009, A. Davies et al. 2009, Bortolotti 2010, Egan 2009, Radden 2011, Young 2011, Mishara and Corlett 2009, Fletcher and Frith 2009.

only when there is some further deficiency (of reasoning) added to an aberrant perceptual experience, on this analysis. And this recognition that delusions may stem from deficits or damage affecting two separate aspects of cognition has prompted particular attention.

Research into delusional thought processes presently being explored, anticipated in the *Anatomy*, includes: (i) how delusions are to be understood in relation to other cognitive states, particularly beliefs and imaginings, and (ii) their causal antecedents. Each question awaits a definitive answer, and each is the source of a range of theories and conjectures.

delusions in relation to beliefs and imaginings

Two present-day hypotheses, against which Burton's account of the relation between imagination and delusion can be examined, are Andy Egan's hybrid notion of "bimagining," and the identification of delusions as imaginings put forward by Gregory Currie and colleagues. The status of "bimaginings" (part belief, part imagining) has been ascribed to delusional thoughts on the grounds that about the objects (or content) of their delusions, deluded people neither straightforwardly believe nor straightforwardly imagine. Thus, "delusional subjects are in states that play a role in their cognitive economies that is in some respects like that of a standard-issue, stereotypical belief that P and in other respects like that of a standard-issue, stereotypical imagining that P" (Egan 2009:268). Egan reasons to this conclusion about delusions because their typical *circumscription* (i.e., except in verbal behavior, they are only weakly behavior guiding), and *evidence-independence*, makes them unlike paradigmatic beliefs (more circumscribed and evidence-dependent) and yet also unlike paradigmatic imaginings, which are less circumscribed and evidence-independent. As a characterization of all delusions, this may be incomplete, since these are at best typical features.[21] But that aside, Egan also points to a methodological assumption required for his account. We must suppose that, as he says, belief

---

21. Radden 2011.

and imagining roles are not "package deals" that would preclude such admixtures.[22]

Burton's faculty psychology is a forerunner of today's functionalist representational theories of mind. Representations are the discrete modules that Egan calls "packages" of content, present in the mind in some functionally appropriate way.[23] While sharing content, separate cognitive states such as beliefs, desires, and imaginings are distinguished in terms of their differing causal interactions with the outside world and other mental states and processes. In the *Anatomy*, a separated functional role is similarly recognized for each of imagination and reason in respect to delusional phenomena. (Burton's model is Du Laurens, on this point: "Seeing ... that *one of these faculties may be hurt without the other*, we must believe that every one of them hath his particular place" [Du Laurens 1599:80, emphasis added].)

To understand how delusions might nonetheless be hybrids between imagining and believing in the way Egan proposes, we turn to the work of Currie and his colleagues. On traditional, "doxastic" notions, delusions are beliefs, or belief-like. Countering this assumption, these researchers have proposed that delusional thoughts are imaginings, *mistakenly identified as beliefs by their confused subject*.[24] The primary basis for identifying something as an imagined thought is that it is experienced as the outcome of our will, or agency, it is argued, and loss of the capacity to distinguish imaginings is related to a more general loss of a sense of agency toward these mental contents. In this "metacognitive" account, the deluded person imagines, rather than believing, a delusional proposition P (while at the same time mistakenly believing that he believes P). A characterization of what is involved in imagining as distinct from believing is analyzed this way:

> when we imagine something, we do not cease to believe things that are inconsistent with what we imagine, and we do not feel any pressure to resolve clashes between what we believe and what

---

22. Egan 2009.
23. Fodor 1975.
24. Currie 2000, Currie and Ravenscroft 2002, Broome and McGuire 2009.

we imagine. Rather, beliefs inconsistent with the imagining move temporarily into the background; they are not available as premises in inferences that involve the imagining but are available as premises in inferences that do not. . . . imaginings are not apt to be revised in the light of evidence; the whole point of imagining is to enable us to engage with scenarios that we know to be non-actual. (Curry and Jureidini 2002:160)

Put in these terms, we can see that Burton's "hurt and misaffected" imagination might be construed as one *unable to recognize and abide by* these respective inferential constraints and freedoms. That one of reason's functions is to recognize and distinguish imagined objects from real ones is evident in a passage that would have been known to Burton. We do not fear a *painted lion*, Du Laurens had explained, because our reason is accustomed to distinguish between the feigned [false] images of the Imagination and the actual objects represented to common sense ("having beheld a painted Lion, it perceiveth that it is not a thing to be feared, and at the same time, joining itself unto reason, doth confirm and make bold" [Du Laurens 1599:75]). With this Laurentian conception of reason's incapacity, likely to have shaped Burton's own analysis, we can see grounds to name the resulting delusions instances of bimagination along Egan's lines. The function of imagining is distinct from that of believing in the normal case. But delusions reflect *dysfunction*. Then, the imagination is in some way unable to recognize and carry out its normal activities. The part of normal functioning that has been lost is precisely the ability to distinguish the painted lion as a "feigned" image.

Similar claims to these have been developed in relation to disorders resulting in verbal hallucination, hypothesized as a hybrid intentional state lying *somewhere between thinking and perceiving*, or even between remembering and imagining. Encompassing phenomenological disturbances are said to "weaken the boundaries between intentional state types" (Ratcliffe, forthcoming). Burton is sparing in his account of the flaw or deficiency that occurs when, as he says "our reason is over-ruled, Will precipitated." But this kind of dysfunctional confusion seems one possible interpretation. Colin McGinn offers another very similar description focused on the likely consequence of such a flaw: "the delusional subject has something *wrong* with the way he forms beliefs ... his irrationality consists in letting his beliefs be driven by what is merely imaginary, since images are the wrong *kind* of thing to base beliefs on" (McGinn 2004:115–6).

Both the first idea, of a compromised capacity to distinguish one's imaginings from one's beliefs, and the suggestion that reason ceases to discern which kinds of thing beliefs should be based on, fit Burton's account of delusional thinking. They also fit his insistence that in the thrall of "fond conceits" the melancholic might be misled, granting his fancies a validity, or prominence, that careful attention to their grounds, *and less fondness for them*, would be sufficient to unseat. That we can be mistaken in, and misled by, the objects of our imagining, Burton wholeheartedly accepts: The ungrounded fears he so often cites as symptoms of melancholy concern imagined or imaginary objects. (His emphasis on the power of the imagination to induce or impede healing, introduced in chapter 2, suggests another kind of misapprehension, not always maladaptive, when the person himself is the witting or unwitting target of the imagination's effects.)

On the hypotheses of Currie and his colleagues, imagining cannot be properly *recognized* by the person entertaining delusions, while on Burton's account, the disabled imagination cannot be supervised and curbed by reason. The idea of a compromised capacity to distinguish between imaginings and beliefs tracks, and seems to be complemented by, Burton's analysis of the disordered imagination marking severe melancholy. When he speaks of the way Reason becomes powerless to monitor and check a runaway imagination, the incapacity is an issue of control—we know we should, but cannot stop or help ourselves from succumbing to it. Arguably though, the failure of reason to curb unfettered imagination—a familiar, and time-honored, if imprecise, metaphor—loses little when reformulated as absence of (a sense of) control. An inability to *distinguish believing from imagining* would also preclude the application of the constraints customarily employed for belief acquisition and maintenance. These normal constraints have been described by researchers in terms of a combination of working memory and executive processes of inhibition. The processes involved would thus include assessment of competing hypotheses that could explain the same phenomena, together with inhibition of the imperatives of "observational adequacy" (when seeing is believing), explanatory adequacy (it makes sense), and conservatism (it requires minimal adjustment of any other beliefs).[25]

Those who are not so seriously affected with melancholy have it within their power to resist. They do not always do so. They neglect the many sensible, practical actions derived from attention to daily habits; the solitary charms of melancholy get the better of them; or they are dealt incapacitating blows by the vicissitudes of life. The person *forming* a delusion may willfully turn from evidence challenging her opinion, avoiding those who disagree, hastening to draw conclusions while knowing that speed can be unreliable, or willfully overgeneralizing, aware that it will jeopardize accuracy. And some evidence from those with delusions confirms this self-control model. On the other hand, first-person accounts of the phenomenology of full-blown delusional thinking indicate that once a delusion is formed, it sometimes presents itself as so uncontrovertibly correct, convincing, or plausible, that nothing can be seen to be a fit challenge for it.[26]

causal antecedents

Burton's emphasis on Reason's deficiencies in cases of severe, delusional melancholy, finds considerable support in contemporary theorizing. Presently the most influential theoretical explanatory model of delusion hypothesizes two distinct deficiencies. Aberrant, confusing, or alarming perceptual experience is one. But only combined with flawed reasoning can aberrant experiences explain the formation and maintenance of delusions.[27] Several aspects of the details of this model follow Burton's conjectures in the passage quoted earlier.[28,29]

25. Davies and Davies 2009.
26. See Radden 2011: 100–108.
27. Davies et al 2001.
28. Although it has also been proffered to explain delusions as they are embedded within syndromal clusters (psychosis), as well as diagnostic disorder categories (particularly schizophrenia spectrum disorders in the work of Roger Frith), two-factor theorizing has been applied to delusions regarded as free-standing symptoms, for example, along the lines of Burton's symptoms-oriented approach.
29. Frith 1992.

Most important is that two factors are involved. A two-way interaction explains how the anomalous experience, and reasoning about it, first form, and then maintain, delusional states.[30] Like Burton, two-factor theorists propose that only after and as a response to the first factor does the cognitive defect convert the anomalous experience into a delusional belief, making up a unidirectional causal sequence. This theoretical model hypothesizes some form of brain damage or dysfunction, which may manifest itself in felt experience, as the first factor. (Likely experiences have been postulated to include heightened perceptual awareness, states of arousal, and the unexpected presence or absence of feelings of familiarity.[31,32]) The second element, corresponding to Burton's (and Avicenna's) corrupted reason, is a deficiency within reasoning.

The demand for a second factor argues that the presence of these experiences (the first factor) may be necessary but cannot be sufficient to explain delusion formation, for there are other discomforting or anomalous experiences that do not result in delusional states. Like Burton and the ancient medical writers he cites, who speak of an additional flaw in Reason itself, this second factor in delusion formation has usually been understood as a cognitive feature affecting a person's belief formation.[33,34] In ordinary belief formation on this analysis, experience triggers a plausible ("candidate") belief, which is subject to a process of critical review ("belief fixation") in light of other information. When delusions form, it is as the result of deficiency or dysfunction in this process of critical review.

Attempts to account for the second factor in cognitive psychology have included bias in the style of attribution (explanations of experiences and events). An "externalizing" attribution style, that ascribes negative

---

30. See Young 2011, Fletcher and Frith 2009.
31. Broome and McGuire 2009: 283–4.
32. Aberrations of perception are also the starting point of prediction error hypotheses, which rest on the idea of a mismatch between prior expectations understood in Bayesian terms and such experience, yielding "neuronal noise" sufficient to engender delusional states (Uhlhaas and Mishara 2007, Mishara and Corlett 2009).
33. Coltheart and Davies 2000, Davies et al. 2001.
34. Others accounts differ in separating the process that leads from the initial deficit or experience to the full state of belief acceptance, proposing instead a three-stage framework that includes hypothesis construction (Davies and Davies 2009).

events to other people rather than to circumstances, has been proposed to partially explain persecutory delusions, for example.[35] Similar claims have been made for the inferential habit known as the jumping to conclusions bias and its allied tendency to ignore alternative explanations.[36] A distorting inclination to privilege the "seeing is believing" impact of the immediate experience (observational adequacy) over as little as possible disturbing the subject's other beliefs, has also been hypothesized.[37]

Construed as (second factor) defects of inference along these lines, delusional belief formation shows close parallels with more normal errors of judgment. Normal and nondelusional reasoners exhibit each of the irrationalities described in this two-factor theorizing: They make unwarranted inferences of every kind and succumb to assessments that are biased and overly hasty.[38] The normal reasoner's irrationalities are customarily assumed to allow remedy through attention, effort, and care, while the delusional person's reasoning errors indicate dysfunction or incapacity that, at least in application to the phenomena constituting the first factor, *cannot* be overcome at all, or can be overcome only with great difficulty. If the delusional person's defect calls for a greater effort than the normal reasoner's, then in one respect, although she may need to try harder, and even seek help in countering her irrational tendencies, the deluded person shares a continuum with more normal reasoners. The difference marking her reasoning deficiency may lie merely with the presence of the first factor affecting it, or with a greater degree of bias and distortion. (These ideas require us to accept that delusional and nondelusional cases are quantitatively, rather than qualitatively distinguishable. Even normal irrationalities are sufficiently subpersonal and extensive to belie the part played there by attention, effort, and care, it is sometimes suggested. We may be subject to such global illusion that what we can and cannot do is actually unaffected by what we fondly think is involved in making an effort. If so, though, the second-factor irrationalities of the delusional patient and the illogic of normal folk will

---

35. Bentall 2003, Blackwood et al. 2001.
36. Stone and Young 1997, Freeman, Bentall, and Garety 2008.
37. Stone and Young 1997.
38. See Fine 2006, Kahneman 2011.

be not merely continuous, but *indistinguishable*—undermining the basis for so construing the second factor. Burton had no doubt that attention, effort, and care could and would make a difference in relation to normal reasoning, however. It is only in severe, intractable Melancholy that such capabilities are lost.)

Two-factor theorizing was developed for the subset of delusions associated with brain damage or disease, and may be limited in its application.[39] Its breadth and flexibility are notable, however, potentially accommodating variations in the first factor (including in being available to subjective awareness or not); in the degree to which the two factors are linked, which may be more or less elaborated, and semantically attenuated; and in the range of illogical and biased forms of reasoning constituting the second factor.[40] The capacity of two-factor theorizing to explain the diversity among delusional states also extends to variations in the assignment of relative explanatory burden. A more alarming first factor may take little beyond the normal degree of inferential error to result in a delusion, whereas matched with more profound inferential deficits, less salient experiences might have the same effect. Combined with the widely held presumption that delusions form a distinct medical class, this breadth and flexibility seem to position two-factor theorizing to apply to a diversity of delusional states, extending even to the kind apparently referred to in Burton's abbreviated cases.[41]

The limited and usually second-hand clinical tales offered in the *Anatomy* are difficult to categorize in any but the broadest terms, it should be added, and give little indication of the types of delusions they might be.[42] A small group of delusions has received attention in contemporary research thus far. Of those neither delusions of misidentification, such as the much-studied Capgras, or of Alien Control, are represented in the *Anatomy*. Persecutory delusions, another subject of recent study, do appear. Even so, the examples in the *Anatomy* are very sparing in

---

39. This has been recognized; see Coltheart 2013, Langdon 2011.
40. Davies and Davies 2009:315.
41. For that range, see Radden 2011.
42. As Babb remarks, there is no evidence that Burton ever actually witnessed the treatment of a demented person (Babb 1959).

their details. It is difficult to know whether some of these cases involve delusional systems (elaborate webs of belief with coherent internal logic), or fixed, single-themed, (monothematic) ideas that leave the rest of cognitive functioning unaffected. Nor can we tell whether these develop slowly, by recognizably inferential steps, or arrive full-blown, out of momentary perceptual experience; or the extent to which they are detached from the rest of the person's psychic life and behavior, or fade and reappear according to the course of recurrent or episodic conditions. None of these variations can be excluded from the case records Burton cites, but nor are they helpfully illuminated.

Today's two-factor analyses employ more complete case material. Such material shows that delusions vary greatly in their degree of elaboration, sometimes taking the form of explanations offered for aberrant experiences, at other times resembling the kind of "endorsements," confidently accepted at face value, from the perceptual experience that is the basis of belief about the external world. Once prompted by the initiating and content-fixing element of aberrant experience, two-factor theorizing has proposed a range of ways the formation and adoption of a delusional idea occurs, depending on the type of first factor involved. Because an aberrant perceptual experience may fully exhaust the representational content of a delusion, it has been pointed out, merely taking hallucinatory experience at face value and endorsing it may be sufficient to produce a delusion. Such perceptual delusions derived from hallucination certainly differ from the more elaborate processes of hypothesis construction and confirmation implicated in other delusional reasoning depicted by two-factor theorizing.[43] And so do delusions apparently prompted as groundless intuitions from unrelated perceptual experience.[44]

---

43. When the Capgras patient proceeds from the sense of something strange about the look of his spouse to "Someone must be pretending to be my wife," the delusional state encompasses what has been described as an *explanation*, as distinct from mere *endorsement* (Davies and Davies 2009:290–1).
44. Some clinical writing also reports what are known as delusional perceptions or delusional percepts: when some idea or train of ideas, accompanied by a sense of significance and meaning, is abruptly and unaccountably triggered by everyday, unexceptional, perceptual experience. (This is the German *Wahneinfall* [delusional intuition].)

Burton sides with Avicenna in controversies over the causal sequence by which delusional thinking occurs: The disease is "first in Imagination, and afterwards in reason," but the "hurt and misaffected" imagination initiates the sequence (1,1,3,2:164–5). And two-factor theorizing also proposes a fixed, unidirectional causal sequence: Only after and as a response to the first factor, does the reasoning defect convert the anomalous experience (or data) into a delusional thought, or assertion.[45] This sequence has been expanded, and a picture of two-way interaction proposed to account for how delusional states are maintained.[46] Thus, although the initial formation of the delusion results from a fixed causal order (from neurological defect, to anomalous experience, to delusional belief formation), the interaction between distorted belief and *continuing misperception* serves to explain why delusional notions are not revised, and are instead tenaciously held.[47] Burton's claims and those of the authorities he cites are not incompatible with this multidirectional sequence. Without the *initially* disturbed imagining, the claim is, the sequence would not occur.

We learn little of the details of how reason is deficient in the two-factor theories described in the *Anatomy*; Burton resorts to metaphor. Yet his overall sense of the way reason can be overcome by an unruly imagination, or weak will, seems to concur with these contemporary

---

45. Perceptions, sensations, and all manner of subjective feeling are affected by expectations, so that these separate cognitive and perceptual elements merge. Unusual perceptual experiences of patients and their sometimes bizarre beliefs have been said to be "part of the same core abnormality," identified as a disturbance in error-dependent updating of inferences and beliefs about the world, so that "it is possible to understand these symptoms in terms of a disturbed hierarchical Bayesian framework, *without recourse to separate considerations of experience and belief*." Recent computational models of perception and learning "suggest that the same fundamental mechanism (Bayesian inference) by which a model of the world is updated by prediction errors, applies to both perception and belief" (Fletcher and Frith 2009:1, emphasis added).
46. Young 2008, 2011.
47. As Young notes, in accounting for why delusions fail to develop in other conditions that seemingly start with parallel deficits (patients with bilateral lesions to the ventromedial frontal lobes): Even if other conditions begin with damage of the kind hypothesized for the delusional patient, only in the delusional case (of the Capgras delusion) are the belief and the experience mutually sustaining in the manner of a feedback loop (Young 2011).

two-factor theories. And far from being distinctive to the deluded reasoner, as we will see in the next chapter, aberrant reasoning patterns, bias and misapprehension, are in the *Anatomy* accepted as an unavoidable part of human nature. Whether or not as the result of the distorting effect of our passions, as Burton thought, bias and error are entirely normal ways of apprehending the world and processing our thoughts. Delusions, in this depiction, are continuous with more ordinary foolishness and mistaken judgment.

This gradualist approach to second-factor theorizing that places delusions on a continuum with normal cognitive processing has its detractors. In a recent analysis, Philip Gerrans has argued for a stronger division between delusions and more normal misconceptions and errors, rejecting as inadequate the doxastic assumptions of the two-factor theorizing described above. In that theorizing, he explains, delusional and normal belief fixation alike mirror the way, on the epistemic model of scientific hypothesis-making, we are thought to understand the world. According to the alternative account offered by Gerrans, however, delusions are produced by, and locked into, the default network engaged in the process of providing "subjectively adequate default response to salient information" (Gerrans 2014:115). Rather than treating particular thoughts or narrative fragments as empirical hypotheses, on analogy with the scientific approach employed by normal reasoners, reduced dorsolateral activity in the deluded reasoner's brain *prevents* "decontextualized supervision." The critical evaluation of the thought as a descriptive statement that may or may not be consistent with other beliefs and relevant evidence is an operation that the subject is unable to undertake. The thought is thus confined within its default system fortress. From there, depending on the nature and degree of the dysfunction in the dorsolateral region, it is accepted and conserved, and may go on to structure the deluded person's subsequent thinking and behavior. (The hypoactivation in right dorsolateral areas widely believed implicated in delusion is offered as support for Gerrans' analysis. The dorsolateral system provides decontextualized supervision for the default system. When that system is lesioned or hypoactive, on this hypothesis, activity in the default system is "unsupervised," resulting in the generation and elaboration of delusional thoughts.)

This is not the only alternative (or supplement) to the standard two-factor theorizing described above. Important work has hypothesized that prediction-error is the source of delusions, for example.[48] However, Gerrans' account has particular bearing for us, since it locates the problem within the same default system to which Burton's faculty of imagination has been shown to largely correspond. Moreover, like Burton, Gerrans also puts forward a two-factor account. Default system thoughts or narrative fragments are triggered by a perceptual or sensory anomaly (the first factor). As an imaginative state not subject to metacognitive supervision, it is uncritically accepted and employed within subsequent cognitive activity. (Gerrans uses the term "incorporation" to describe this process of uncritical acceptance and employment.) How to account for what goes wrong is where Gerrans differs from other two-factor theorists. This is not merely a case of extremely biased and faulty supervision of the default thought; the required supervisory decontextualized processing system is broken and cannot function. In support of this claim, Gerrans points to some preliminary evidence that in patients with schizophrenic delusions the relevant dorsolateral circuitry is hypoactive.[49] More generally, Gerrans' focus on deficiencies in the default system is identified with some findings linked to schizophrenia. Even when attending to external stimuli and directed tasks, those diagnosed with schizophrenia exhibit greater levels of default system activity. From this it is concluded that the default network system is in this group "hyper-connected and hyperactive" (Whitfield-Gabrieli et al. 2009).[50]

---

48. See Fletcher and Frith 2009, Mishara and Corlett 2009.
49. Gerrans 2014:148.
50. This study examined the default network in patients diagnosed with early phases of schizophrenia and their young first-degree relatives, using functional MRI, while patients and controls alternated between rest and performance of working-memory tasks. The controls exhibited task-related suppression of activation in the default network. Patients and relatives exhibited significantly reduced task-related suppression in medial prefrontal cortex, and these reductions remained after controlling for performance. Also, during rest and task, patients and relatives exhibited abnormally high functional connectivity within the default network, and the magnitudes of default network connectivity during rest and task correlated with psychopathology in the patients. The study concluded that "hyperactivation" or reduced task-related suppression of default regions and hyperconnectivity of the default network likely contribute

This finding, that the default mode cannot be "turned down," resonates both with Gerrans' hypotheses and with Burton's suggestion that the imagination is somehow overly active in those with melancholy.

At first sight, the success of cognitive therapy and the hypothesis-testing described in first-person accounts of successful self-analysis by those who have been afflicted with delusions appear to preclude Gerrans' alternative understanding of how delusions are acquired. Yet the fact that delusions sometimes remit in the face of hypothetical reasoning does not show that they *originate* as the result of (erroneous) hypothetical, empirical science-style reasoning, Gerrans (rightly) insists.[51] For several reasons, however, Burton would diverge from Gerrans in rejecting the hypothesis-testing model of how delusions are initially acquired. First, he acknowledges that bias and other reasoning faults are present in nondelusional reasoners to a lesser degree. Indeed, because of the spell cast by the imagination, they are an endless temptation and hazard for all reasoners. In addition, as we saw, his account of how friends can help with delusions includes a process of rational persuasion and analysis that (loosely) follows the epistemic model that is analogous to scientific inquiry. But more importantly, Burton's is, for better or worse, a habituation model of severe melancholy. These delusional states are an outcome of the bad cognitive habits of the *akratic* melancholic, they are the dire cost any of us might have to pay for neglecting to monitor the unruly activities of an overactive imagination and the dangerously intense feelings they engender.

In its broader themes also, the *Anatomy* seems more consonant with the standard two-factor theorizing. Burton stresses the commonality between melancholy as disease and the more normal responses that make us human. With the Stoics, his focus is on the errors and failures of reason, to which we are all heir. The hypothesis-testing model is not wholly his. But more importantly, nor is it wholly complete, since it omits feelings and passions. (The exclusion of emotions from most contemporary models of delusion, which Burton would deplore, has recently

---

to, and enhance the risk for, thought disturbances in schizophrenia (Whitfield-Gabrieli et al. 2009).
51. Gerrans 2014:159.

been recognized.[52]) He would suppose delusions formed through some combination that included at least three factors: (i) neglected or errant hypothesis-testing, (ii) a raging imagination, and (iii) unregulated passions. We cherish our "fond conceits," and it is those inclinations and feelings that engender and *motivate* the errors and biases in our reasoning.

DELUSIONS AND DREAMS

We saw in chapter 2 that Burton accepts a long tradition in which the imagination produces dreams as well as delusions. Du Laurens makes the same connection: It "happeneth all alike" to melancholike persons as to those which dream, he says, and "dreames have recourse into the imagination as well as melancholie" (Du Laurens 1599:99). The link is of special importance since disturbed and troubling dreams are frequently alluded to as symptoms of melancholy.[53] These, and all dreams, Burton says, are brought about by "a concourse of bad humors" (I,2,3,2:250). Elsewhere, he explains further:

> The affections of ... [the] Senses are Sleep and Waking, common to all sensible creatures ... [when] the common sense resteth, the outward senses rest also. [Then] The Phantasie alone is free ... This ligation of Senses, proceeds from an inhibition of spirits, the way being stopped by which they should come; this stopping is caused by the vapours arising out of the stomacke, filling the Nerves, by which the spirits should be conveyed. When these vapours are spent, the passage is open, and the spirits perform their accustomed duties. (I,1,2,7:153)

Despite its humoral language and presuppositions, this description of dreaming actually corresponds to several aspects of contemporary analyses. First, the Imagination is the central factor in dreaming, a time-honored

---
52. See Ratcliffe, forthcoming, and Cratsley, forthcoming.
53. On the "terrible dreames" afflicting the melancholic, see I,3,1,1:383; also I,3,2,2:411.

position still adhered to by some contemporary thinkers debating whether dreams are some form of belief.[54,55] In addition, the parallels between dreams and delusions in Burton's account match those contemporary analyses, including Gerrans'. As described in the above passage, sensory functions *rest* when we dream (in this, it reflects default system functioning); imagination is entirely free, and the "customary duties," which include the supervisory efforts of reason, are temporarily stopped.

In each of these elements, Burton's account corresponds to Gerrans' portrayal of dreams as an extreme case of hyperassociative default processing. Delusions are not dreams, but "they have some of the properties of 'normal' waking cognition" (Gerrans 2014:69). Dreams and delusions share important properties of default thinking inasmuch as they "involve the activation of components of a network that simulates a stream of personally relevant experiences and thoughts *in the absence of actual perceptual input or supervision by decontextualized thought*" (Gerrans 2014:152–3, emphasis added). There are differences between dreaming and delusional thinking: Only in the latter, while the interplay between the default system and normal cognition is compromised, the functioning of the default system remains "embedded in the overall functioning of the mind" in still receiving input from sensory and memory systems (Gerrans 2014:151–2).

Aside from Gerrans' more informed science, it seems clear that the emphasis on dreams as default system activity more thoroughly divorced from normal sensory and supervisory functions, does not differ substantially between the two accounts. And as we saw earlier, the parallels are also reflected in the absence, or deactivation, of the supervisory feature with delusional thinking. In addition to their obvious differences, night dreaming, the day dreaming of mind-wandering, and delusional thought processes share similarities.

The many tales of misapprehensions and implausible notions in the *Anatomy* correspond loosely to the categories of hallucination and delusion in today's psychology, although Burton provides us with thin, and

---

54. On that debate, see Gerrans 2014:153.
55. See also Gerrans 2014, McGinn 2004, Gendler 2011.

perhaps even misleading, symptom and case depictions. By contrast, his theoretical account is rich and full of substantive claims, several of which share assumptions and principles with the important recent work on delusional states coming out of contemporary science. His acceptance of the view that a disordered or deficient imagination is the source of such aberrant thinking is one of these, along with a conception of imagining that corresponds to the default attentional system. The parallels he draws between delusions and dreams are another. And finally, his elaborated two-factor causal model, we saw, aligns his analysis to standard approaches within cognitive psychology.

In some respects, the two-factor account most closely resembling the *Anatomy*'s is one in which normal supervisory functions are *entirely* dysfunctional or, in Burton's word, "corrupted." That failure may still be a product of cognitive bias, and correspond to scientific models, however. Based on the ease with which they can be imagined, or brought to mind, what is known as the imagination or simulation bias distorts judgments about the probability of hypothetical occurrences. And these limitations on imagining may yet be so stringent as to entirely *prevent* imagining alternative explanations, rather than merely making imagining them *difficult*. The process by which more realistic or plausible hypotheses can be brought to mind may be not merely impaired, but broken. Thus, Burton's two-factor account from Avicenna is compatible with present-day standard two-factor theorizing. It need not relinquish the parallels, maintained in the *Anatomy*, between more normal, flawed reasoning on the one hand, and the errors of the person harboring delusions on the other.

Chapter 7

who labors not of this Disease?

Some melancholy is unavoidable, Burton has insisted. Not to be confused with the notion of melancholy as disease strictly so-called are the ideas in the *Anatomy* about melancholy as our universal human fate. Speaking of melancholy this latter way (melancholy as universal), he concedes his usage to be a misleading one, an "equivocal and improper sense." Yet it rests on an important observation. The distinctive phenomenology of melancholy finds parallels in feelings and emotions that are so inescapable in every human life as to be "the very Character of Mortalitie." These two ways to view melancholy, as disease and as a part of our shared humanity, are not always easy to separate within the pages of the *Anatomy*, but they call for separate analyses.

To the idea that melancholy is unavoidable is added a parallel theme in Democritus Junior's Letter to the Reader. Not only is humankind inexorably subject to melancholy, Democritus Junior asserts, but also we are all deranged:

> Folly, Melancholy, Madnesse, are but one disease. Delirium is a common name to all . . . t'was an old Stoicall paradox, *omnes stultos insanire*, all fooles are mad, though some madder than others. . . . Who is not touched more or lesse in habit or disposition? . . . Fooles are sick, and all that are troubled in mind. . . . Who is not touched, more or lesse in habit or disposition? If in disposition, all dispositions beget habits, if they persevere, saith *Plutarch* habits either are, or turne to diseases. And who is not sick, or ill disposed, in whom doth not passion, anger envie, discontent, feare & sorrowe raigne? Who labours not of this disease? . . . So that take Melancholy in

what sense you will, properly or improperly, in disposition or habit, for pleasure or for paine, dotage, discontent, feare, sorrow, madness, for part, or all, truly, or metaphorically, 'tis all one. (I:25)

Commentators often dismiss these assertions as jesting or ironic, and point, rightly, to their incompatibility with the rest of the *Anatomy*.[1] The separate themes that we are all melancholy and all mad are not unrelated. By a round of equivocations and conflations, they can be linked through the "old Stoicall Paradox." Democritus Junior here anticipates other, more recent connections from our own era, moreover, when feelings are not understood as intrinsically undesirable. And neither theme is far from the interests of contemporary mind sciences.

Some claims about the tie between universal suffering and the characteristics associated with melancholy cannot be expressed in today's naturalized terms; others can. And these must be separated. For themes about the melancholy and madness afflicting all humankind, we return to their classical origins, and to some of the ways melancholy is distinguished and subdivided in the *Anatomy*. The aberrant feelings constitutive of melancholy suffering begin as the normal afflictions experienced by everyone; only later, and only sometimes, do they eventually give rise to derangement. In addition, Democritus Junior's insistence that we are all mad is an exaggerated foreshadowing of the findings of psychology from the last decades of the twentieth century, where attention has been drawn to the bias and inaccuracy built into the very structure of normal thought patterns.

Melancholy understood as a universal condition, together with the parallel theme of our universal want of reason, thus make up the subject of the present chapter. These ideas anticipate debates and findings in contemporary mind sciences, where they correspond to the claims that sadness and cognitive error are each typical for humans. The chapter begins with a review of the several different kinds of melancholy introduced in the *Anatomy*, and of the legacy of Stoicism in Burton's ideas. Then we look at Burton's conviction that melancholy was growing to

---

1. The Letter is an a priori mockery of the rest of the work, according to one commentator (Fish 1972); a "myth," to another (Vicari 1989:190).

epidemic proportions. The assertion that melancholy is unavoidable has echoes in contemporary debates about sad and distressed states. Within psychiatry, psychology, and philosophy, in particular, the relationship between "normal sadness" and depression as disorder has been contested. In addition to these debates about the universality of sadness, moreover, contemporary findings seem to offer some degree of confirmation for Democritus Junior's overblown ideas. If not outright mad, they suggest, we are all at least endlessly flawed reasoners, and are so as the result of our feelings. All the world may not be entirely deranged, but all the world sometimes exhibits something surprisingly close to derangement—just as we are all, sometimes, melancholy.

KINDS OF MELANCHOLY

Among the kinds of melancholy identified in the *Anatomy*, some are more easily extracted than others from humoral language, we have seen, and two of the former type have been the focus of our particular attention. First, Melancholy in Habit, or habituated melancholy, is chronic, severe, and intractable. This is melancholy as disease, strictly so called. Second is the melancholy associated with temperamental tendencies. There is consistent acknowledgment that some melancholy tendencies are innate, in contrast to melancholy symptoms brought about by experiences or other external effects on the body, that are said to be "adventitious" (I,3,1,3:397). These temperamental "complexions" or traits are not inherently unhealthy. In many, but not all cases, however, they function as diatheses for unhealth. Allied with adventitious effects, they bring about the symptoms of melancholy. Burton may seem to confuse those with healthy but melancholy temperaments and those suffering melancholy as disease. But assuming the habituation model, his analysis works. The melancholy temperament is a predisposing factor, increasing the likelihood of the disease state arising through habituation. Alone, it is not unhealthy. But triggered by other factors, it is transformed into an ingredient of disease.

Less easily separated from humoral language is the category of unnatural, adusted melancholy. "Adust" or burnt melancholy results when the overheated black bile sends smoky fumes to the brain, serving to obscure and distort reasoning. Similarly, Melancholy as disease proper is "unnatural," because the black bile has undergone some qualitative change. (Natural black bile aids bodily functioning.) The humors each vary in degree, according to the temperature, bodily location, naturalness or unnaturalness of the humors, and whether they are simple or mixed (I,3,1,3:397). Although described in these humoral terms, adusted melancholy seems to more or less correspond to the more severe and diseased condition (Melancholy the Habit). A milder *sanguine melancholy* is also distinguished.[2] Then, in yet another taxonomy, reference is made to a three-part classification: head melancholy (the "sole fault of the brain"), melancholy affecting the entire body (when "the whole temperature is Melancholy"), and hypochondriacal or windy melancholy, that arises "from the Bowels, Liver, Spleene, or Membrane" (I,1,3,4:169).

Because they are not easily disengaged from humoral assumptions and anatomy, these further differentiations will not be considered here. And indeed, Burton himself expresses skepticism over the various taxa identified within the medical canon on melancholy. When the matter is diverse and confused, as he says,

> how should it otherwise be, but that the Species [of melancholy] should be divers and confused? ... If natural Melancholy be adust, it maketh one kinde; if blood, another; if choler, a third, differing from the first; and so many severall opinions there are about the kindes, as there bee men themselves. (I,1,3,4:168)

Moreover, what physicians say of distinct species of Melancholy, it matters not, since in the bodies of their patients, they are "commonly mixt." How difficult it is, he exclaims rather testily, "to treat of severall kindes apart; to make any certainty or distinction among so many

---

2. Melancholy men, Burton says in an allusion to sanguine melancholy, "have the most excellent wits but not all; this humour may be hot or cold, thick or thin; if too hot they are furious and mad; if too cold, dull, stupid, timorous and sad; if temperate, excellent" (I,3,3,1:421–2).

casualties, distractions, when seldom two men shall be like affected *per omnia?*" (I,2,1,1:171). The sheer variety of ways melancholy affects individual sufferers shows the folly of applying any hard and fast divisions in practice, it is suggested. This disorder of Melancholy is "super particular . . . all those Geomentricall proportions are too little to expresse it" (I,3,1,4:404–5). "Some dote in one thing . . . To some it is in disposition, to another in habit . . . *It comes to many by fits, and goes*: to others 'tis setled and fixed" (I,3,1,4:404–5).

Among the differentiations noted above, the primary one between melancholy as habit and disposition is expressed in the key passage we have encountered before:

> In which Equivocal and improper sense, we call him Melancholy, that is dull, sad, sowre, lumpish, ill disposed, solitary, any way moved, or displeased. And from these Melancholy Dispositions, no man living is free, no Stoicke, none so wise, none so happy, none so patient, so generous, so godly, so divine, that can vindicate himselfe, so well composed, but more or less some time or other, he feeles the smarte of it. Melancholy in this sence is the Character of Mortalitie. (I,1,1,5:136)

Melancholy as disease is properly only understood as chronic melancholy, the habit. (Burton uses "habit" as we do today, when habits are said to produce a response directly without depending on further motivation.) This distinction also occurs in the Letter, where Democritus Junior dismisses as "*improperly* melancholy" those who are melancholy in disposition only (I:109), and distinguishes the unavoidable, passing distresses as mere melancholy "provocations" (I:138). Since no one fails to feel the smart of melancholy of this kind at one time or another, melancholy suffering is universal, and no living man is free. And the "smart" and pain of melancholy here includes the whole range of negatively toned feelings and downhearted moods enumerated above, that may be very short-lived: being dull, sad, sowre, lumpish, ill disposed, solitary, any way moved, or displeased.

The severe, habituated condition was discussed in chapter 6. Even when we have set that condition aside, however, less severe melancholy symptoms can be viewed as (i) widespread but mild illness and also as (ii) part of the human condition, and *so not illness at all*. Although the separation is sometimes blurred, the *Anatomy* contains reference both to the ubiquity of melancholy in the latter sense of (ii) and to its universality in the former epidemiological sense of (i), and these are—in principle, if not in actuality—entirely distinguishable ideas.[3] We begin with the elements of Stoicism in these contrasts, then proceed to the melancholy Burton takes to be a widespread and growing disease in the manner of (i) above. This epidemiological reading of the ubiquity of melancholy must be dealt with, and dismissed, at the start.

THE "DIVINE SENECA"

The long passage quoted on page 215 continues with a line from scripture: "Man that is borne of a woman is of short continuance, and full of trouble." And the entire passage exemplifies the *Anatomy*'s blend of observations about human nature—things distress and upset us—with religious doctrines about sin. Yet like so many of Burton's ideas, the origins of each of these tenets lie further back than Christianity, as we'll see, in Stoic philosophy.

Scholars have stressed that Burton offers secular and religious healing in equal measure, which he does.[4] But within secular healing, the *Anatomy* also addresses two forms of distress, the abnormal as well as the

---

3. Whether Burton intentionally blurred, or merely failed to recognize, these separations, his conflation of melancholy with madness served a purpose, it has been observed, permitting him to establish the "collective melancholic madness of humanity by surveying its viciousness, sinfulness, and foolish susceptibility to passions" (Gowland 2006:16).
4. Until the late seventeenth century, moralists and physicians are said to have "viewed their aims as compatible and complementary," and Burton was no exception (Schmidt 2007:186). That said, this position on melancholy, sin, and healing was not a static one. Historians have observed real shifts during the early modern period and differences between the ideas about, and consequent pastoral care of, melancholy by Dissenting divines and those of Burton's Church of England. See Schmidt 2007, Gowland 2006.

normal. Because he was a humanist as well as a cleric, the work seeks to be "a cure for the melancholy that is life" (Fox 1976:267), as it has been put. Like his beloved ancient philosophers, Burton demonstrates a recipe for how to live well in the face of sad and apprehensive states *regardless of their source*. In emphasizing this link between melancholy as a state of disorder and the inevitable sufferings, large and small, prolonged and passing, that are our human lot, he reflects Hellenistic attitudes. And by acknowledging the normal sadness and sorrow inherent to melancholy, Burton recognizes the special place assigned to these distressing mood states and feelings in Western cultural traditions, where they ground important social, moral, and aesthetic norms. Here, his touchstone is none so much as Seneca, with his introduction of "consolatory" writing, and his stress on "sickness of the soul" as the human condition.

Seneca's work had played a large part in the revival of Stoic ideas during the renaissance, spurred by the efforts of Lipsius. And the "divine Seneca" was Burton's favorite philosopher. It is the particular focus and range of Seneca's ideas that make his writing so pertinent to Burton's, however. Like all the Stoics, Seneca saw the passions as a central idea for philosophy. (Even his tragedies show concern over the destructive effects of excessive and inappropriate feelings.[5]) Among the passions, moreover, certain feelings drew Seneca's particular attention: those that plague the human spirit, and bring about misery and distress, making us "lose our minds" as he puts it, by eclipsing rationality. His three consolatory letters (*consolata*) concern fear and grief.[6] These letters themselves, directed in a personal way to a particular recipient with whose troubles he sympathizes, are echoed in the style and tone of the *Anatomy*, with its sympathetic, personal form of address. And Burton apparently models his style on Seneca's, which he defends against more systematic writing. Quoting others, Democritus Junior names Seneca "that Superintendent

---

5. Seneca's tragedies differ from those of the Greeks, it has been observed, in that their object seems to be to demonstrate *the limits of intense passion* rather than questions of necessity and moral choice (Haddad 1958:14).
6. He addresses Marcia on the loss of her son; his mother Helvia over their separation, and the freedman Polybius on the death of his brother.

of Wit, learning, Judgement ... the best of *Greeke* and *Latine* writers." In his own writing, he says, he "jumbles up many things together immethodically, after the Stoicks fashion" (I:15). Also, Seneca's work is deeply practical in its goal, like that of other Stoics: we must fashion our own lives through diligent habits directed toward caring for the soul. And these purposes also form part of the *Anatomy*. Like Cicero, Seneca recognized life's suffering as inevitable and an aspect of the human condition that looms too large to be entirely divorced from the particular travails of the madman or the melancholic.

Following other late-sixteenth-century writings to provide spiritual comfort, Burton adds a lengthy Consolatory Digression modeled on these works of Seneca and Cicero (particularly the *Consolatio seu de luctu minuendo*), but also on the medieval Christian forms (Boethius's *De consolation philosophiae*, for example), and the extensive consolation discourses found in renaissance humanist writing.[7] More generally, Burton's immediate Christian influences on these matters were also great. Affective states of feeling and emotion lie at the very center of the *Anatomy*, linking its goals and concerns: As "simultaneous determinants of sinfulness, virtue or vice, and health or disease," the emotions held a special place at the point of intersection between moral theology, moral philosophy, and medical psychology, it has been explained.[8] Burton lavishly employs consolatory platitudes from each of these sources, quoting Chrysostom's plea that "a good hour may come upon a sudden, expect a little" and reminding his readers of the value of hope: "despair not, but hope well.... Cheare up, I say be not dismaid ... hope refresheth, as much as misery depresseth" (II,2,3,3,1:167).

---

7. These works of consolation were designed to give comfort for the writer as well as the reader, it is emphasized. They reflect the deep concern with the nature of despair and the proper response to it accompanying the Reformation and Counter-Reformation, a burgeoning literature of spiritual comfort that has been described as "a 'purified' adaptation of the *consolatio*, which had incorporated Christian elements from the Church Fathers onwards" (Gowland 2006:251).
8. Gowland 2006:133.

"AN EPIDEMICALL DISEASE": EPIDEMIOLOGICAL ISSUES

Burton saw melancholy all around him, increasing to the point of becoming an "epidemicall" scourge. And certainly, his were fearsome times, as he himself depicts them. Democritus Junior says,

> I heare every day of War, Plagues, Fires, Inundations, Thefts, Murders, Massacres, Meteors, Comets, Spectrums, Prodigies, Apparitions, of townes taken, cities besieged in France, Germany, Turkey, Persia, Poland, &c. daily of musters and preparations, and such like, which these tempestuous times afford. Battles fought, so many men slain, Monomachies, Shipwracks, Piracies, and Seafights, Peace, Leagues, Stratagems, and fresh Alarums. (I:4–5)

Like everything in the Letter, this description is intentionally, and comically, exaggerated. Yet the early seventeenth century was a time of religious upheaval throughout Europe, with changes and upsets of the kind that, on the *Anatomy* account, were included among the precipitating causes of melancholy distress. And the common perception that increasing religious warfare across post-Reformation Europe reflected a world degenerating into chaos seems to have been shared by Burton, who speaks of "lamentable cares, tormentes, calamitys & oppressions" as signs of *"mundus furiosus,* a mad world" (I:30).[9] The discontents noted above are reiterated in the more soberly written Consolatory Digression, moreover, where "discontents and grievances" are divided according to the general and the particular, or more personally affecting:

> *generall* are warres, plagues, dearthes, famine, fires, inundations, unseasonable weather, Epidemicall diseases which afflict whole kingdoms, territories, cities: or *peculiar to private men,* as cares,

---

9. Burton apparently felt these concerns quite personally. Indeed, it has been observed that the attraction of Seneca's version of Stoicism for him lay in its emphasis on the virtue and independence secured by leaving politics for the seclusion of a more private life (Gowland 2007:274).

crosses, losses, death of friends, poverty, want, sicknesse, orbities, injuries, abuses,&c. (II,3,1,1:126, emphasis added).

Whether or not, as Burton apparently supposed, his were times when there was a correspondingly greater prevalence of melancholy symptoms, is a complex question for historians. It has been pointed out that melancholy did not leave its mark on the historical record in the manner of other plague epidemics in Europe. And in a careful analysis of the evidence, at least for England, the existing casebooks have been judged to indicate only weak support for any significant increase in the number of diagnoses of the condition. The seeming increase Burton fearfully observes has been explained by a range of factors: the increased attention to occult aspects of natural philosophy and medicine that stimulated additional learned interest in melancholy, and the nature of melancholy as an emotional condition that gave it prominence within religious, moral-philosophical, and political discourses on the passions, so that the apparently high incidence of the disease may to some extent reflect the increased domain in which the concept of melancholy could be applied.[10]

Just as are estimates about mood disorder in our own time, claims about the prevalence of melancholy are complicated by the element of relative severity. Melancholy symptoms and effects range from severe to mild. And mild melancholy, treatable with homely remedies, is evidently intended, or at least included, in many of Burton's assertions. Added to that, melancholy had been a central motif from Elizabethan drama and literature, as well as a subject of pictorial traditions, and may have often been as much artifice as real suffering by the time of the *Anatomy*. It was a condition also seen as "sinful, vicious and debilitating" (Gowland 2006:114). Yet equally, it had become an affectation, adopted to create an impression.[11,12] So the difficulty of

10. Gowland 2006:81–4.
11. Melancholy was "*à là mode* in Jacobean England," it has been pointed out (Macdonald 1981a:148–9). Melancholy as affectation during the late sixteenth and early seventeenth centuries is reviewed in Bamborough 1952:103–8.
12. On the vast literary and dramatic backdrop to Burton's melancholy, see Babb 1959, Skultans 1979, Lyons 1981, Heffernan 1995. That Burton himself read widely in English literature and knew at least some of Shakespeare is well established, although he may

discerning real from imagined melancholy symptoms must confound any estimate of actual numbers. Instead of asking why people were afflicted with melancholy, we must ask "why people described themselves or others as melancholic," at the very least (Gowland 2006:83). An increased awareness of mental suffering, together with greater concern over the issue of prevalence, and of self-murder, observed by Napier, and a stronger interest in irrationality and self-identity, might in addition have brought about a perception of prevalence at odds with the facts, it has been noted.[13] But epidemiological facts would also be obscured by the quicksilver quality of melancholy. Melancholy symptoms could be engendered, increased, or heightened by exercises of the imagination alone: Merely dwelling on it could make it so. (This is the dangerous power of the imagination that Burton alludes to when he suggests that for those prone to melancholy, it will not be wise even to read his book.)

Very similar epidemiological puzzles beset today's efforts to find accurate numbers of those afflicted by depression. Alleged discrepancies between diagnosed and actual cases are much debated, their validity challenged. Some have charged underdiagnosis, others overdiagnosis. Each of these, in its way, is a matter of concern. Stigmatizing and negative societal attitudes over every kind of mental disorder, including depression, are widely acknowledged to have made people reluctant to seek the clinical help they may need; thus, the problem of underdiagnosis. Overdiagnosis "medicalizes" or "pathologizes" normal feelings and behavior, with comparably severe social and personal consequences. But overdiagnosis, not underdiagnosis, is of special importance here. The idea is that normal states of sadness and responses to loss have been unwarrantedly subject to medical diagnosis and treatment and inappropriately labeled as instances of depression when they are more normal reactions. Burton's recognition that there are forms of sadness that are unavoidable, normal, and indeed the very "Character of Mortalitie,"

---

have disparaged plays and stories (Lyons 1981). The mutual influence of popular medicine and literary conceptions of melancholy at this time are more generally evident, moreover. See Heffernan 1995.

13. Macdonald 1981a:2.

renders this concern over normal sadness is a particularly pertinent one for our discussion.

In light of other remarks about the dangerous ways melancholy might infect a person, there is a second sense in which the "epidemicall" quality of the melancholy Burton observed can be understood: as a contagion. With remarks about the way a yawn, or even the sight of disease, can be transferred from one person to another, and about the power of charms due merely to "a strong conceit and opinion," Burton's idea that "the forcible imagination of one party, moves and alters the spirits of the other" (I,2,3,2: 254), is a recurrent theme. Yet, such ideas are dangerously close to the occult causes theorized by contemporaries (Paracelsus, for example) from whom Burton seems careful to distance himself. One person's melancholy could be conveyed to another through a process that might be regarded loosely as contagion, but must be understood as naturalistically (if mysteriously) caused.

NORMAL SADNESS

In contemporary times, it is widely recognized that some states of sadness, such as grief, are akin to, but not, depression. Yet the processes undergone by the person with depression are thought by many to be indistinguishable from those of the person who mourns the death of a loved one, to use Freud's particular, famous example.[14] More recent psychiatric lore has sometimes made a place for sadness that is an appropriate response to the loss of loved ones on precisely these grounds. In appearance, it may not differ from the symptoms of depressive illness, but at least for a stretch of time after the death, grief was exempted from the attribution of "disorder," and not diagnosed as depression.

---

14. Stressing these similarities, Freud insisted that mourning *does not seem pathological*, only because, as he says, "we know so well how to explain [it]" (Freud 1917:153). And following Freud, others have judged that the mourner is in fact ill, explaining that, "only because this state of mind is common and seems so natural to us, we do not call mourning an illness" (Klein 1935:354).

This exception was stated in two earlier editions of the *Diagnostic and Statistical Manual of Mental Disorders* (DSM; American Psychiatric Association 1980 and 1994).[15] Excluded from the category of mental disorder were the expectable and culturally sanctioned responses to particular occurrences.[16] Of such occurrences, grief is the only example provided. Yet in everyday life and clinical lore alike *normal*, adaptive, even appropriate responses to other, comparable sources of distress are widely acknowledged.

Revisions to the fifth edition of the DSM and the eventual elimination of the bereavement exclusion brought widespread debate over "normal sadness." Bereavement sometimes initiates depressive episodes, it was pointed out, and from history of past depression the length and probability of future depressive episodes following bereavement can be predicted.[17] The actual parallels between grieving and depression symptoms were challenged.[18] So were the grounds on which the eventual decision was made to eliminate the bereavement exclusion from the revised diagnostic manual. A seemingly arbitrary privileging of grief among the many normal sadnesses encountered as the result of life's vicissitudes, and the impracticality of exempting them all, were one consideration. The risk of "false negative" cases of grief, and suicide, among

---

15. These were the third and fourth editions of the manual. No such exclusion occurred in the World Health Organization classification (1992).
16. APA 1994. When the sadness of grieving exceeds the usual norms governing duration, its status as pathology is considered: "if the symptoms begin within 2 months of the loss of a loved one and do not persist beyond those 2 months, they are generally considered to result from Bereavement . . . unless they are associated with marked functional impairment or include morbid preoccupation with worthlessness, suicidal ideation, psychotic symptoms, or psychomotor retardation" (APA 1994:323).
17. Lamb, Pies, and Zisook 2010, Zisook and Kendler 2007.
18. Several differences were noted: "In grief, painful feelings come in waves, often intermixed with positive memories of the deceased; in depression, mood and ideation are almost constantly negative; In grief, self-esteem is usually preserved; in MDD [major depressive disorder], corrosive feelings of worthlessness and self-loathing are common" (APA 2011:1). Other research pointed to the presence of resilience and grit in as many as 50 percent of those who grieve, where there is no observed diminution of functioning (Bonanno 2004, Stix 2011).

the untreated grieving, that could and should be provided specialized care, were another.[19,20]

Writ larger, it has been pointed out, the debate over the bereavement exclusion concerned nothing less than the proper role of science in society and the authority given psychiatry to define disorder.[21] Mental states are so entwined with every aspect of our lives, this is an unavoidable and unique challenge for mind sciences; they are deeply implicated in value norms surrounding their endeavors, and have reason to address them.

Anticipating and influencing these debates leading up to the revision of the DSM in 2013, was new scholarly attention directed at the fraught category of normal sadness. A whole range of depression-like responses comparable to those in grieving (responses to marital dissolution, unemployment or status loss, chronic stress, and such experiences), have been pointed to, classified as loss of attachments, and sorted. (They relate to power, status, resources, respect, ideals, goals, and meanings, on one such taxonomy).[22] The sources of such emotional distresses are confirmed by social science and are widely supposed to be universal.[23] Among the many sadnesses that come from these other losses, the sadness of grief was not judged exceptional—but nor was it judged to be appropriately diagnosed as depression. There must be something that distinguishes true depressive disorder from the sadness that constitutes a normal reaction to loss, Allan Horwitz and Jerome Wakefield reasoned. Emphasizing the conceptual difference between

---

19. "[T]he grief exclusion criterion [either] needs to be eliminated or extended so that no depression that arises in the setting of adversity would be diagnosable. This latter approach would represent as a major shift, unsupported by a range of scientific evidence, in the nature of our concept of depression as epidemiologic studies show that the majority of individuals develop major depression in the setting of psychosocial adversity." (Kendler 2010:1).
20. See Kendler 2010, Tekin 2013, Zachar 2014, Frances 2010, Wakefield 2012, Demazeux and Singy 2015. Tekin refers to the presupposition that grief and depression are indistinguishable and would eliminate the bereavement exclusion as "grief erosion" arguments (Tekin 2013).
21. See Zachar 2014.
22. Horwitz and Wakefield 2006:30–38.
23. The likelihood of episodes of depression has been linked to preceding job loss or comparable personal setbacks within the previous twelve months (Kendler, Gardner, and Prescott, 2002, 2006, Kessler 1997).

(pathologically) depressive suffering and more normal responses to life's vicissitudes, "normal" or "nondisordered sadness" has thus been characterized as a healthy, and *adaptive* response to loss. Diminishing with time, in the case of mourning, or with the cessation of the source of stress in the case of other losses and setbacks, this is part of our human makeup.

Why normal sadness might be regarded as an adaptive aspect of that makeup is, these authors recognize, a puzzling question. Because of the prevalence and persistence of depression, however, speculations (including theirs) about the adaptive aspect of *normal sadness* have not been separated from speculations put forward to account for *depression*, some of which were raised on pages 172–3. For sadness to have been naturally selected, there must once have been circumstances where it enhanced the likelihood of survival. (Summing up such speculations, Horwitz and Wakefield point out that differing situations may have elicited the distinguishable sadness responses confirmed by social science to invite depression: "The communication of low affect after losses of attachment can attract support and sympathy from others, and sustain relationships. The submission of depressed people in subordinate positions can prevent punishment from dominants and promote survival. Lowered motivation and physiological slowness can disengage people from unproductive forms of activity and allow them to reengage in more productive endeavors" [Horwitz and Wakefield 2007:51].) Confident that neuroscience will eventually uncover the mechanism distinguishing normal sadness, these researchers have thus posited the existence of dysfunction in a mechanism designed to deal with loss, dubbed the "loss response mechanism." There are some structures in the person, they explain, that are "biologically designed to produce such [grief-like] responses at appropriate times." In cases of depression, those structures have failed (Horwitz and Wakefield 2007:25).

With their emphasis on the way real disorder reflects breakdown of the loss-response mechanism, a mechanism thus far identified by appeal to states that remain unaffected by the cessation of the stressor, these authors employ the concept of a "sustaining cause" (Gert and Culver 2004). Despite its applicability in other contexts, the sustaining cause criterion is ill-suited to depression, however. Profound experiences sometimes permanently mark a person's outlook and responses, even on the cessation of the stressor and despite the passage of time, and even in a normal psyche; they *make a lasting impression*.[24] These exceptions may be rare.[25] But they indicate that we must await the discovery of some biological or neurological marker to enable us to identify the hypothesized loss-response mechanism that would allow us to distinguish normal sadness from pathological depression.

Grieving is statistically *normal*, and so predictable. To this extent, the bereavement exception and the presence of other typical or normal sadnesses are the obvious concern of the mind sciences, where empirical study can tell us much about them.[26] In addition, however, as Burton would readily have recognized, normal sadness is often *normative*, when what is normal may or may not be normative, and what is normative may or may not be statistically normal. This is particularly evident in grieving. The straightforwardly empirical study of grief will tell us in what way, how intensely, and how long we might expect to grieve, but not what is *proper* about grieving. But that normative aspect of moral psychology is also inescapably connected to the mind sciences.

The critique that normal sadness has been unwarrantedly medicalized, ignoring or occluding the unavoidable and normal suffering that is ordinary living, is often expressed in a charge of overdiagnosis, and overtreatment.[27,28] Problems with undertreatment are as frequently voiced in relation to other mental disorders as to depression. And within the

---

24. See Radden 2009:107–8.
25. Other insufficiencies of the sustaining-cause criterion have been noted. See Zachar 2014:173.
26. On the science of grieving, see Stroebe et al. 2008.
27. For example, "The conclusion is inescapable that the great majority of distress-inducing conditions that sociologists study appear to involve normal distress that arises because of social circumstances and endures roughly as long as those circumstances persist" (Horwitz and Wakefield 2007:203). And the elimination of the bereavement exclusion alone can be expected to "massively pathologize normal grief responses" (Wakefield 2012:335). This matter is often focused on overtreatment in primary care, particularly. Rates of prescribing of antidepressant medication doubled in the UK between 1998 and 2010, and in the United States 11 percent of the population aged over eleven now takes an antidepressant. People without evidence of major depressive disorder are being prescribed drug treatment, it is complained (Dowrick and Frances 2013).
28. See also Frances 2013.

debate over normal sadness, concern was expressed that those in need of treatment for their bereavement-induced depression were deprived of it by the exclusion.[29] The issue of overtreating depression seems to have a significance not shared by the overtreatment of other disorders, however. (It is also much more commonly voiced than concerns about overtreatment of other mental disorders.) This is presumably because of the point that Burton emphasizes: Some forms of normal emotional suffering are unavoidable and universal. That depression so closely echoes the sufferings to which we are all heir as human beings, makes overdiagnosis and overtreatment of depression uniquely urgent concerns.

These challenges surrounding normal sadness point to contrasts that are largely unchanged since the seventeenth century. We still regard some suffering as unavoidable, and the character of mortality. However they are separated, these differences between normal or typical sadness and genuine depression nonetheless diverge between then and now in some notable respects. In the early seventeenth century diagnostic classifications were vague and incomplete, expert medical treatment was limited in both its availability and success, and homely measures made up the commonest response to any despondent moods. More importantly, the distinction is not consistently depicted as a categorical one, at least by Burton, as it is by theorists such as Horwitz and Wakefield. Melancholy is sometimes identified with the distinctive underlying adusted humoral state, suggesting a closer parallel with these theorists' postulation of a discoverable underlying mechanism distinguishing pathological depression from normal sadness. For the most part though, Burton describes a looser separation, relying on a habituation-based continuum marking degrees of severity.

Habituation underlies Burton's notion of how passing melancholy sadnesses and fears are transformed, through time and repetition, into chronic and intractable disease states. This point is expressed quite

---

29. Thus, "in recognition of the fact that bona fide major depressive episode could be triggered by the loss of a loved on in susceptible individuals, in order to avoid false negatives the bereavement criterion includes explicit guidelines for what would constitute a pathological grief reaction that should be diagnosed and treated as a major depressive episode" (First 2011:5–6). See also Carey 2012, Shear, Simon, and Wall 2011.

unequivocally throughout the *Anatomy*, as we have seen. And we also find it in the Letter, where, quoting Plutarch, Democritus Junior says,

> ill dispositions *beget habits, if they persevere* . . . habits either are or turne to diseases. (I:25)

Also emphasized by Burton is that melancholy habits begin with entirely normal, inescapable sadnesses and worries. Thus, appealing to Austin [Augustine] for support, he explains of the perturbations from which "no mortall man is free" that are "the most frequent causes of Melancholy":

> if they be reiterated, as the raine (saith Austin [Augustine]) doth a stone, so doe those perturbations penetrate the minde: and . . . produce an habit of Melancholy at the last, which having gotten mastery in our soules, may well be called diseases. (I,2,3,1:248)

Not all feelings will be so dangerous: Those that are said to be "light, easie, and . . . seldome" will not cause harm.[30] Nonetheless, there is an inexorable quality to these effervescent passions. Persisting over time, and repeated, they will eventually "penetrate" the mind to produce "an habit of Melancholy" (I,2,3,1:248). With all its accompanying sadness, sorrow, fear, and imbalanced passions, that habit is the end result of repeated melancholizing and bodily and psychic neglect.

FEELINGS AND NORMATIVITY

Separate from the general recognition that some feelings are unavoidable and so statistically normal are familiar normative claims associated with philosophical and religious traditions in which sadness and sorrow are at the center of evaluative appraisal. To be human is to experience sadness, certainly. But to suffer in the right way, in response to one's life experience is to possess the preconditions for character and

---

30. I,2,3,1:248.

right action, or to find favor with a deity, according to these respective traditions. Feelings are in this respect normative. The sad mood of the mourner is not only normal; it is morally appropriate (Solomon 2004). To fail to grieve would be deeply wanting, showing not only a callous disrespect for the deceased, other mourners, and for the solemnity of the occasion, but a want of feeling reflecting an immature or deficient moral character. This distinction between what is normal and what is normative is employed in assessments of moral virtue. The distinctiveness of melancholy and depressive subjectivity thus seems to hold lessons about these states as aspects of morality and moral psychology, not merely as symptoms. In the passage quoted at the start of this section, Burton apologizes for the loose usage by which melancholy extends to cover all human suffering—it is an "Equivocal and improper sense" of Melancholy, only. Rather than a failed attempt to avoid such broader implications by focusing as promised on melancholy understood as a disease, however, the whole work, drenched in Aristotle and the Romans, is a demonstration of melancholy's ineluctable tie to the social attitudes around human suffering through these shared states of sadness.

Such normative associations are aesthetic as well as moral, within our Western cultural traditions derived from Aristotle, moreover. A bleak gravity marks the "tragic" style, content, and framing, of—as well as what are judged *appropriate responses to*—much great art, most especially tragedy. In the *Poetics* and *Rhetoric* Aristotle identifies features that explain the process of catharsis. Observing the undeserved ill fortune of others depicted on stage, the audience is moved by feelings of pity and fear: pity toward the other's suffering, and fear of enduring a similar fate. Tragedy, then, is defined as an imitation of an action that is "serious and complete"—it must be undeserved ill fortune—which "has some greatness about it . . . It achieves, through pity and fear, the catharsis of these sorts of feelings" (*Poetics* 1449b21–29). Through catharsis, we come to understand the inevitability of human suffering.[31]

---

[31]. Tragedy's accomplishment, if not its goal, has been construed as providing through the arousal of pity and fear "a clarification (or illumination) concerning experiences of the pitiable and fearful kind" (Nussbaum 1986:290).

Whether or not Aristotelian psychological insights into tragedy are accepted today, Western intellectual traditions reflect the attitudes of gravity and respect for these ideas about individual suffering, and these ideas in turn frame and direct our understanding of human sadness in all its forms. These social norms serve as a reminder that the manifestations of melancholy make up a cultural category applying equally to disorder and to those melancholy dispositions from which, as Burton says, no one living is free.

Sometimes, the sad and apprehensive feelings associated with melancholy and depression are themselves accorded special resonance within philosophical views about human existence. The tragic view of life may be the proper one to adopt in the face of our human predicament, it is postulated. William James likens our awareness of our own mortality to a worm at the core of all our usual springs of delight. It is one that might, at any time, turn us into "melancholy metaphysicians," as he puts it. Coloring our every response and perception (all our usual springs of delight), the dejection this brings will be fitting and appropriate. Arguably, then, sad and dejected moods are fitting responses for anyone acknowledging human mortality.[32] As what has been called the grand hypothesis of melancholy, this position "describes our place in the universe" (Kramer 2005:227). The isolation that one feels in depression, Peter Kramer says of this view (which he does not share), is the isolation people "*ought to feel* in a mechanical, chaotic, and uncomprehending universe" (Kramer 2005:224, emphasis added). That "ought to feel" is not a prediction, it is prescriptive.

Kramer criticizes what he takes to be an unwarranted valorization of melancholy and depression in these traditions, predicting that the elimination of the disorder of depression will bring an end to such attitudes about the suffering and sadness it engenders. We mistakenly treat depression as the substitute for suffering in general, he notes, and we should not. A confusion in the order of things is properly emphasized

---

32. Almost as broadly focused is Søren Kierkegaard's critique of modernity. Certain facts about the modern world *warrant* particular, dark moods, on his account. When modernity is its object, such distress is reasonable, even proper. For other analyses of the relation between melancholy and aspects of modernity, see Bell 2014, chapter 4.

by this last remark, however. It is suffering in general, not depression (or melancholy before it) that leads the way, here, and is the more appropriate subject of these normative attitudes.

Aided by glamorous associations that stretch from the text in the *Problems*, attributed (if mistakenly) to no less than Aristotle, extolling the brilliance of melancholy men, through Ficino's exultant writing in the renaissance, to well after Burton's time in the romanticism of the nineteenth century, Melancholy has often eclipsed normal sadness as the preeminent and valorized affection.[33] Yet with its traditional normative connotations, normal or typical sadness alone can account for the special significance attributed to these states of affective disorder.[34] Whether it is melancholy or depression, the valorization associated with such disorder has led to the confusion of the two very similar themes. Melancholy's natural fit for the human condition derives from its link to normal or typical sadness and sorrow, not the reverse, however. If not always, then at least with regularity, Burton recognizes this. The *Anatomy* account almost entirely avoids the more glamorous connotations of melancholy. In that respect it anticipates some present-day acknowledgment that post-nineteenth century Romantic Melancholy, at least, is a different feeling altogether—a form of sadness in which, as it has been described, the negative emotion is an occasion for "self-exaltation."[35] Omitting any glamorizing link with brilliance and sensitivity, Burton does not describe such exalted and self-referential feelings. The states he sees as our unavoidable fate and the Character of Mortalitie are normal sadness and sorrow.

Despite the intimate link between sorrow and fear, and the seeming universality of apprehensive states of fear, anxiety, and worry as part of

---

33. Long believed to be Aristotle's own writing, the passages in the *Problems* are today recognized to be by a follower.
34. Feelings of sadness are shared by different cultures. But the guidelines for how long and intensely, and in response to what experience, such sadness is felt are, of course, culturally shaped.
35. The subject "looks at himself in his loss or deprivation and in the sufferings that this causes his sensitive soul, and he sees himself as ennobled, as beautiful, as extraordinary." This state, it is concluded, is thus "an emotion about an emotion, a pride or self-admiration in sadness. The experience partakes of both emotions, so that the suffering is real enough even if the sadness be not quite authentic" (Roberts 2003:243).

the human condition, Burton seems to recognize that because of its cultural inheritance, sorrow in some ways stands alone here. It is emblematic of our humanity, while the apprehensive states of fear and worry that are just as common and universal, are not.

The origins of these references to melancholy as the very character of mortality in the "divine Seneca" and Cicero allow us to discern their particular link to Democritus Junior's second assertion—that "We are all mad." That we are all mad, all melancholy, all diseased, also finds its original expression, and rationale, in Stoic thought. The Stoics' unceasing attention to the passions lay in the conviction that the passions lead us astray in our thinking. They result in error, misjudgment and bias. The remedy against these dangers involved regulating or even expunging the passions, together with a form of medicine for the soul that resembles what we might today call cognitive therapy. By curbing the passions that are responsible for these errors of judgment and at the same time critically evaluating all our reasoning to seek out and correct these misapprehensions, we can each be our own physician. The reasoning concluding that we are all mad relies on this set of ideas. We all experience passions. Such perturbations serve to distort our judgment, which is inextricably bound up with them. Distorted judgment is a form of madness. So, in a way, we are all mad.

WE ARE ALL MAD

While allowing Burton to reveal his distinctive, playful side through the persona of Democritus Junior, the Letter is jarring in seeming to contradict much of the rest of the *Anatomy*. Conflating madness, folly, and melancholy, Democritus Junior makes appeal to Tully (Cicero) through the thought that any false belief is a form of derangement. We all entertain false beliefs, therefore we are all sick. Hence, the passage introduced earlier:

> Folly, Melancholy, Madnesse, are but one disease.... Who labours not of this disease? (1:25)

To the extent that the *Anatomy* is regarded as a work of satire, Democritus Junior's Letter will have a different standing than those in the body of the text and should not perhaps be expected to fit them. In most of the *Anatomy*, certainly, a distinction is maintained between melancholy and madness, as we have seen, with melancholy symptoms less violent, quieter, and more given to sadness and fearful states than those of madness.[36] It is a distinction of degree rather than kind, granted. But this is unequivocally a distinction, nonetheless.

This contradiction, and the seeming incompatibility between the Letter and the more sober contrast separating melancholy from madness has been explained in terms of the overarching scope and purpose of *The Anatomy*. In addition to demonstrating the destructive effects of melancholic passions on the individual, and the external world, and providing an encyclopedia of medical knowledge, that purpose can be construed as nothing less than to establish the collective madness of humanity, it has been asserted.[37] The expansiveness of this purpose cannot be doubted. Burton's book is many things: a religious work, a medico-philosophical compendium, a self-care manual, a response to the troubled political context he saw around him, a reflection on the state of all knowledge in his time, and an example of humanist skepticism. Each of these aspects has implications for, and must be included in, a complete account of the *Anatomy*, although several exceed what could be of interest to our contemporary mind sciences. Nonetheless, the message from the Letter about the collective madness of humankind has bearing on that science. Following the Stoics, Burton accepts that our judgment goes awry as the result of our passions. The imagination provides an endless goad to misjudgment as well, both through its effects on the passions and their effects on it. Error, bias, distortion, false conclusions, logical flaws—these are the cognitive outcomes.

Human reasoning is thus inevitably flawed and irrational. And within today's cognitive psychology we find the same acknowledgment

---

36. I,1,1,4:132.
37. This aim included a political response to societal disharmony, according to Gowland, a "a perception of turmoil afflicting the external world" (Gowland 2006:17). For an account of each of these overarching aims, see Gowland 2006: 1-32.

of ways our thought and reasoning fail to comply with rationality as it can be ideally understood. Since powerful empirical studies have shown the bias and error in all judgment, it has been widely accepted that inconsistency is "built into the design of our minds" (Kahneman 2011:385).[38]

The answer to Burton's rhetorical question ("Who labours not of this disease?") is indeed: We all do. "Thou thyself," as he says, "art the subject of my Discourse" (I:1). Naturally, and irremediably, contemporary research has shown, our judgments are irrational, illogical, biased, and endlessly distorted by our mental laziness and blinding self-love.[39,40] We resort to time- and energy-saving heuristics, shortcuts that allow us to make decisions in the face of uncertainty, yet often lead us into error. Rather than examining evidence even-handedly, we succumb to confirmation biases that allow us to remain undisturbed by new and unsettling information. We perceive, believe, remember, and selectively acknowledge what is agreeable to our feelings and attitudes.

Humans have at least been supposed to exhibit consistent preferences and to know how to maximize them. But even this aspect of what is familiar as the rational agent model (or *homo economicus*) has been upended by such empirical findings. And our reasoning has been shown the outcome of an uneasy, although productive, tension between mental systems that are rapid, easy, unreasoned, decisive, and often wrong and those that are more accurate, but laborious, slow, and fatefully indecisive. As Daniel Kahneman puts it, that first, intuitive system "is ... the origin of much that we do wrong, but it is also the origin of most of what we do right—which is most of what we do." (Kahneman 2011:416).

The identification of cognitive biases has proliferated since the original findings that showed a tendency to misjudge conditions under uncertainty (future events, and hypotheticals of every kind) identified with famous research by Tversky and Kahneman toward the end of the twentieth century. The different biases include attribution errors of various

---

38. See Kahneman and Tversky 1983.
39. Fine 2006, Kahneman 2011, Ariely 2008.
40. Irrationality for Kahneman connotes "impulsivity, emotionality, and stubborn resistance to reasonable argument" (Kahneman 2011:411). So rather than concluding that humans are irrational, he prefers to say that they are not well described by the rational agent model.

kinds (also called correspondence biases), which involve the tendency toward mistaken explanations of events and motivations; confirmation biases, which favor selecting information supporting previously held assumptions and beliefs; and rather misleadingly termed "self-serving biases," which distort information to favor the person's own interests. It is widely supposed that cognitive biases *can be adaptive*. Like the heuristics also identified by Tversky and Kahneman, which provide swift shortcuts to deal with large amounts of information, and the cognitive processing limitations of all humans, many are thought to be necessary. Particular forms of bias become the individualized and characteristic cognitive styles, the case of attribution bias illustrates. When magnified, the normal errors described above constitute the attribution style postulated as one factor in the formation of, and continuing adherence to, delusional ideas, in some contemporary models. (As a particularly salient aspect of reasoning, for example, the "externalizing" tendency to attribute negative events to other people rather than to unfortunate circumstances, partly explains why some people form persecutory delusions.) The category of *emotional or affective biases* sometimes assigned to a subset of errors in thought and judgment is not a helpful one, it must be added. All biases are affective biases. Any breakdown between emotional and nonemotional biases spells an implausible bifurcation of affection from rationcination. Self-love is a kind of emotion, and it explains attribution and confirmation biases just as much as emotional ones. Similarly, desire to avoid the painfully hard work of nonintuitive inference is another emotion; so is the desire to swiftly reach a conclusion; and, albeit that they work below the surface of conscious awareness, so are the triggers of selective remembering and deficient imagining. Sometimes, it is true, our puny cognitive systems may lead us to inaccurate conclusions due to the processing "noise," produced by deviations in memory-based information processes converting objective observations into subjective estimates.[41] Yet all other biases and heuristics must be deemed emotional biases—even those involving selective memory

41. Mishara and Corlett 2009.

and imagination that lie beyond any *direct* power to remedy through attentive effort.[42]

Among the many biases identified by social science, those affecting inference and decision-making, judgments under uncertainty, and those that are indicated by variable capabilities around imagining and remembering are the ones important for our discussion.

In Western traditions, thought processes are subject to normative evaluation not unlike the way feelings are. Stricter, codified constraints governing correct and appropriate ways to reason make up what is known as *regulative* or *procedural rationality*. That such procedures do not describe actual human reasoning processes, but rather an *ideal*, is a fact whose recognition within the science of economics has been somewhat slow.[43] Procedural rationality viewed as a supreme, and sole, ideal has itself been challenged by the findings about normal and typical reasoning just described, however; procedural rationality is applicable to some tasks and not others, it is increasingly presupposed. Moreover, because we all "labor from this disease," human reasoners differ only by degree in their procedural rationality. In comparison with the extent to which all reasoners diverge from the ideal, the differentiations are small separating wildly inaccurate or merely lucky judgments, from those that are closer to the ideal.

These parallels between contemporary findings and Democritus Junior's extreme claims are less than complete in two ways: (i) There is not widespread recognition of the role of imagination so important to Burton's account in these findings; and (ii) nor is the part played by emotions within cognitive processing always emphasized.

(i) Contemporary mind sciences do not as consistently place the reliance Burton does on the relation between and effects of *imagining* as the source of these ubiquitous cognitive errors. Here, too, however, the empirical findings of psychology are catching with the *Anatomy*. Identifying the "biases of imaginability" (Tversky and Kahneman 1974),

---

42. Exceptions are again those stemming from real limitations to human thinking and the processing "noise," noted above.
43. The assumption that agents are rational, is no more than an abiding but unwarranted *faith* in human rationality (Kahneman 2011:411)

that have become known as *simulation biases*, is one example. Assessing the frequency of a class whose instances are not stored in memory, it has been explained, a person typically generates several instances imaginatively, and evaluates frequency or probability by the ease with which the relevant instances can be constructed. And this estimation procedure, though commonly used, has been shown to result in systematic errors.[44] Recently, as we saw, researchers examining this simulation bias in relation to depressive pessimism, have postulated that those who are depressed are better able to imagine or simulate negative outcomes, and so explain them.[45]

(ii) The extent to which cognitive error involves feelings and affective states is also increasingly recognized. Of such recognition, for example, Kahneman observes that "emotion now looms much larger in our understanding of intuitive judgements and choices than it did in the past." We saw in chapter 1 the centrality accorded to affective elements in all cognitive activity within one prominent neuroscience model; those elements form, as Damasio puts it, a running polyphony, that "underscores and punctuates specific thoughts in our minds and actions in our behavior."[46] An *affect heuristic* has been hypothesized, where "judgements and decisions are guided directly by feelings of liking and disliking, with little deliberation or reasoning" (Kahneman 2011:12). But that category is also misleading: Affective states also motivate "irrational" reasoning more generally understood, as we have seen. What is easy, swift, and effortless *appeals to us, it is pleasing*.

Without explicitly acknowledging this way our reasoning style reflects our feelings, inclinations, and affective tendencies, some psychologists have depicted every reasoner in terms of a relationship, in tension, between two contrasting systems. System 1 operates automatically and quickly, with little or no effort and no sense of voluntary control; System 2 allocates attention to the effortful mental activities that demand it (such as complex computations), and its operations are often associated with the subjective experience of agency, choice, and

---

44. Tversky and Kahneman 1974:426–7.
45. MacLeod et al. 1997a, Koster, Fox, and MacLeod 2009.
46. Damasio 2010:43, quoted on page 41.

concentration. On this account, System 1 has been said to contribute the emotional element in the person's deliberations, to take over in emergencies, and assign total priority to "self-protective actions" (Kahneman 2011:35). Emotions here are often understood to be pancultural, short-term, stereotypical responses involving automatic nervous system arousal, that are not susceptible to modification by higher cognitive processes.[47] In this, they bear only loose resemblance to Burton's passions. But even in those limited terms, by emphasizing the emotional and motivating aspect of the System 1 reasoning, this account obscures the way feelings, inclinations, and affective tendencies also direct us when unpleasant and difficult cognitive tasks are undertaken. We concentrate, and exert effort, because we want some reward—just not an immediate one. And in that respect, the mind's reward system is equally engaged, whichever reasoning system prevails.

COGNITIVE THERAPY AND SADDER BUT WISER

The inseparability of feeling and thought is emphasized in the tenets of cognitive therapy, whose practices rest squarely on the notion that distorted judgments are the cause of imbalanced or dysfunctional emotions like depression, and so can be corrected through a critical reevaluation of one's beliefs.[48] Affect and cognition "have a mutually reinforcing relationship that contributes to the evolution and maintenance of depression symptoms," it has been explained, so that "Pessimistic or negative conditions can trigger and perpetuate negative affect, and negative affect can lead to a tendency to focus and ruminate on negative conditions" (Biegler 2011:67).

---

47. A group has been identified comprising the core emotions of "anger," "fear," "sadness," "enjoyment," "disgust," and "surprise." (They correspond roughly to occurrences of what we usually mean with those terms.) See Griffiths 1997.
48. Although recent critical analysis questions the validity of the widely assumed tenets underlying cognitive therapy, Burton would have entirely agreed with them. See Varga 2012a.

Making use of cognitive habits that are also found in normal reasoners, Paul Biegler illustrates these mechanisms with mood-congruent processing biases and the availability heuristics introduced earlier. First, there is evidence that those with depression are better able to process mood-congruent information, so that there is easier recall of information with negative content, leading to an increased frequency of negative thoughts and, it is hypothesized, the subsequent reinforcement of negative mood. Then, there are the availability (including simulation) heuristics. These come into play when (all) reasoners reach judgments of frequency, as we saw: The events and examples that are easiest to imagine or recall are inaccurately granted greater probability. From studies to test these several hypotheses, it has been concluded that mood congruency, attentional biases, availability, and simulation, provide "a useful way of conceptualizing the negative information-processing biases that typify depressed thinking." The data presented indicate that "depressed people attend more closely to negative information and accord it greater weight when determining the likelihood of future events." These biases are a mechanism explaining the tendency of depressed people to make pessimistic predictions, it is conjectured (Biegler 2011:71). The extent of reliance on specific heuristics and biases serves to differentiate those people with depression from others. It explains their negative, pessimistic cognitive habits. And some of these reasoning flaws, because they occur below conscious awareness, may be inaccessible to direct, effortful amelioration. Yet even the person whose reasoning is inaccessibly hampered by mood-congruent recall of information can anticipate and make conscious efforts to compensate for such limitations, as she can the blinders imposed by availability biases, once they are understood. And there lies the hope, and approach, of cognitive therapy.

Those supporting this thesis about the relationship between emotions and cognitive habits in depression, and the role played by availability heuristics in reinforcing depressed moods, must explain, or explain away, the depressive realism of the mildly depressed, who are famously "sadder but wiser," in approaching the ideal of procedural rationality more closely than the majority of normal reasoners.[49] This "wisdom"

---

49. Alloy and Abramson 1988.

has been widely challenged, and is, at the very least, limited: The sadder and wiser correlation did not hold up as well with predictions about the future, for example.[50] But other studies have also suggested that artificially induced low mood enhances accuracy.[51] The original research has been criticized, based on methodology and alternative interpretations of the findings, whose limited scope has been stressed: This was an advantage in self-knowledge only, and did not extend to greater accuracy in predicting events that are in no way related to the person; predictions of future events were less, not more, accurate; and whether the original subjects were all suffering diagnosed depression was questioned.[52] That the presence of overconfidence in control groups of nondepressed reasoners has been deemed a confounding factor was another (although apparently question-begging) criticism. Yet the possibility that the overlapping desiderata of (procedural) rationality and mental health might diverge has been recognized. Erroneous misbeliefs in the form of positive illusions are often taken to have adaptive advantages over more accurate ones, for example.[53] Within limits, they would likely be judged an indication of mental health and stability. Thus, at the least the sadder but wiser studies point to the need for care in theorizing about the relation of erroneous belief and mood in depression—*as well as caution in ranking mild depression as pathology*. Moreover, because any predictions about the future would be confounded by self-fulfilling prophecy, the possibility of fruitful research to determine the facts of the matter may be limited. And predictions and speculations about future states of affairs are a form of thought so elemental as to discourage us from alluding to "wisdom" at all in relation to these observed contrasts between normal and depressive reasoning. Our conception of wise judgment involves complex, on-balance assessments, and in these, at least, we can suppose that reasoning biases in the mildly depressed will serve to temper any isolated advantage yielded by the accuracy of one limited range of conclusions.

50. Dunning and Story 1991.
51. Forgas 1997.
52. Biegler 2011:72–3.
53. See McKay and Dennett 2009.

Both Stoic thinking and Christian attitudes during Burton's time show a notable abhorrence for affective states, and our contemporary mind science is ostensibly free of that attitude. Contemporary studies do not always grant the close tie between emotions and reasoning accepted by the Stoics, which is put forward in the *Anatomy* (let alone the emphasis on imagination in relation to the those feelings) and made evident in the presuppositions underlying cognitive therapy for mood disorder. Yet the appeal made to mechanisms that doom all reasoning to fall short of procedural rationality belies the separation of the affective from the cognitive. Most cognitive biases are, at bottom, affective biases, inseparably entwined with our affections. Burton's choice of the passions as his starting point was, in this respect, a prescient and fortunate one.

"Disease" and "diseased" are as much attributed to states and traits that are psychic as bodily, in the *Anatomy*, and are unabashedly normative. Moreover, disease lies in mistaken judgment as much as bodily ills. If we can accept those tenets, then the seemingly overstated claims in Democritus Junior's Letter might be read as confirmed, in some respects, by contemporary science. The Stoics whom Democritus Junior follows reached these observations through an attitude toward the passions that we do not share today. But the observations themselves have been borne out within empirical study. Even normal reasoners are endlessly flawed. Cognitive bias and error are also normal, and equally our human lot. And the question of what it is normal or typical to *feel*, has parallels in how it is normal or typical to *reason*.

Burton's intention to limit his discussion to Melancholy as disease is sabotaged by the feelings and moods at the center of melancholy. These states have a universality, and a normative force derived from Western cultural traditions, that cannot be contained within what was intended to be a thoroughly medical analysis. Although it introduces aspects of moral psychology and philosophy that have no place in a naturalized science, melancholy as the Character of Mortality is unavoidably connected to melancholy the disorder, through the contested divide between the normal or typical and the pathological. As the remarkable debate about the bereavement exclusion so recently demonstrated within psychiatry, moral psychology and philosophy are thus inescapably linked to science.

When Melancholy has become a chronic condition it is almost, if not entirely, beyond remedy. In contrast are passing states that, *if neglected*, may become the more dangerous, habituated disease. While unavoidable, these passing states can be somewhat reduced, as well as averted, and even expunged, through sensible management, and we turn next to the extensive program of preventive self-care Burton recommends to that end.

Chapter 8

remedies

Understood as disease or ill health, melancholy is best seen as a collection of habits. And as habits, melancholy symptoms differ from the symptoms understood within the models of disease found in most of today's medicine, as we have seen. These presuppositions about Burtonian "diseases" and "symptoms" frame the conception of his "cures" - the remedies that are the subject of the second Partition of the *Anatomy*. (The use of "cure" and "cured" in describing these treatments is confusing to our modern ears, when cure has come to indicate completed and successful treatment. But for Burton they are simply remedial attempts.) In spite of parallels between them, these ideas also serve to separate the homely emphasis on melancholy as a collection of tendencies and bad habits from today's mood disorders, so often depicted as assailing and disarming us the way bacterial infections do. As habits of mind, moreover, melancholy invites a range of remedies that are themselves largely behavioral and cognitive habits, preeminent among which is unremitting attention to one's bodily and psychic states. Few require the attention of medical practitioners. They are to be undertaken entirely alone, or with nonmedical, and nonauthoritative, assistance—including the distractions, counsel, and ministrations provided by friends. Daily habits and self-control are mainstays, together with commonplace aid from those around us. Holistically and eclectically understood, these recommendations are offered with a spirit of cautious optimism:

> our passions are violent, and tyrannize over us, yet there bee meanes to curbe them, though they be head-strong, they may be tamed, they may be qualified, if he himself or his friends, will but

use their honest endeavours or make use of such ordinary helps, as are commonly prescribed. (II,2,6,1:101)

The wide-ranging recommendations enumerated in the Second Partition are derived from presuppositions about the nature of melancholy laid out earlier in the *Anatomy*. Those presuppositions can be grouped around three principles: First, these remedies largely involve agency; second, they are preventive in their aim; and third, they form a holistic approach calling for a collection of complementary responses, none of which will likely be effective alone. Some implications for treating today's mood disorders can be surmised from Burton's assorted remedies and the principles underlying them. But first, the principles themselves must be examined. Analogies with contemporary treatments from our own time are introduced in chapter 9, while here, Burtonian remedies enter only in reference to the seventeenth-century setting, within which, by contrast with the care of today, medical help was relatively ineffectual, and its authority limited.

Burton's theoretical tenets and treatment recommendations can be summarized, answering the question, Who is the melancholic? First, he, or she, is all of us. Buffeted and saddened by the vicissisitudes of the world around us, by temperamental tendencies, or by neglect of the obvious, homely ways we should protect against the dangers of melancholy habits, as well as by the unruly passions that distort reasoning and engender bias, any person might succumb to the lure of a prodigious and undisciplined imagination. The melancholic is one who fails to attend to the insidious charms of solitary and idle mind wandering, of loose speculations and uncritical conclusions, and who neglects the obvious preventives found in productive activity, social exchange, critical thinking, and attentively instilled daily habits.

SELF-CARE AND THE SIX NONNATURALS

Humoral lore about the preventive, self-care *regimen sanitatis* through adherence to the six "nonnaturals," and the "therapeutics of the passions" (Hadot), had been preserved through medieval and renaissance times.[1] The remedies found in the *Anatomy* reflect their origins in Galenic medicine, and Stoic philosophy, respectively, as well as their elaboration and development through medieval Christianity. In equal measure though, these remedies are shaped by the vaunted place of the imagination in renaissance and early modern times and recognition of the strengths and vulnerabilities of that supremely powerful faculty, as well as the role assigned to aberrant imagining by renaissance thinkers such as Weyer.

About the place of personal agency in healing, Burton is adamant:

> from the Patient himself, the first and chiefest remedy must be had ... if he be willing, at least, gentle, tractable, and desire his owne good. (II,2,6,1:101)

We must heal ourselves: The person can and should become his own physician. In all Melancholy, "thou *tenderest thine owne welfare* ... the good health of body and minde" (III:4,2,6:445, emphasis added). This is not going to be easy, it is emphasized:

> 'Tis a natural infirmity, a most powerfull adversary, all men are subject to passions, and Melancholy above all others, as being distempered by their innate humors, abundance of cholar adust, weaknesse of parts, outward occurrences.

Even the wisest men and greatest Philosophers regularly fail here, he goes on,

> unable to moderate themselves in this behalf ... Stoicks, Heroes, Homers gods, all are passionate, and furiously carried sometimes. (II,2,6,1:101)

The "good rules and precepts" from the ancients followed by Burton in his recommendations presuppose that conditions of bodily and psychic

---

1. They had been reintroduced to Europe through Avicenna's *Canon* and other works.

health are entwined in ways not so easily recognized in later, more dualistic psychology, it will be remembered. Health and unhealth were as much attributes of the nonbodily soul or psyche, as the body; the sick mind, Galen had insisted, was as appropriately healed by doctors as was the body. Marcus Aurelius speaks of envy as an incurable disease; Epictetus of the school as the *dispensary* for the soul. These analogies and parallels were reinforced by the medical involvement in the cultivation of the self, it has been pointed out, so that "the ills of the body and those of the soul can communicate with one another and exchange their distresses: where the bad habits of the soul can entail physical miseries, while the excesses of the body manifest and maintain the failings of the soul" (Foucault 1986:55).[2]

In his emphasis on agency and self-healing, Burton follows his Stoic guides as well as Galen. The cultivation of self-care in Stoic thought has been described as growing out of a cluster of newly adopted attitudes, an emerging individualism that included "cultivation of the self," where the relation of oneself *to oneself* was intensified and valorized.[3] With these themes, Seneca and Epictetus defined the person as the being who was *destined to care for himself*.[4] Concurring with these attitudes, as we saw, were Christian ideas in early modern times: Self-government had come to be increasingly valued.[5] This emphasis and attitude is also explained by the state of medical knowledge and treatment in the early seventeenth century, moreover. The person can and should become his own

---

2. Such interpenetration of soul and body make up what has been called the "medical model" of Hellenistic philosophy (Nussbaum 1994). They bear little resemblance, however, to what is known as the medical model underlying today's psychiatry, whose emphasis is on "value-free" concepts linking psychic with bodily states and processes to accommodate the causal presuppositions guiding other sciences. Burton's model was not reductionistic, nor was it value free, so his is merely a medical model is the classical sense.
3. Foucault 1986:43.
4. The care of the self for Epictetus is "a privilege-duty, a gift-obligation that ensures our freedom while forcing us to take ourselves as the object of all our diligence. 'Spend your whole life learning to live' was an aphorism Seneca quotes, which asked people to transform their existence into a kind of permanent exercise" (Foucault 1986:46).
5. The significance of agency in the *Anatomy*, and this prominence accorded to self-government and the ethical perspective, is judged to have been undeservedly neglected (Tilmouth 2005:525–6).

physician since *he cannot rely on doctors to do better*. While respectful of the ancient medical learning cited throughout the *Anatomy*, Burton shares with the renaissance humanists some considerable skepticism over the efforts of the physicians and other healers of his own time.[6] About them, he says,

> in every village, so many mountebanks, empirics, quacksalvers, Paracelsians, as they call themselves *causifici et sanicidae* [makers of pretexts and killers of healthy people] . . . wizards, alchemists, poor vicars, cast apothecaries, physicians' men, barbers, and goodwives, professing great skill, that I make great doubt how they shall be maintained, or who shall be their patients. (II,1,4,1:11)

Several contrasts with healing today emerge from this passage. Before the organization of self-regulating professionalism and the expertise it entailed, surgeons *were* barbers, and barbers sometimes surgeons. Medical men were as likely as not the "mountebanks, empirics, quacksalvers [quacks]" so disparaged by the humanists.[7] Moreover, other authorities received comparable respect: including the goodwives or country women, whose knowledge of herbal remedies and "kitchen physic" Burton elsewhere praises.[8] (This recognition of the authority of nonmedical experts was not uncommon: Thomas Hobbes, according to a near-contemporary, "had rather have the advice, or take Physique from an experienced old Woman, that had been at many sick people's Bed-sides, than from the learnedst but unexperienced Physitian" [Aubrey 1949:154].) One could also appeal to the prognostications of

---

6. Montaigne's opinions on this point are well known: "Why do doctors work on the credulity of their patient beforehand with so many false promises of a cure, if not so that the effect of the imagination may make up for the imposture of their deconcoction? They know that . . . there have been men for whom the mere sight of medicine did the job" (Montaigne 1957:73–4).
7. Among medical experts, historians point out, surgeons were accorded less respect than physicians during this era because of these associations.
8. His mother, he acknowledges to have "excellent skill in Surgery, sore eyes, aches, &c. and such experimentall medicines, as all the country where shee dwelt can witnesse, to have done many famous and good cures upon diverse poor folks, that were otherwise destitute for helpe" (II,5,1,5:254).

astrologers—and, of course, there were the clergy, including those "poor vicars."[9] (Even the poor vicars were known to double as surgeons, to eke out their livings.[10]) In spite of all these competing authorities, expectations about effective remedy were low, compared with our modern-day ones. Indeed, the era's faith in the healing capacities of the imagination has been attributed to this dearth of effective treatments. The concept of psychosomatic disease, it has been asserted, "was wider in the seventeenth century than it is now.... Such notions ... drew strength from the numerous instances of psychosomatic healing in an age when the potentialities open to purely physical remedies were very limited" (Thomas 1997:209–10).

Following ancient medical sources, the categories of remedy are sorted into three parts: Diet or Living, Apothecary, and Chirurgery [Surgery], and these are followed in the arrangement of the Second Partition.[11] In his discussion of apothecary and surgery, Burton qualifies the negative attitudes expressed toward doctors (above), in several important ways.[12] For some kinds of remedies, including concoctions in the form of herbal and other medicines, it is made clear that expert knowledge is safest—from whatever source. (His own mother, Burton grants, was a skilled dispenser of "experimentall medicines."[13]) But required are practitioners who are honest, careful, and not predatory. In applying for help from physicians and surgeons, we must seek not any, but a *good*, doctor.[14]

> It is not therefore to be doubted, that if we seeke a Physitian, as we ought, we may be eased of our infirmities, such a one I meane as is *sufficient, and worthily so called*. (II,1,3,1:11, emphasis added)

---

9. See Macdonald 1981a, Thomas 1997.
10. Thomas 1997:275.
11. II,1,4,3:18.
12. "it is required that the Patient be not too bold to practice upon himself, without an approved Physitians consent, or to try conclusions, if he read a receipt in a booke; for so many grossely mistake, and doe themselves more harme then good" (II,1,4,2:16).
13. II,5,1,5:254.
14. "Thus much I would require, Honesty in every Physitian, that he be not over carelese or covertous, Harpy-like to make a prey of his patient" (II,1,3,1:12).

There are other, equally important, qualifications on seeking medical help. The patient must have "sure hope that his Physitian can helpe him." (Hippocrates himself was so fortunate in his cures, Burton wryly observes, because "*the common people had a most strong conceipt of his worth*" [II,1,4,2:16].) Added to this confidence, the patient must be persevering, obedient, and constant, not replacing his physician on a whim.[15] And whatever the source of healing, there is one final qualification. The patient must be

> willing to be cured, and *earnestly desire it* . . . wish his owne health; and not to deferre it too long. (II,1,4,2:14, emphasis added)

Herbal remedies for preventing, averting, and healing melancholy reflect a combination of expert (if not always medical) knowledge with self-care. These remedies include hellebore and borage, "The best medicines that ere God made."[16] The particular value of these two plants is indicated by their place in the engraved frontispiece Burton had designed for the 1632 edition, where they appear in two of the eleven scenes. Both white and black forms of Helleborus or Hellebore (a herbaceous perennial flowering plant from the botanical family of *Ranunculaceae*) were included in ancient and medieval medicine, although the white hellebore is in our day recognized to have been a different plant. White hellebore was a "strong purger upward" (II,4,2,1:228), while "that most renowned plant," black hellebore, is described as a "famous purger of melancholy, which all antiquity so much used and admired" (II,4,2,2:231).[17] Borage (*Borago officinalis*) is acknowledged to have similarly ancient origins as a remedy, known for its cooling properties and its use with mood regulation and mental disorder.[18] These two plants were part of a much larger

15. II,1,4,2:16.
16. Argument of the Frontispiece (I:xii).
17. The use of black hellebore, attributed to no less of an authority than Hippocrates, is taken to confirm that, employed carefully, this plant is a strong and effective remedy against melancholy when used as a purgative. What is now believed a misattribution to Hippocrates has been traced to Pliny's *Naturalis Historia*.
18. The astrologer and herbalist Nicholas Culpeper, in his comprehensive and authoritative volume on herbal medicine first published in 1653, speaks of hellebore as the "herb of Saturn," noting that "The roots are very effectual against all melancholy diseases,

number recommended in the *Anatomy*, from which range, herbal treatments used every part of each one. In addition to conserves and syrups derived from them, Burton notes, were "substance, juice, roots, seeds, flowers, leaves, deconcoctions, distilled waters, extracts, oils, etc." (II,4,1,3:216).

The primary purpose of these herbal remedies was purgative, as it was of the several chemical substances and metals similarly employed. These remedial substances—simple and compound, gentle and violent, "upward" (to produce vomiting) and "downward" (as enemas) in their purgative effects— are here all carefully explicated and illustrated in the second volume of the *Anatomy*. In one graphic example, Burton describes the effect of a large amount of the purgative substance Antimony or Stibium on a melancholy parish priest in Prague (remarking as an aside that it was a quantity of medicine fitter for a horse than a man):

> hee was purged of a deale of blacke choler, like little gobbets of flesh, and all his excrements were as black blood ... yet it did him so much good that the next day he was perfectly cured. (II,4,2,1:229–30)

The purgative function of such treatments, it has been pointed out, was symbolic quite as much as actual.[19] Purging purified—and did so within the body and psyche equally. "Averters" served the same literal, and symbolic, purpose. Made up of herbal and other compounds, averters took the form of clysters (enemas) or suppositories, each used to "draw this humour from the braine and heart, to the more ignoble parts" (II:5,1,4:244).

---

such as are of long standing, as quartan agues, and madness" (Culpeper 1985:154). Similarly, all or any of the leaves, flowers, and seeds of borage (an herb of Jupiter, another of the planets linked to melancholy), Culpeper says, "are good to expel melancholy" (Culpeper 1985:53).

19. Michel Foucault speaks of the "thick, overloaded blood of melancholics, heavy with bitter humours," replaced with "the light, clear blood whose fresh movement would dissipate delirium" (Foucault 2006:310).

There remains a place for medical intervention in the employment of these remedies. Induced vomiting and strong enemas were best overseen by those with some experience or expertize. Even herbal remedies and homemade concoctions could be misused. Recognizing the dangers of ignorantly self-administered treatment, Burton omits from his text the many recipes and doses lest, as he says, they should "give occasion thereby to some ignorant reader to practice on himself, without the consent of a good physician" (II,4,2,3:236). Some other treatments (also broadly purgative in their aim) are clearly intended to be not only supervised but also undertaken by a "good physician" or surgeon, as is indicated in the separate subsection of the *Anatomy* devoted to "Chirurgical [surgical] Remedies."[20] Blood letting, either by opening the vein with a sharp knife, cupping, horse-leeches, or the use of cauteries (searing with hot irons) were all included here—although the primary *physical* remedies appear to have remained the largely self-administered herbal and medicinal purges.

The best remedy of all lies with the comforts, distractions, and healing qualities of friendship. The help of friends when reason fails in severe cases was described in chapter 6. But friends can also be important in more everyday efforts. A friend's counsel is a charm, like mandrake wine, Burton explains:

> Friends' confabulations are comfortable at all times, as fire in Winter, shade in Symmer . . . good words are cheerfull and powerfull of themselves, but much more from friends, as so many props, mutually sustaining each other like Ivy and a wall . . . the simple narration many times easeth our distressed minde, and in the midst of greatest extremities, so diverse have beene relieved, by exonerating themselves to a faithfull friend: he sees that which we cannot see for passion and discontent, hee pacifies our mindes, he will ease our paine, asswage our anger. (II,2,6,1:105)

---

20. II,4,3,1:237.

A friend provides the speediest way to avert incipient melancholy and can sometimes do so very quickly, ensuring that many "are instantly cured, when their minds are satisfied" (II,2,5,2:107).[21] With severer disorder, by contrast, when the melancholic's "weakness be such, that he cannot discerne what is amisse, correct or satisfie," friends have more to do. With such advanced cases, the role of friend is an important and demanding one, as we saw.

In the historical setting of the early seventeenth century, help was often inexpert and unreliable. This seems to warrant Burton's stress on aid provided by nonmedical, and nonauthoritative, sources, particularly friends and companions. The emphasis on self-healing and preventive care can also be tied to underlying ideas and assumptions about disease, as we'll see. But these practical limitations, imposed by the state of medical knowledge in the period deserve special emphasis today in light of transformed social attitudes about seeking help. In our era, the appearance of mood disorder is regularly greeted with the admonition to seek help from a medical authority. In the early seventeenth century, "Help yourself!" was the likely response to the signs of melancholy—not today's "Get medical help!" And the availability of medical expertise and authority in our present-day setting points to another very apparent difference: "Get medical help!" obviates "Let your friends and companions help you." For better or worse, the importance accorded to friends in the *Anatomy*, in supporting, aiding, and in severe cases managing melancholy, have few direct parallels in present-day settings. (Peer-support initiatives like those associated with twelve-step programs are the closest, although for the most part they occur well outside the sphere of orthodox clinical care.)

Melancholy has an illimitable number of causes, as we have seen: behavioral and mental habits, and passing and more fixed humoral fluctuations springing from individual temperament, tendencies, and bodily changes, as well as all manner of experiences, even astrological signs and demonic influences. Remedies in the *Anatomy* reflect a

---

21. The same point is reiterated in the Third Partition: "Which cannot speedier be done, then if hee confesse his griefe and passion to some judicious friend . . . that by his good advise *may happily ease him on a sudden*" (III,25,2:208, emphasis added).

comparable array. To our contemporary eye, the sheer number of preventive and treatment measures prescribed is almost laughably immense—nothing less than a whole "lifestyle," of recommendations, that take up 266 pages of the whole work of 1,500 pages. Similar advice is found in less scholarly writing from those times, popular works such as Elyot's *Castel of Helth* (1539), for example.[22] Likened to today's self-help manuals, these books provided simplified humoral ideas to explain prescribed regimens, and Burton's writing in the Second Partition seems to mirror them—more especially Elyot's very Galenic one.[23]

Among the multitude of measures enumerated in the *Anatomy*, a prominent place is assigned to the regimen for maintaining healthy humoral balance (the *regimen sanitatis*), prescribed through the six nonnaturals of Galenic medicine.[24] These nonnaturals are listed by Burton as exercise, fresh air, sleep, diet, evacuation, and perturbations provoked by the passions. The distinction between the "naturals" and "nonnaturals," is also Galenic: The body's constituents, or inherent properties, were natural (its qualities of heat, cold, warmth, and dryness, for example, and the humors themselves, along with the animal spirits). The nonnaturals affected those constituents.[25] While not constitutive of the body, the nonnatural properties altered its humoral balance. Attention must be paid to each one of these aspects of a daily regimen. About the nonnaturals and melancholy, Burton says,

---

22. On the prevalence of such self-help texts in that era and variations between them, see Tilmouth 2005, Lund 2010. Often written by, and always intended for, laypeople, these works on the prevention of illness claimed to equip a patient to deal with the event of it. Thus, the intent of Elyot's book was that "every manne may knowe the state of his own body, the preservation of helth, and how to instructe welle his physytion in syckenes that he be not decyved," it has been explained (Lund 2010:88–9). Widely reprinted and popular, Elyot's book focuses attention on the nonnaturals and is itself is modeled on the Galenic *Ars Medica*.
23. Drawing on traditions of medieval medical regimens, works such as these early modern ones promote the health-giving properties of moderate *laetitia*, or cheerfulness, it has been observed—an attitude in some tension with Burton's ambivalence over how far real peace of mind is sustainable. See Lund 2015.
24. The Galenic regimen was one of several put forward by medical authorities at the time. See Tilmouth 2005, 532–4.
25. For a thorough discussion of these aspects of humoral medicine, see Arikha 2007.

The six non-naturall things caused it, & they must cure it. (II,2,1,1:19)

Underlying this emphasis on the daily regimen, it has been pointed out, the idea that ill health can be cured or prevented by *strengthening the host*, rather than weakening an invader, is the guiding motif. It lingers today in the principles of homeopathic medicine, where the goal is to strengthen the body's ability to heal itself, and is also a key tenet of public health policy and practice. Moreover, through the nineteenth and the first half of the twentieth centuries, physicians still prescribed nonspecific treatments they believed would augment the patients' constitutions and inherent homeostatic mechanisms, to allow them to regain their equilibrium.[26] In early modern times, however, when medical knowledge and authority were relatively limited, strengthening the host was the primary goal, and of paramount concern.

Since it entailed everyday mental and behavioral habits, attention to the nonnaturals lay within any person's grasp. These habits could be acquired and exercised, at home, and alone, through nothing more— or less—than regular practice, close attention, and self-control. With its *regimen sanitatis* for daily self-care, Galenic medicine placed significant emphasis on self-mastery, and it is a priority and value ringingly endorsed throughout the *Anatomy*. This is as much a moral as a practical value: We can, and *should*, maintain our health this way. Failure to adhere to the regimen, Burton deems a "want of [self] government," and he warns that by such failure we not only engender Melancholy, but

degenerate into beasts, [and] transforme our selves. (I,1,1,1:128)

Personal agency, and self-government are highly valued in Stoic thought. More specifically, Stoicism stresses identifying and taking charge of those things within our control, and practicing serene acceptance of things that lie outside that sphere, such as matters of fortune, or immovable facts of our situation.[27] Not all of these ideas are evident in

---

26. Callahan and Berrios 2005:73.
27. This is an aspect of the Stoic theory of value separating virtue from "indifferents," those spurious benefits and detriments (such as health, property, wealth, and sickness),

the *Anatomy*, Burton adopts Stoicism selectively, as we have seen. As a source of distress and disturbance, value judgments must be expunged, for the Stoics, and this abhorrence is foreign to Burton's religious beliefs.[28] But the Stoic emphasis on self-government, autonomy, and self-mastery were reinforced by Christianity, and always to be encouraged. They were general, and very important, Christian virtues in addition to classical ones. Burton strongly approves.

The first five nonnaturals are amply illustrated in the *Anatomy*. Since each one brings about humoral changes in the body that would in turn affect every element of psychic health, each also plays a part in ensuring the sixth (regulating the passions). In this respect, Burton's dualistic but embodied model differs not at all from that of our contemporary medicine's uncompromising materialism. The first five nonnaturals are of less interest to us today, however, because, like many of the remedies proposed, they are so inextricably bound to humoral lore. (The emphasis on purgatives and averters illustrates this, but so do the copious instances of what seems to us today random and arbitrary advice on particular practices.[29])

Of special importance to our mind sciences is the sixth of the nonnaturals. The other five pertained to health in more general terms. Regulating the passions was an indispensable element of health and healing regardless of the particular ailment involved, it is true. But melancholy was primarily a disorder of affect, and the sixth nonnatural was most immediately directed toward the perturbations of the mind, or passions.[30]

---

mistakenly apprehended to be genuine goods and evils. The wise person is not mistaken this way, and avoids the pleasures and pains, desires and fears prompted by these erroneous assessments. See Gill 2010:151–2.

28. On the Stoic view a sharp separation must be made between external things, which we are powerless to change, and the judgments we make about them, which we may withhold or adjust.

29. How many different foodstuffs to eat at one meal is an example: "A great inconvenience comes by a variety of dishes, *which causeth the precedent distemperature*" (II,2,1,2:25, emphasis added).

30. The length of the section on the passions has been pointed to in confirming this special status, explained by Burton's "unwavering preoccupation with the emotions" (Tilmouth 2005:533).

The effects of the passions on the imagination, and its on them, each engender melancholy, and regulating the passions is thus the immediate goal of the whole *Anatomy* project. By giving reign to such feelings (Lust, Anger, Ambition, and Pride are those named in this instance), we

> follow our owne ways, wee degenerate into beast, transforme our selves, overthrowe our constitutions ... and heap upon us this of Melancholy. (I,1,1,1:128)

General ideas such as these about the need to regulate the passions originate in Stoic thought and the neo-Stoicism of the renaissance, as we have seen, where the passions combine with false and distorted beliefs to prevent contentment and tranquility. Fused with medieval Christianity, the same concerns are also directed toward temptation and sin. Thus, avoiding the twin fates of the distressing unease abhorred by the Stoics, and sinfulness condemned by Christianity, was an overarching goal of Burton's extensive recommendations.

Philosophy, for the Stoics, was an ethical concern, devoted to learning how to live.[31] This philosophical and ethical purpose also frames Burton's recommendations for averting and curbing melancholy.[32] Undertaking philosophy meant not theorizing but rather practicing how to live, freely and with self-awareness, in pursuit of self-care, keenly attentive to all of one's thoughts, feelings, and actions. It involved engaging in regular exercises designed to establish habits to free oneself from worries, feelings, and desires, those incessant hindrances to

---

31. This traditional ethics of self-mastery, it has been observed, follows a juridical model of possession: Seneca speaks of one's belonging to oneself, being one's own master, and exercising authority over oneself (Foucault 1986:65). And the task of testing oneself, examining oneself, and monitoring oneself in a series of clearly defined exercises, makes "the question of truth ... concerning what one is, what one does, and what one is capable of doing—central to the formation of the ethical subject" (Foucault 1986:68).
32. The *Anatomy*'s emphasis on the therapeutics of the passions arises from Stoic philosophy, rather than Epicurianism—although the aims, exercises, and practices, were in many cases shared by each. The influence of Epicurianism in Europe came later, during the second half of the seventeenth century (Long 1986:242).

tranquility.[33,34] Since these passions were associated with things past (memories, and deeds), or future (hopes and fears), emphasis should be on the present, the here and now.

The exercises involved in regulating the passions, attributed to Chrysippus, Epictetus, Seneca, and Marcus Aurelius, are not contained in any systematic treatise (among those remaining to us), but drawn from several texts with which Burton has shown himself familiar.[35] They are alluded to so frequently in subsequent periods, including the Stoic revival during the renaissance, that it has been assumed that they were well known and had been part of daily life in the philosophical schools.[36] Several aspects of these inner exercises have particular bearing on preventing and treating melancholy. First, their goal: seeking truth though clarity, coherence, and logical validity of reasoning and thought. As depicted in the *Anatomy*, this involves attentive, rigorous assessment of evidence and inductive reasoning patterns.

The potentially misleading appearances of things had been the particular object of Stoic critical assessment. Burton dispenses with the details of the Stoic epistemic process of belief acceptance, however, in favor of a simpler focus on evidence and evidentiary reasoning.[37] An illustration of this approach occurs where he admonishes the person who claims to see signs of demonic influence (not uncommon in those times, when the Devil's presence and influence in worldly things were understood

---

33. Hadot 1995: 86.
34. "Philosophy, in antiquity, was a spiritual exercise . . . philosophical theories were either placed explicitly in the service of spiritual practice, as was the case in Stoicism and Epicurianism, or else they were taken as the objects of intellectual exercises" (Hadot 1995:104).
35. Seneca's *Letters*, Epictetus's *Handbook* and *Moral Discourses*, and the *Meditations* of Marcus Aurelius.
36. Hadot 1995:83–4.
37. Epictetus advises challenging every impression. This vigilant attitude he refers to as a nightwatchman one, and he speaks of being a tester of coinage, an assayer, who evaluates all representations or appearances and only then gives, or withholds, assent. "[We] ought not to accept a mental representation unsubjected to examination, but should say, 'Wait, allow me to see who you are and whence you came'" (*Discourses* III:xii:85).

literally). The claim is not entirely dismissed here: It was not *necessarily* untrue, but likely mistaken:

> Thou thinkest thou hearest and seest divells . . . 'tis not so, 'tis they corrupt phantasy, settle thyne imagination, though art well. Thou thinkest thou has a great nose, thou art sicke, every man observes thee, laughes thee to scorne, *perswade thy selfe* 'tis no such matter: this is feare only, and vaine suspition.

One must "persuade" (or dissuade), oneself to be rid of these mistaken ideas. Describing the exact technique required for such an exercise, Burton then speaks of moments when one is "discontent . . . sad and heavy," and goes on that, in such a situation, "we must ask *why*, and *upon what ground*?" Consider of it, he admonishes,

> *examine it thoroughly.* (II,2,6,1:103 emphases added)

We must pay attention to dejected moods and fears and their underlying beliefs, assumptions, and inferences, subjecting them to critical assessment and skeptical review, and thereby dissuading ourselves from accepting them. This attitude of wariness, maintained even in moments when self-control is weakest (in dreams, drunkenness, or melancholy, as Epictetus says), seems to be how we must approach our passions. Melancholy symptoms are a form of bad habits. To "cure" them, we adopt and try to instill another set of habits, including cautious, critical attention directed toward our every thought and feeling. Attentively employed, these habits will help to avert, dispel, and heal melancholy symptoms, Burton implies.

Flights of the imagination will be the special subject of these daily cognitive exercises aimed to eliminate unwarranted belief and ill-formed judgment. Pleasing and seemingly innocent as it often is, the unfettered play of the imagination is dangerous because imaginings and feelings are an endless goad to one another, as we have seen. Imaginings and errant beliefs prompt feelings, feelings in turn foster misleading and potentially harmful imaginings. To curb unruly and overweening passions and keep melancholy at bay, we must monitor and correct all conceits, fantasies, willful blindness, and exaggerated fears resulting from the solitary, careless, self-indulgent ruminating or "melancholising." These "phantastical and bewitching thoughts," so urgently, so continually set upon, creepe in, insinuate, possess, overcome, distract and detain ... [some people] they cannot I say go about their more necessary businesse, stave off or extricate themselves, but are ever musing, melancholizing, and carried along ... in this labarinth of anxious and solicitous melancholy meditations. (I,2,2,6:243)

Like the Stoics before him, Burton also proposes other methods to regulate and avert the passions in addition to these forms of self-directed cognitive therapy. We are to engage our imaginative capabilities by constructing alternative explanations, conjuring up different scenarios, and employing memory to reframe new perspectives, for example. Distraction is essential, and sums up many of these maneuvers. The Stoics had introduced techniques such as re-labeling to bring about a changed perspective; and reminding oneself of others' misfortunes to regain a sense of proportion about one's own.[38] Parallels drawn between physical and spiritual exercise encouraged the repeated recitation of action-guiding maxims. Burton does not explicitly recommend each of these practices, yet his frequent references to using the imagination to regulate the passions suggest he would have had them in mind, and he does reiterate the need for the careful introspective supervision of thought, feeling, and action that the Stoics called *prosokhe*.

With his attention on quelling excessive and inappropriate imagining (these "phantastical and bewitching thoughts") the emphasis on the imaginary objects in the *Anatomy* can also be traced to the Stoic stress on the here and now (*hic et nunc*). Attention to the present moment in Stoic thought, it has been observed, "frees us from the passions, which are *always caused by the past or the future*" (Hadot 1995:84–5, emphasis added)[39] Burton's description of the lure of melancholising points to "such pleasant things ... present, past, or to come" (I,2,2,6:243). This

---

38. For a review of recent research examining and explaining the neuroscience of such "reappraisal" aimed at altering affective states, see Buhle et al. 2013.
39. Contemporary cognitive therapy has developed this emphasis on the here and now, focused around the practice of mindfulness. A state of mindfulness is in the moment, and the Stoic term *prosokhe*, it has been pointed out, may also be translated as "self-awareness" or "mindfulness." See Kuyken et al. 2008, Robertson 2010, Williams and Kabat-Zinn 2013, Mars and Abbey 2010.

enumeration also is incomplete, however, in failing to capture all the dangers surrounding the imaginary. The *here* and *now* is also the *actual* rather than *hypothetical*. And as we have seen, it is our endlessly inventive imaginary creations—not merely the objects of memory (the past) and anticipatory states (the future)—that are the products of the imagination. A passage from Epictetus's *Discourses* where he speaks of being afraid, not of death or exile but of fear itself, seems to capture exactly the apprehensions running through the *Anatomy*:

> we are ever going out of our way to heap up terrors and make them out greater than they actually are. For example, whenever I go to sea, on gazing down into the deep or looking around upon the expanse of waters and seeing no land, I am beside muself, fancying that if I am wrecked I shall have to swallow this whole expanse of waters; but it does not occur to me that three pints are enough. What is it, then, that disturbs me? The expanse of the sea? No, but my judgement. Again, when there is an earthquake, I fancy that the whole city is going to fall upon me. . . . What . . . are the things that weigh upon us and drive us out of our senses? Why, what else but our judgements. (Epictetus *Discourses* II:xvi:327–29)

Danger lies in all these objects. Those that are unchangeably past or hypothetically future are *not now*; and those that are merely imaginary are *not here*. Worries and fears such as those described by Epictetus all disturb the passions. Whether Burton knew such troubling concerns from personal experience, from his observation of others, or from descriptions like this by the ancients, he does seem to entirely concur with this depiction of the inner life of imagination-fostered worry: this "labarinth of anxious and solicitous melancholy meditations . . . winding and unwinding themselves, as so many clocks" (I,2,2,6:243), as he says.

As these examples of Stoic strategies suggest, the exercises inherited by Burton reflect the intellectualistic focus of classical philosophy, where the passions were seen as unworthy, dangerous, and disruptive elements in our psychic lives. Yet Burton would merely quell and regulate the passions, not extirpate them. And his recommendations in the Second Partition are less narrowly and less intellectually focused than these Stoic ones for that reason. Attention to all the nonnaturals could not alone avert and avoid melancholy, other activities are also required, and many pages of extra activities are recommended.[40] Primary among them remain the use of distraction and diversion. Keeping busy, enjoying the soothing effect of music, dance and exercise, seeking the company of friends—Melancholy may be treated or at least mitigated, by *"some contrary passion, good counsell and perswasion."* Contrasting ideas, real as well as imagined, are especially valuable here. Set prosperity against adversity, we are advised:

> as wee refresh our eyes by seeing some pleasant meddow, fountaine, picture, or like: recreate thy minde by some contrary object, with some more pleasing meditation divert thy thoughts. (II,2,6,1:102, emphasis added)

These distractions can also be undertaken by friends, who can set the melancholic about "some businesse, exercise or recreation, *which may divert his thoughts*" (II,2,6,1:102, emphasis added). Friends also owe uninvited, and even unwelcome help in ensuring these distractions and diversions, and issuing warnings. If they see a man given to melancholy,

> solitary, averse from company, please himself with such private and vaine meditations, though he delight in it, they ought by all meanes to seeke to divert him, to dehort him, to tell him of the event and danger that may come of it. (II,2,6,2:109)

Regular conversation with others is recommended, for example, particularly those who, because they are close to us, offer the extra candor and insight of friendship.[41] Solitary pursuits and idle habits must be avoided, as we have seen, for nothing "begets [melancholy] sooner, increaseth and continueth it oftener than idleness" (I,2,2,6:239). Such "behavioral"

---

40. Only a broad interpretation of the sixth nonnatural allows that the cure of melancholy lies entirely and exclusively with "willpower and dietetics" as it has been asserted (Tilmouth 2005:536).
41. II,2,6,2.

means must also be sought to turn us away from the thoughts, moods, and dangerous imaginings that would unsettle our feelings. If the melancholy person may not otherwise be accustomed to "brook . . . distasteful and displeasing objects, the best way . . . is generally to avoid them" (II, 2 6 2:108). If "hee have sustained a great losse, suffered a repulse, disgrace, &c.,"

> if it be possible, relieve him. If he desire ought, let him be satisfied, if in suspence, feare, suspition, let him be secured, and if it may conveniently bee, give him his hearts content; for the body cannot be cured till the minde bee satisfied. . . . If that may not be hoped or expected, yet ease him with comfort, chearfull speeches, fair promises, and good words, perswade him, advise him. (II:2,6,2:109)

When the "Patient himself is not able to resist, or over-come these heart-eating passions," his friends or physicians "must all join" he says, appealing to Hippocrates:

> First they must especially beware, a melancholy discontented person . . . never bee left alone or idle: but as Physitians prescribe physicke *cum custodia*, let them not bee left unto themselves, but with some company or other, least by that meanes they aggravate and increase their disease. (II2,6,2,:106)

As this variety of remedial responses from the patient himself and his companions and physicians indicate, Burton's is a holistic account. Every person carries the diathesis for melancholy to some degree, since we are all as humans prone to suffer from the vicissitudes of living. Because every person, and every element of everyone's lives, is a party to this effort of keeping melancholy at bay, remedies must be correspondingly *eclectic*. Melancholy is a collection of symptoms, or bad habits; to treat it requires many different remedies rather than a single one. Whether we count them all as part of the sixth nonnatural, or as independent measures, the range of these measures is vast.

PREVENTION, BY PARING THE NAILS BEFORE THEY GROW TOO LONG

Attention to the six nonnaturals, and to the many other remedies and recommendations detailed in the Second Partition, was primarily preventive medicine. Melancholy is a progressive disorder, stubbornly resisting treatment once it becomes habituated, or chronic. It must be avoided and averted before it sets in—not merely treated when it occurs: "withstood *in the beginning*," as Burton insists. Like so much else, Burton's emphasis on early prevention is also found in Du Laurens. But the focus on prevention is attributed to ancient medical lore. Of the good rules and precepts we learn from physicians, the first is to "withstand the beginning." This, Burton declares, quoting Ovid, is a precept "which all concurre upon" (III,2,5,2:208), for,

> he that will but resist at first may easily bee a conquerer at the last. (III,2,5,2:207)

The primary emphasis within these efforts is prevention that is early. Melancholy may be treated or at least mitigated, as he says, by "some contrary passion, good counsell and perswasion,"

> if it be withstood in the beginning, maturely resisted, *and as those ancients hold, the nayles of it be pared befor they grow too long.* (III,3,4,1:306)

We must practice habits that will avert and avoid melancholy when, triggered by life's inevitable setbacks, the tendency we all possess places us in danger of succumbing to "an Habit of Melancholy." Paring the nails refers to *averting the onset of melancholy symptoms*—as well as reducing their severity.

"Prevention" is an elastic term.[42] It may mean reducing the likelihood of initially developing melancholy-inducing habits. With disorders that are

---

42. Recent reports from the Institute of Medicine and the National Research Council and Institute of Medicine Committee on the Prevention of Mental Disorders and Substance Abuse among Children, Youth, and Young Adults have recommended that

episodic or recurring, it also means slowing the return, or reducing the severity, of subsequent phases after the initial one. There is little in the *Anatomy* to suggest that melancholy is an episodic disorder, the way today's depression appears to be; it seems closer to a gradually worsening low, dysthymic mood, that is repeatedly triggered into states of more particular distress by either imaginatively generated fears and thoughts or external events and experiences. Nonetheless, the analogy with paring the nails before they grow too long allows Burton to intend each of the above interpretations through the self-care and healing advocated in the *Anatomy*. Melancholy can be entirely averted, delayed, or lessened in its effects through the preventive measures he recommends. With greater effort on their part, prevention can also be effective in those whose inherent temperament of melancholic character types strongly predisposes them toward melancholy. All these endeavors, even when they depend on advice from experts, remain importantly self-initiated and self-administered. Because of the value placed on autonomy and self-government in the era, these efforts are thus also preventive in a final sense: They serve to avert the ministrations and interventions imposed by others. Others may have to help, but Burton shows a strong preference for being independent in one's self-care.

"THERE IS NO CATHOLIKE MEDICINE TO BE HAD"

Just as the causes of melancholy are illimitable, so an almost infinite range of treatments, preventatives, and remedies will also likely be needed to counteract it. There is no Catholike medicine to be had, for,

> that which helps one, is pernitious to another. (II,5,1,5:252)

> prevention be defined as those interventions that occur prior to the onset of a clinically diagnosed disorder, that is, the *initial onset of what is taken to be a single, chronic disease*. See O'Connell, Boat, and Warner 2009. Conformity with this usage is uneven across clinical and research settings, however, and measures of prevention have included those of severity as well as chronicity (the number and length of episodes and the length between reoccurrences, for example). To reduce confusion over the elasticity of the term "prevention," one suggestion has been that programs designed to avert initial incidence of disorders be deemed "anticipatory" (Anderson 2010:777).

Mixed diseases, he says, "must have mixt remedies." Different remedies will address different properties of the sufferer, and all will be required. Added to prayer and other religious practices, comforting words, amulets, and astrological advice must be more ordinary remedies, as we have seen: herbal draughts, bleeding, purges and vomiting, behavioral and social adjustments (such as avoiding solitude and idleness), daily exercises using the imagination to manage the passions, and careful attention to the other five nonnaturals of diet, air, excretion, sleep, and exercise. Burton's insistence that only in combination can remedies be expected to succeed is supported by his assertion that "seldom two men shall be like affected *per omnia*"[43] and recognition that a therapy that is "conducing to one" may have the opposite effect on another (see II,5,1,5:252, above). This position has been attributed to Montanus.[44] It also reflects his holistic notion of health, however, as made up of many elements. Again echoing Galenic medicine, ill health, with all its causes, must be treated with a comparably eclectic set of remedies. This is reasoning found when multifactorial interventions are advocated today. A multifactorial etiology for depression, it has been observed, argues for a multipronged approach to intervention.[45] No one of these might alone be sufficient, Burton indicates, but *together they may succeed*.

> if not alone, yet *certainely conjoyned* [they] may do much. (III,2,5,2:207)

So these remedies are notable not only for Burton's themes of prevention and self-healing but also for his emphasis on the necessity of their combination, in a form of what might today be called holistic healing. Purgative doses, fresh air, busyness, and cognitive exercises to regulate the passions may each do little by themselves, but as truly complementary medicine, and self-wrought healing, this passage suggests, they will at least be less likely to fail.

---

43. I,1,3,4:171.
44. See Tilmouth (2005:534), who also attributes to the influence of Galenism Burton's recognition that the management of health is an art.
45. See Jacob 2012.

Associated with today's common-cause, etiological disease model, where a single causal factor is assigned to account for the symptoms or symptom cluster relied on for medical diagnosis, is a tendency to think in terms of a single, isolated treatment response directed toward a specific, local ill. Such responses, we saw, made up the etiological stance invited by the new medical knowledge that allowed the causes of many diseases to be identified and targeted with precision. For coherent disease entities such as bacterial infections, whose causal properties were entirely understood, a single, specific remedy could be found—the magic bullet that would be entirely sufficient to effect cure. But neither the medical knowledge of causes, nor that kind of disease model, is available to Burton. Knowledge of causes was limited. And Melancholy is nothing over and above a multitude of endlessly differing symptoms, only loosely united by the characteristic moods of groundless fear and sadness. Understood within a network model of disorder, any melancholy, whether it be incipiently chronic or more passing, reflects a shifting cluster of symptoms with only relative stability and coherence. From this we can recognize some of the force of Burton's treatment eclecticism—his insistence that nothing less than the totality of remedies may be necessary to effectively treat any given instance of melancholy. To accommodate this range of symptoms, a comparable range of remedies will be required. Indeed, given the illimitable nature of causes and symptoms of melancholy, there must be variations between symptoms and symptom clusters—among different individuals, as well as through time within the same individual. And perhaps no specific remedy can be expected to be effective for all cases; the symptom clusters making them up are not sufficiently uniform. (This eclecticism can also be attributed to the part played by expectation (or placebo) effects. No specific remedy can be reliably effective for all melancholy symptoms because of the vagaries of expectation effects that, as Burton says, might allow one individual to be entirely healed merely by a strongly held idea.[46])

In the *Anatomy* focus is on the daily habits directed by the six nonnaturals *as they, through time, work together* with other factors, such as

---

46. Sometimes, nothing more than "a strong conceit or apprehension ... will take away Diseases," he observes (I,2,3,2:252).

experiences and temperamental tendencies. Avoiding and averting melancholy is adopting and maintaining habits, and this longitudinal perspective acknowledges the effect of each element on each other element understood within a temporal sequence. We must adhere to every one of these habits, not merely because all might be required in any given instant but also to maintain and reinforce them through stretches of time—in short, to habituate them.

While preventive self-healing and eclectic remedies have very apparent bearing for milder states of disorder, they will be ineffectual with more debilitating and severe cases, Burton willingly concedes. It is precisely this that explains the urgent need to anticipate and prevent severe melancholy before it sets in. The failure of his remedies with more severe cases can be expected not because such cases represent disease of a different order, as it would usually be understood today, however. (It is depicted this way, for example, in efforts to differentiate true melancholic depression from other kinds, as we saw in chapter 4.) That way of thinking is allied to the common-cause etiological model Burton avoids, and it overlooks his differentiation between passing and habituated, or chronic, forms of melancholy. Those more severe cases of disorder result from repeated feedback loops linking symptoms to causes. Unchecked repetition is in this respect an indicator of severity, so that more severe and chronic forms of melancholy are distinguished by resisting personal efforts at prevention. When we neglect, or can no longer adhere to, the required behavioral and cognitive regimen and need to seek outside help, our melancholy has advanced to become a recalcitrant and dangerous disease. Rather than his network-style assumptions being applicable only to milder forms of melancholy, Burton offers a criterion of severity accommodated by those assumptions.

SUCCESSFUL PREVENTIVE, ECLECTIC, SELF-CARE

What limits does Burton envision for preventive self-care? Perhaps in practice not all melancholy can be dispelled through self-directed, preventive medicine. The tendency toward *akrasia* must undermine and thwart such efforts. We are endlessly lured to melancholise, and to lapse from careful, critical monitoring of our thoughts and feelings and sensible behavioral habits. Quite aside from our doomed moral state of original sin, unmitigated tragedy and bad luck, or an inveterately dark temperament, will affect our ability to heal ourselves. Burton is not optimistic on this point. No promises or predictions are or can be made as to successful or long-lasting cure. True, the successes of the ancients in preventing Melancholy are cited:

> Many are fully cured when . . . [they are] secured and satisfied in their mindes; Galen . . . brags . . . that he for his part hath cured diverse of this infirmity . . . by right settling alone of their mindes. (II,2,6,1:100)

If Galen did it, then perhaps we can be guardedly hopeful, this suggests. By avoiding the situations and mental habits that are likely to disturb our feelings, by seeking help from friends, and by slowly establishing healthful habits, Burton seems to think much lies within our power to change and improve, and that—as long as we start early—*unaided*. Potentially, all habituated melancholy can be averted this way—except, as he says, that sadness which is our human lot, which is not melancholy at all, strictly so called. At other times he strikes a more somber note. Even while it includes the ministrations of good doctors and companions as well as self-care, the Second Partition ends on a cautious note, hedged with qualifications:

> These in briefe are the ordinary medicines which belong to the cure of melancholy, which if they be used a right, no doubt may do much good . . . [and] must needs ease, if not quite cure: not one but all or most. (II,5,3,2:265–6)

If *used right*, must *ease, not cure*, in *most, not all*. This is not a very optimistic outlook.[47]

---

47. And indeed, Burton's disposition was not an optimistic one: Speaking for himself as well as those around him, he judges that "if there bee true happinesse amongst us, 'tis but for a time" (I:2,3,10:275).

Untreated, melancholy admits of a degree of severity leaving the sufferer beyond the help provided by preventive measures, and incapable of self-directed healing. The kind of preventive, self-administered treatments described above will thus have limited application. But the confusing ambiguities surrounding the notion of prevention also complicate the matter of treatment with more severe cases. Preventive effectiveness can be measured in a range of different ways, and these variations will be an impediment to determining how many instances of severe disorder may have been averted by such earlier interventions. If properly adhered to before it becomes a chronic condition that is unresponsive to any remedy, and given willingness on the part of the sufferer, Burton's preventative steps *could in principle* unfailingly avert melancholy. *In practice*, by contrast, human nature leaves melancholy unavoidable.

The burden of melancholy tendencies undoubtedly falls more heavily on some than on others, moreover. This will be due to individual variations in *akratic* weakness, or traumatic life experience, as much as to native humoral temperament. Among the humorally based character types, those with the melancholic temperament possessed the strongest diathesis or risk factor, for succumbing to melancholy; they will have to try harder than those blessed with a sunnier character, it is implied. Not suggested, however, is that these tendencies so strongly determine melancholy mood states that the individual is completely at the mercy of his inherent temperament. Through neglect and a failure to adopt and follow healthy habits, he may find himself such a helpless victim. But melancholy as disease, at least, unlike that sadness which is the Character of Mortalitie, is never our immovable fate until *after we have ourselves made it so*.

> Perditio tua ex te: thou hast lost thy selfe willfully, cast away thy selfe, *thou thy selfe art the efficient cause of thine owne misery, by not resisting such vaine cogitations, but giving way unto them.* (I,2,2,6:245)

A faith in free will lies beneath this optimism, and it leaves somewhat tepid Burton's acknowledgment of the causal role played by the naturally melancholy temperament. Inborn tendencies are at most incomplete and weak effects. Perhaps they "incline without compelling," in such a way that their influence can be resisted, as Burton puts it, describing astrological sources of Melancholy. Of Starres as a Cause, he concludes,

> they doe incline, but not compel; no necessity at all ... and so gently incline, that a wise man may resist them. (I,2,1,4:199)

This passage has been taken to be an equivocation, apparently widely adopted during the renaissance, serving to protect its adherents against the seemingly deterministic implications of astrology.[48] Yet, it equally fits the case of the person whose temperament works as an especially powerful diathesis, *inclining but not compelling him* toward the melancholy that, acting wisely and early, *he may resist*. Even those whose inherent temperament strongly predisposes them toward melancholy retain sufficient agency to prevail over their temperament, as they are depicted here.

This position on Burton's part has bearing on the passive role often assigned to the depression sufferer today. The blame and shame once thought helpfully reduced through recognition that the psychiatric patient is powerless in the face of a debilitating disease has been particularly emphasized for depression, where depleted agency, a diminished sense of autonomy, and reduced motivation, are characteristic aspects of the symptom picture of depressive disorder. In his cursory case descriptions, Burton does not emphasize these traits. (Arguably, they are implied in his use of untreatability as an index of severity, as reflected in the person unable to help himself.) But nor are passivity and inertia incompatible with his habituation-based analysis of melancholy. If severe disorder brings diminished agency, he would presumably insist, then so much more urgently should the person strive to avert its *initial* onset. Those with advanced melancholy deserve our sympathy. Those whose habitual melancholy has been allowed to become an entrenched, chronic, and seemingly incurable condition correspond to the passive and pitiable victims of depression—but they do not start out that way.

---

48. Kocher 1953.

As we saw in chapter 3, the *Anatomy* account has parallels with the symptom-focused network models today proposed as alternatives to more traditional conceptions of mood disorders. To recapitulate: The interaction Burton describes cannot be entirely captured in any set of unidirectional, body-to-mind, causal sequences. And contrary to much that has been asserted or assumed about causation in humoral medicine, no regular pattern of causation can be traced from bodily "temperature" to melancholy symptoms. What is more, the inherent tendencies or risk factors associated with the melancholy temperament are not an exception to this. It is clear that the number afflicted with melancholy potentially far exceeds the number of those who are temperamentally prone to it. According to the geometrically balanced classical ontology, this should be one-quarter of the total, since there are four humors. But melancholy was widespread and *growing*—to epidemic proportions.

The temporally extended natural history of melancholy as disease at the center of Burton's analysis is similarly fitted to a network model. The examples used in chapter 3, where symptoms (sadness, solitariness) become in their turn causes of further symptoms, illustrate a temporal sequence. Following that sequence makes it possible to attribute disorder. And, in a final parallel, entrenched and more severe forms of the disorder result from repetition. The extent of the network and the number of repeated feedback loops linking symptoms together contribute to severity.

In light of the suffering and severity of the mood disorders we see in our own era, it is difficult to accept these apparently simplistic admonitions. They seem insufficient, superficial, moralistic, and unfeeling. Moreover, there is another concern: The symptoms of depression, particularly, are often observed to include reduced motivation and a diminished sense of agency. Asking the victims of such conditions to make an extra effort, and marshal self-control for daily self-help exercises seems inappropriate and ineffectual as a treatment measure.

Yet from the confusing ambiguities in the notion of prevention can be discerned substantive grounds why we should not dismiss Burton's prescriptions as hopelessly, and unfeelingly, optimistic. These ambiguities must impede efforts to measure the extent and severity of disorder, since the application of Burton's remedies in particular cases may have prevented melancholy before it became an entrenched, chronic condition. Had they been tried, they may have *reduced the number of severe cases of melancholy*, altering the balance of more to less severe. (That reduction, certainly, was Burton's aim.) And therein lies the particular force of these recommendations. Averting more severe forms of melancholy through the practice of preventive self-care and healing may suggest a model for reducing the number of cases of severe mood disorder in our own time.

Chapter 9

from the *Anatomy* to the clinic and lab

"Depression" may be understood as depressive disorder, mixed anxiety and depressive disorder, melancholic depression, or simply as depressive symptoms, including those associated with other conditions entirely. Whichever way they are taken, however, the disordered moods and symptom clusters of today are different from the states Burton calls Melancholy, and several reasons, some historical, others medical and conceptual, have been shown to discourage drawing any simple equations between them. Yet, at the same time, telling analogies and commonalities link Burtonian Melancholy to the mood disorders we see today. The implications of some of those parallels for approaching our contemporary disorders are the subject of this last chapter.

Basic structural elements were our starting point. From Burton's humorally inspired analyses, it has proven possible to extract an underlying cognitive architecture that is in some respects quite consonant with several of the models, findings, and preoccupations of the contemporary mind sciences. Because, and perhaps only because, the *Anatomy* account is compatible with the mind construed on a broadly cognitivist model, it is plausible to think about whether it might contribute to the understanding and care of today's mood disorders, and how it might generate, or add to, research hypotheses regarding them. Burtonian psychology is fundamentally divergent from that associated with much modernist psychology and philosophy of mind. But the cognitive turn,

I have argued, invites a reconsideration of the earlier conceptions of mind so long eclipsed by the particular forms of mind–body dualism that came to replace Burton's.

In this chapter we turn first to the treatment principles derived from Burton's underlying architecture, principles shown to guide his many remedies for avoiding, averting, and easing melancholy symptoms. These principles have obvious bearing on approaches to mood disorder in—and beyond—the clinic. And, more directly, so do many of those recommendations themselves. Today, in scattered places, both principles and remedies are already employed in clinical care, as well as in more homely, and in public heath, initiatives. In most settings, however, at least within the United States during the second decade of the twenty-first century, they are not. They hold potential as valuable *additions* to, or *replacements* for, current practices. After introducing brief examples illustrating where these recommendations and principles are found and might be used, I note implications of Burton's psychology for generating new research hypotheses. These pick out three features: the underlying model of mind itself; the conception of disease; and ideas about the part played by the Burtonian faculty of Imagination that so closely corresponds to present-day conceptions of simulation. Each feature of the *Anatomy* account points to research directions with bearing on our understanding of today's mood disorders.

TREATMENT

Today, an inchoate assortment of data and clinical endeavor make up efforts to prevent or treat depression and related affective disorders. From these, a handful can serve to illustrate these points of connection with the *Anatomy* account. They are (i) the use of the imagination in healing work; (ii) the application of cognitive exercises in treatment settings; (iii) recent attempts to employ multifactorial and eclectic treatments; (iv) early prevention to combat the apparent epidemic of depression; and (v) an emphasis on agency in relation to self-care.

harnessing the imagination

Recognizing and using the power of our own imagination is the prescription for healing ourselves, Burton emphasizes; it is a faculty that can be employed in a range of ways to restore and regulate our aberrant moods. Imagining, or simulation, plays a part in affect regulation through the increasing use of guided imaging for the treatment of mood disorder, for example.[1] Similarly, the hypotheticals of imagining are variously employed within cognitive therapy. They counter the negative, "catastrophic" thinking about future outcomes associated with mood disorders, for example, when a more realistic and less dire appraisals of future outcomes are achieved through a process of repetitive *rehearsal* called "imaginal exposure," in which the worst outcome is imagined and reimagined. By reviewing what is feared, it has been explained, "the patient is able to start to accept the possibility of the feared event" (Beck et al. 2005:250). More far-reaching implications of Burton's imagination-centered remedial principles might expand treatments using expectation effects. The use of open placebos within formal treatment settings has been proposed for the treatment of depression, for example, where it is pointed out that properly handled, the placebo effect can be regarded as an efficient tool for clinicians and their patients.[2] Not all such innovations will be successful. (Employing open placebos so as to entirely avoid deception has proven a challenge.[3] And earlier findings apparently supporting the effectiveness of such practices have been subject to

---

1. The use of *guided imaging*, and its effects on stress levels, immune system functioning, and mood, was described in chapter 2. In a closely parallel example, a "mental contrasting" procedure has been employed to overcome addictive behavior, involving two imagining exercises to attain a goal. The subject is first required to entertain a positive fantasy of the achievement of the goal and all the positive consequences that could be expected to follow; second, this positive fantasy is imaginatively contrasted with the negative reality of the subject's present distance from achieving that goal, and the obstacles in the way of its attainment. See Oettingen et al. 2010, Oettingen 2012. See also Pictet et al. 2011.
2. The frequency and circumstances of placebo use in clinical practice remains elusive, due to lack of agreement over definitions. See Andrews 2001, Fassler et al. 2010. Its potential is increasingly recognized, however. See Kaptchuk and Miller 2015.
3. See Jopling 2008, Justman 2013.

methodological critique.[4]) Nonetheless, recognition that the Burtonian imagination and its allied expectation effects hold the potential for promoting self-healing, is a profound one, whose practical implications and applications would appear promising and likely to be far reaching.

cognitive exercises

Many of the activities and regimens involved in today's cognitively based treatments (such as cognitive-behavioral therapy, or CBT) employ the capabilities of the imagination along the lines just sketched. By engaging in forms of self-talk, or even something approaching self-hypnosis, or practicing mindfulness-related exercises, the person may ward off the negative moods, distress, and despair of depression and anxiety states. Some of these cognitive approaches acknowledge their commonalities with the Stoic instructions for regulating the passions that guided Burton. And variations on those ideas have already been integrated into cognitive therapeutic exercises and practices.[5]

multifactorial and eclectic treatment

To be effective, we saw, the various remedies for melancholy must work together, as complements; no single one will alone be effective beyond the individual case, yet together they might be sufficient. Every imaginable

---

4. For misleading consent language and *double-entendres* in the way the effect has been described to research subjects, see Jopling 2008, Justman 2013.
5. About these links, it has been explained that cognitive therapists "behave within a stoical tradition when they help their patients to change situations which are inherently negative by increasing their sense of control and of coping so they may make all changes that are possible." To illustrate, this passage goes on: "if alternative interpretations and beliefs are not possible and situations cannot be changed, a certain indifference or forbearance is fostered. An analogy would be: "You cannot change a cold, wet summer day into a warm, sunny day. Strong negative emotions in such circumstances would be unhelpful. What would be helpful would be to look for ways of making such an eventuality tolerable—through alternative activities, looking forward to a better day, etc." (Blackburn 1997: 293–4). For further acknowledgment of the Stoic legacies underlying cognitive approaches, see Robertson 2010.

remedy and resource, including those involving daily habits and personal responsibility for healthcare, may be required for effective prevention in any given case. These more eclectic and multifactorial treatments are particularly apt for conceptions of mood disorder that avoid assumptions of the etiological disease model. If there is no single underlying cause, then more eclectic and less specific remedies recommend themselves. Successful as magic bullets have proven with many medical complaints, this implies, there may be no magic bullet for mood disorder. It is a holistic disorder calling for a wide range of separate responses, likely effective only when working together.

Since the last decade of the twentieth century, a worldwide increase throughout medicine in what are known as complementary and alternative medicine approaches (CAMs) has been reported.[6] Parallels between the approaches and practices prescribed in the *Anatomy*, and this endorsement of complementary and alternative forms of medicine are there—although within these contemporary medical settings "complementary medicine" is often merely construed as a replacement or substitute for more traditional approaches.[7] Closer to Burton's ideas, perhaps, are integrated and holistic medicine, which emphasize the emergent properties arising out of the combination of an assortment of remedies. (In a typical definition, "integrated medicine" is said to be a combination of mainstream biomedicine with complementary and alternative medicine, so that such synergistic effects can be attained.[8])

Complementary, alternative, integrated, and holistic approaches are found in many parts of medicine, and research studies have begun to

---

6. The prevalence of CAM therapy use in the United States has increased steadily during the last half of the twentieth century (Kessler et al. 2001). For a wider perspective, Frass et al. (2012) reviewed the use of CAMs from 1990 to 2006, and found an increase in western European countries and the United States, with prevalence rates ranging from 5 to 74.8 percent. (Chiropractic manipulation, herbal medicine, massage, and homeopathy were the therapies most commonly used; and depression was among the ailments most often associated with CAM use.) See also Bodeker et al. 2005. For a critical assessment of such studies, see Eardley et al. 2012.
7. See Rhead 2014, Eardley et al. 2014, Frass et al. 2012.
8. Dobos and Tao 2011:11.

assess their effectiveness.[9] For example, data on lifestyle and mental health is being assembled that apparently confirms the treatment effectiveness of what have been called "therapeutic lifestyle changes," and these correspond quite closely to the *Anatomy*'s recommendations for averting melancholy. (Lifestyle here encompasses elements of the Galenic *regimen*, as well as other factors Burton assumed, or would have gladly included had they occurred to him.[10]) More generally, healthy habits around exercise, diet, and sleep are increasingly recommended for psychiatric disorders, including depression.[11] With the sole, and notable, exception of those combining psychopharmacology and some form of psychotherapy, however, holistic and integrated approaches still often remain outside the treatment repertoire of modern psychiatric medicine and psychopharmacology.[12] They are found within several less medically oriented practices, and many consumer-driven movements. The recovery and rehabilitation models, for example, clearly embody such holistic approaches.[13]

---

9. Research on patients seeking treatment for anxiety and depressive disorders (SADD), designed to measure the effectiveness of more holistic approaches, found them comparable to the effects of conventional (and homeopathic) medicine (Grimaldi-Bensouda et al. 2012).
10. According to one definition, lifestyle comprises exercise, nutrition and diet, time in nature, relationships, recreation, relaxation and stress management, religious or spiritual involvement, and service to others (Walsh 2011:579).
11. In one recent study, the coaching of older adults in healthy dietary habits using cognitive therapy and the Internet was effectively employed to lower the risk of depression (Stahl et al. 2014).
12. For a review of the effectiveness of these combined treatments for depression symptoms, see Pampallona et al. 2004. These researchers' conclusion was that psychological treatment combined with antidepressant therapy is associated with a higher improvement rate than drug treatment alone.
13. In a standard work on this approach, the term "recovery" refers to *a combination* of internal conditions such as attitudes and experiences and external conditions, that together, with reciprocal effects, produce the process of recovery (Jackobson and Greeley 2001). One early example of this recovery paradigm was the Boston University Center for Psychiatric Rehabilitation, whose model for recovery-oriented services includes services directed at symptom relief, crisis intervention, case management, rehabilitation, enrichment, rights protection, basic support, and self-help. See also the emphasis on eclectic responses in the *rehabilitation* model for mental health, measured in terms of "steady progress towards a more systematic, relational and effective application of principles and techniques that presently lie in separate, often isolated, domains." The need is for "systems-wide coherence" in which "all its *disparate values, principles and*

prevention

Understood to include avoiding the onset of illness altogether, preventive medicine is well established today and regularly employed to avert other chronic medical complaints such as heart disease and certain cancers. In contrast to *treatment* for depression once it occurs though, and despite considerable stress on the prevention of reoccurring episodes (or "relapse"), regimens aiming to entirely avoid initial episodes of depression have received less systematic and sustained research attention, and correspondingly little acknowledgment in public health policies.[14] Some explanations for this are perhaps not difficult to guess at. The causes and triggers of mood disorder are at once various, as Burton recognized, and idiosyncratic to the sufferer. Its primary symptoms, subjectively identified and readily concealed, can often be effectively hidden from others, as well as remaining unrecognized by their own sufferer. (Recently developed "depression literacy" public information campaigns attempt to address this last feature.)

Social attitudes compound this. So does the elastic concept of prevention, introduced earlier. Among assessments of preventive efforts, some blur or disregard the distinction between first and subsequent depressive episodes, while others have focused exclusively on later, rather than initial, ones. The accumulating data on preventive measures for mood disorder thus remains difficult to evaluate. Each point is important, along the course of depression (understood as a single, but episodic condition), for the apparently epidemic proportions of initial episodes of unipolar depression persist with subsequent ones.[15]

---

technologies coalesce to provide . . . the effective rehabilitation of people who live with disabling mental illness" (Spaulding et al. 2003:4, emphasis added).

14. Prevention has long been "an important target of intervention in psychology and psychiatry," it has been pointed out, but although effective preventive interventions directed toward high-risk groups have been developed, they have thus far had "poor reach and sustainability in the community" (McLaughlin 2011:361). For these lacunae in one nation's setting (Australia), see also the conclusion that resources have been focused on "reducing the duration of mental disorders through provision of more *treatment* and. . . neglected reducing the incidence of disorders through *prevention*" (Jorm 2014:795, emphasis added).

15. Estimates are inexact, but on one the relapse rate of symptoms during remission and recurrence after an episode of untreated depression is between 50 and 80 percent (Biegler 2011:153).

If today's affective disorders were to be approached according to Burton's recommendations for melancholy, a most obvious practical implication would follow. The present allocation of resources for research and treatment of these disorders would be revised. A shift of attention would occur: *away from* the present focus on idiopathic causes and treatment of late-stage disorder, and *toward* both the identification of all causes, exogenous as well as endogenous, shared as well as idiosyncratic, and early preventive efforts. As well as the acknowledgment and elimination of particular triggers in the external environment, these initiatives might be expected to emphasize individual responsibility for affect regulation and recognition of the care and promotion of mental health as a personal goal.

Toward the prevention (as distinct from the treatment) of mood disorder, attitudes have recently changed, and a trend looks to have begun in some of these directions. In the 1990s, projections drew widespread attention to the magnitude of depression as a serious and growing public health problem, measuring and predicting the cost of untreated depression in terms of mortality and morbidity.[16] In the public health sense of maintaining health and averting and avoiding illness through early intervention and preventive measures, "prevention" has become a watchword.[17] The public health perspective has brought new terminology and analogies, and stress on early intervention. "Behavioral vaccines" are proposed for mental, emotional, and behavioral disorders in young people. "Behavioral vaccine" is a telling phrase, capturing the connotations of epidemic proportions, general risk, and early and effective control that are all hallmarks of public health approaches.[18] With depression construed as a public health issue, screening has followed,

---

16. See Murray 1997. The Global Burden of Disease Study's predictions that depressive disorder would rise to second among the causes of disability were confirmed for developed countries by 2002, by which time it ranked first in developing countries (Mathers et al. 2008).
17. See Cuijpers et al. 2012; also Jorm 2014, McLachlan 2014.
18. See also: "if major depressive episodes can be prevented, the health care system should provide routine access to evidence-based depression prevention interventions, just as it provides inoculations for other common and debilitating health problems" (Munoz et al. 2012:285).

as has increasing research attention. (None of these approaches has proven without problems, it should be added. The metrics for depression symptoms depend on rating scales that have been associated with false positives and confusion over where disorder gives rise to "normal sadness."[19]) That preventive measures can be effective is at last being subject to systematic study, moreover.[20] And the foundations of applying a preventive approach to mental disorders are being explored with awareness that such disorders bring distinctive ethical features.[21]

One of the most comprehensive applications of preventive principles to policy is Australia's "beyondblue" program, launched in 2000. As part that nation's federal National Mental Health Strategy, this organization was to direct attention and resources to mood disorders, primarily depression and anxiety.[22,23] Based on the tenets of cognitive behavioral therapy, its preventive pedagogies associate depression with maladaptive beliefs and cognitive processing styles (thought patterns that are unwarrantedly global, absolute, and past-oriented, particularly, and beliefs that are inappropriately self-critical). For example, beyondblue's SenseAbility program for high-school-age students involves a style of learning aimed to enhance the "protective factors" and "resilience" of students through emphasis on positive psychosocial

19. See Horwitz and Wakefield 2007.
20. For efforts to measure prevention, see Kupfer et al. 1989, Merry et al. 2011, Von Zoonen et al. 2014. In a Cochrane review, Merry and colleagues found fifty-three studies of psychological and educational depression-prevention measures directed toward children and youth, involving fourteen thousand participants; they concluded that a number of studies showed decreased episodes of depressive illness over a year. The Von Zoonen study showed it possible to reduce the incidence of depressive disorder at the rate of prevention carried out with twenty people to avert each new case.
21. The principles guiding a public health approach in relation to mental, emotional, and behavioral (MEB) disorders, it has been asserted, emphasize factors such as the universality of risk, the reduction of stigma, and cost-effectiveness (Embry 2011:3–4).
22. Another, complementary Australian initiative, launched in 2002, the Black Dog Institute, differs in several respects from beyondblue but shares its emphasis on preventive measures undertaken within educational settings.
www.blackdog.org.au
23. As well as promoting early intervention strategies, initiatives are focused around raising awareness and reducing the stigma of depression, supporting consumer and carer advocacy, facilitating training for carers, and funding strategic and applied research related to mood disorders.

adaptation, "depression literacy," self-awareness, and training in self-talk to expunge overly negative cognitive attitudes. An Essential Skills module employs the Stoic-inspired separation between eventualities beyond our power to change, and attitudes toward those eventualities that can be within our control. Through role-play, video, and a range of other techniques, students are taught to recognize negative and unhelpful commentary (in others and also in themselves as self-talk), identifying cognitive errors such as all-or-nothing thinking; overgeneralization; "mind reading" beyond the evidence; exaggeration, in the form of both magnification or minimization; and "catastrophizing" (Irwin, Sheffield, and Holland-Thompson 2010). Emphasis is placed on self-awareness as monitoring and critically evaluating one's thoughts. And, evoking Burton's own approach, students are also subjected to explicit warnings about the risk of disorder associated with uncritical inferences and neglect of these "neuroprotective" forms of self-care.

With its emphasis on prevention and education, this is public health, rather than treatment and care. And it is an approach hearkening back to the ancient practice of maintaining health through efforts to strengthen the host rather than attacking an invader. In keeping with the epidemic metaphors associated with these policy efforts, which speak of establishing "herd immunity" through universal inoculation, those at particular risk for depression are nowhere identified in these pedagogies, and idiopathic risk factors (such as genetic traits) are not stressed. (Depression does have such idiopathic risk factors, and corresponding to the data on prodromal symptoms found to auger the onset of schizophrenia, we might expect to see data on prodromal or subthreshold symptoms for depression. Certainly the usefulness of this approach to the prevention of other disorders has been emphasized.[24,25] Yet prospective studies of affective disorder have been few, and successful primarily in identifying the harbingers of bipolar, not unipolar, depression.[26] Explaining this

---

24. McGorry et al. 2002.
25. Prodromal symptoms have been observed to precede the full syndrome by weeks or months, and "if these symptoms are detected, recurrences of affective disorders ... could be treated earlier and perhaps more effectively" (Fava et al. 1991:149). See also Fava and Tossani 2007.
26. Jackson et al. 2003.

dearth of positive findings, it has been pointed out that with its large individual variability, the prodromal phase of unipolar depression lacks sufficient diagnostic specificity to be of use.[27] And prospective study from prodromes through to the point of fully developed disorder, it has been observed, would similarly involve assessment of an unwieldy collection of variables.[28] Too many causes, as Burton pointed out for melancholy.)

Public health as we know it was not a concept understood or available in the early seventeenth century. Yet in these recent initiatives aimed at "strengthening the host" afforded by today's public health structures, we seem to be seeing the start of a welcome redistribution of resources, policy and research attention toward preventive mental health.[29]

agency and self-care

Burton's habituation model finds its obvious correlate in an increased emphasis on personal agency and on the importance of healthy habits and whole "lifestyle" approaches to affect regulation, together with their implications for personal self-care and early prevention. Attention is directed toward daily habits and other aspects of everyday life. In taking responsibility for their health, those with disorder are self-determining agents, on this analysis, appropriately in charge of regulating their own moods. Rather than states that assail us, against which we are powerless, those moods are here conceived more as aspects of the selves we actively construct, and must tend, in the manner of classical care of the soul.

---

27. Fava et al. 2013. Thus, Fava and colleagues identified as unhelpfully generic the prodromal features of anxiety, irritability, impaired work and interests, fatigue, and insomnia.
28. At the least, these include personality, neurotic traits, and their interaction in the evolution of affective disorders (Fava et al. 2001). Prodromal symptoms have been identified for the subcategory of unipolar depression known as hopelessness depression, where symptoms of hopelessness predominate, followed by self-blame, brooding, decreased self-esteem, dependency, and decreased appetite (Iacoviello et al. 2013). And patients have been shown able to monitor such moods, with subsequent clinical usefulness (Jackson et al. 2003).
29. Although welcome, it will require close scrutiny and monitoring from bioethics as it proceeds. See Radden 2016.

Within the range of responses to untypical mood states and even to diagnosed mood disorder today, it is possible to find many instances where assumptions such as these have already been embraced and put into practice. Outside of mainstream psychiatry, for example, several consumer-driven movements, including the recovery and rehabilitation models, strongly emphasize agency and personal responsibility for healthcare.[30]

Burton's stress on early prevention for melancholy anticipates the collection of changed attitudes described above. When responsibility is put in the hands of the individual early, the condition is still amenable to such an approach. If neglected at the start, according to the *Anatomy* analysis, self-care will likely prove too little, too late. When melancholy has become an entrenched habit, agency is lost, and the sufferer must submit to the care of others. Today, the person with depression is often depicted as powerless in the face of her disorder and, when the disorder is severe, too disabled to help herself. How much this reflects a confirmation of Burton's ideas, because the helpless and passive depression patient exhibits a degree of severity that *would have been averted* earlier by preventive measures, is a puzzling counterfactual about which, without empirical data, we can only speculate. Nonetheless, given the stakes, such speculation—and research—seem worthwhile.

Medical psychiatry's slow recognition that depression may be a fully or partially preventable condition suggests an underlying perception that the salient risk factors are beyond the individual's control: temperamental patterns and other genetic tendencies that, if not complete predictors of depression, function as inexorably powerful diatheses, to

---

30. An emphasis on agency is integrated within the rhetoric and principles of the recovery movement, where the aim of the recovery model is said to be "to have consumers assume more and more responsibility for themselves." Particular responsibilities include developing goals, working with providers and others to make plans for reaching these goals, taking on decision-making tasks, and engaging in self-care. In addition, responsibility is stressed a factor in making choices and taking risks: "full empowerment requires that consumers live with the consequences of their choices" (Jackobson and Greenley 2003:3). A similar emphasis on agency is found in models emphasizing rehabilitation over treatment. Unlike treatment, their purpose is "to overcome disabilities that are barriers toward realizing one's own wishes and aspirations. The role of all participants is to identify goals and work towards them" (Spaulding, Sullivan, and Poland 2003:17).

be triggered unavoidably, by the inevitable slings and arrows of everyday life.[31] The study of prevention in relation to mood disorder often employs rhetoric (such as reference to recognizing and *monitoring* symptoms), with the rather somber implication that monitoring is the best we can do. And certainly, self-awareness must be a first step in self-care. Yet "monitoring" sometimes suggests an end, rather than a step toward, and precondition of, agency. And language, of course, matters—both as an indication of underlying assumptions on the part of the speaker, and in its effect on its hearer.

Common-cause etiological disease models, and their allied magic bullet conceptions of remedy for depression exemplified within psychopharmacology, also reveal an attitude toward the agency of the sufferer that may be overly deterministic. By contrast, cognitive psychotherapies seem to position the subject more actively, as capable of not only monitoring but also adjusting and regulating her own affective states. (This approach has a ready aid and an obvious application in the Internet, which has been noted, bringing new models for the self-directed patient.[32]) Those who are depression-prone can learn to recognize and avoid stressors, even with causal models wherein the initial vulnerability remains their immovable fate.[33] These are matters of degree, nevertheless. The depressed patient who faithfully adheres to the often tedious and discomforting process of acquiring suitable medicine, and observes her pharmaceutical regimen faithfully, is exerting agency also.

Our reluctance to attribute responsibility for mental health care to the individual may not all lie in our unwarrantedly deterministic

---

31. In one hypothesis, such unalterable factors have been identified with abnormalities in the serotonin transporter gene and unchecked cortisol damaging the hippocampus linked to a lack of underlying "neuroresiliance" in the face of stressors, that result in vulnerability to depression (Kramer 2005). Another hypotheses, as we saw, posits dysfunction or even breakdown in a mechanism designed to deal with loss, the "loss response mechanism" (Horwitz and Wakefield 2007).
32. See Hollandare et al. 2011, Van Voorhees et al. 2011, Van Staten, Cuijpers, and Smits 2008, Valimaki et al. 2012.
33. The relative merits of antidepressants and CBT in promoting patient autonomy have been analyzed in terms of reduced rumination, negative attribution, and enhanced problem-solving capability. Because it provides better self-understanding in relation to stressors, CBT has been assessed to be a preferable treatment (Biegler 2011:119–141).

rhetoric, nor yet in the misapplication of a disease model more appropriate for bacterial infections. For example, knowingly undertaking preventive measures such as Burton suggests requires us to *imagine future states of pain and suffering* as likely, if not inevitable. And perhaps the affliction is not so much an unmovable fate too obdurate to avert through prevention, as too distressing for us to imaginatively anticipate. Knowing the distress and trouble that life will inevitably bring, we may not easily entertain those imaginings during times of more carefree happiness or contentment, or want them to dampen the exuberant joys of youth by introducing early preventive measures. The halting progress of attempts to plan for the occurrence of mental disorder more generally, even in the case of predicted recurring episodes, suggests that this may be so for other conditions as well. For more organic symptoms, including the reduced psychological function of degenerative diseases, we plan through living wills and other advance directives. By contrast, we are perhaps more reluctant to anticipate unipolar mood disorders.

The *Anatomy* is in many ways a fearful and gloomy work. Yet to his credit, Burton faces the prospect of Melancholy unblinkingly—and more squarely than we seem inclined to do our own potential future suffering. "Thou dost now flourish," he warns, with goods of body, mind, and fortune. Yet,

> thou knowest not what stormes and tempests the late evening may bring with it. Be not secure then, be sober and watch. (I, 2,5,5:380)

RESEARCH HYPOTHESES

Three ideas arising out of the *Anatomy* are sufficiently significant as to deserve research attention. The first is the relationship between severe and mild states of melancholy; the second is the conception of disease applied to affective disorders and their treatment; and the third is the role played by the functions of the Burtonian Imagination, or default system processing, in affective disorder and affect regulation.

severity

The relationship between severe and milder states of disorder is established in the *Anatomy* on a habituation model, we saw. The more advanced and entrenched these feelings and thought patterns become, the more severe, and difficult to treat—so that eventually, they may have been incrementally transformed into the chronic, probably incurable condition Burton calls Melancholy the Habit.

Its reliance on the practical criterion of treatability leaves this model orthogonal to the familiar distinction by which disorders are either continuous with, or categorically distinct from, normal functioning, we also saw. Melancholy is a disorder of the kind best described as "practical," in that the different forms it takes depend on such practical questions of treatability. This status as a practical kind leaves any analogy between melancholy and the mood disorders of today difficult to assess, whether our focus is less severe types of depressive disorder, or subtypes distinguished within contemporary disease taxonomies, such as melancholic depression. Rather than bearing a relation of type to subtype, the differences today cited between these two forms of depression have sometimes instead been taken to indicate the presence of two distinct categories, one the underlying, endogenous state of melancholic depression marked by its relative severity. This sounds somewhat like Burtonian Melancholy, and has been explicitly identified with melancholy of old. But, on Burton's account Melancholy is a progressive disorder: severity comes from repetition. If this habituation analysis has any force, depressive disorder and melancholic depression may reflect *less* and *more advanced stages*, respectively, of a single type of progressive (habituated) condition.

In the first decades of the twenty-first century, the standard classificatory systems hitherto employed by clinical and research psychiatry have been subject to a radical critique, in which their validity and usefulness as research tools has been challenged.[34] With classificatory psychiatry subject to such unprecedented new scrutiny and revision, the hypothesis that a habituation model may allow us to conceive of

---

34. Cuthbert et al. 2013.

and subdivide mood disorders differently seems not out of place. And the above suggests that three alternatives are distinguishable. One hypothesis is that depressive disorder and melancholic depression are entirely separate disorders; a second is that they are type and subtype of one disorder; and a third is the Burtonian alterative, that they are *different stages of a single disorder*, viewed longitudinally. Until subject to some form of empirical testing to establish their relative explanatory and predictive advantages, none of these alternative hypotheses can be counted out, within the current disarray that is contemporary psychiatric classification.

disease concepts

About the conception of disease best applied to mood disorders, we saw that the *Anatomy* can be read to make use of the symptom-focused model widely employed before the nineteenth century, which emphasizes a disorder's natural history observed through time. Although not entirely foreign to Galenic medicine, the bacteriological or germ theory conception is a product of a later era, and of vastly greater medical knowledge. With its single, localized causes, and explanatory fecundity, yielding effective, specific antidotes for so many illnesses, the bacterial model postdates Burton. But mood disorders may not resemble bacterial infections as closely as many other diseases do. And the bacterial disease model may not be as applicable to the treatment of mood disorders today as has been widely supposed. Burton did not construe Melancholy in common-cause etiological terms; and perhaps it may also be misleading to so construe depression. Such is the position urged by Kendler, Borsboom, and colleagues, as we saw, whose revised thinking casts depression as a network of many separate causes that are interrelated and reinforced in looping subinteractions. In another variant on standard common-cause etiological disease models, there is also growing employment of diathesis-stress conceptions of mood disorder, where inherent tendencies are triggered by setbacks and adverse life experiences.

Following these recent, revised models, disordered depression (and anxiety) would better be understood in one of two ways, each familiar from the *Anatomy*. They might be construed as a network of symptoms resulting from any number of causes, external and internal, and loosely linked together through interactive subnetworks of causally related symptoms. Alternatively, they might be taken to result from the interaction between stable internal diatheses or risk factors combined with external triggers to produce symptoms. On either interpretation, they diverge from the common-cause etiological model guiding much contemporary psychiatry. Recent efforts that compare the results of common-cause and network models of depression are just the kind of hypothesis-testing science that Burton's analysis of melancholy would seem to demand.[35]

Misleading presuppositions are shared by the common-cause etiological disease models and the "magic bullet" thinking associated with many of today's ideas about treatment. Forming the basis of psychopharmacology, these ideas presuppose that the underlying cause should be subject to a specific, targeted response. If not all disorders involve a single, specific, discoverable underlying dysfunction, however, and no such cause is to be found for mood disorders, then older treatment approaches that emphasize strengthening the host may be a more appropriate than those employing the newer tropes, with their emphasis on vanquishing invaders.

From a rejection of bacterial models for mood disorder, it also follows that temporally separated episodes of symptoms are not ipso facto to be counted as parts of one discrete, disease entity. On an etiological model a relation of identity unites earlier and later episodes of a single disorder, and this is by conceptual necessity. With mood disorders understood as networks of causally interacting symptoms, the relation between earlier and later episodes is merely empirical. Whether disorders such as melancholy and depression are unitary entities will be determined by the symptom pattern they exhibit through time.

But that said, the Burtonian picture is not one in which the symptom picture of melancholy could have changed so radically as to be unrecognizably different from one decade, or era, to the next. The

---

35. See Cramer et al. 2011, discussed in chapter 3.

symptoms of melancholy may be infinite in variety; and sadness and fear are not depicted as unfailingly present, essential features. But the relation of sadness, particularly, to normal affections, together with their interactive link with the imagination, leave unwarranted and excessive fear and sadness permanent, rather than passing, characteristics of melancholy. As the "nature of Mortalitie," states of sadness and sorrow remain integral to normal human experience, as Burton recognizes. One implication of this, as we saw, is that the contested boundaries of "normal sadness" remain an unavoidable issue for contemporary mind science. Determining the boundaries of normal affective response in relation to feelings as resonantly human and normatively weighted, however, renders any negotiation over sorrow and sadness one between science and society, not merely an issue of psychiatric classification.

imagination (simulation)

The role of the imagination in affective disorder and affect regulation points the way toward further research hypotheses. One of these concerns medical epistemology, the other, risk factors for depression.

Today, as never before, new technologies allow scientists to observe and measure aspects of default system functioning, including the mind-wandering states that have been shown correlated with depressive disorder. The meaning of those correlations, and whether the close and iterative relationship between imagining (or simulating) and feeling, proposed in the *Anatomy*, offers an accurate picture of cognitive processing, is a matter that science is now better positioned to confirm or dismiss. With such findings in hand, support for the ancient approaches to affect regulation laid out in the Second Partition can become the subject of testing.

A more controversial implication of the part played by the imagination relates to the powerful expectation effects Burton takes to influence whether melancholy becomes severe in any given case. The vulnerability of the imagination to negative ideas with nocebo effects, together with the intimate link between imagination and affective states, we saw, encourages Burton to suppose that even exposure to a book about melancholy might serve to cause it, in a person already so predisposed. If exposure to ideas about melancholy invites it, then a form of social contagion will be a serious risk.

We do not generally regard depression as a contagious disorder. (Although little studied, psychological contagions are loosely judged to include the transfer of "memes," themes, and ideas in ways that bypass the flow of ideas from one person to another in what is known as normal social learning, when both are cognizant of its occurrence.) Yet robust placebo effects are recognized to influence the course and severity of milder depressive symptoms. And if there are parallels between placebo and nocebo effects, we can expect that nocebo effects might be similarly powerful. Exposure to others suffering from depression, for example, might be a risk factor, increasing the likelihood of comparably negative outcomes. Whether through contact with peers, exposure to advertising, social media, or a combination of those, individuals today are subject to many influences bearing similarities to the person-to-person contact that brings epidemics. Burton's idea, in that case, is not so far-fetched. At the least, it seems to suggest a hypothesis deserving further attention. Along the lines of attempts to identify clusters of other disorders and behavioral syndromes (like suicide), the evidence for such contagion can be sought empirically. If there are no depression clusters, then that aspect of Burton's speculations can be put to rest.

It would be a mistake to yearn for Burton's times, attitudes, or beliefs, as we confront the "epidemicall" mood disorders of today. Yet the corner of today's mind sciences engaged with the study, treatment, and care of such disorders is an arena so important; so filled with incomplete knowledge, unexplained phenomena, and unresolved challenges; and so central to all cognition and, indeed, much human endeavor, that even Burton's *Anatomy* might be able to help. The selective and interpretive reading undertaken here invites few sure answers, but it does raise a number of fundamental questions. Might it be helpful to relinquish orthodox conceptions of disease for mood disorders? Could greater emphasis on the role of early prevention alter the course of such complaints? Might an understanding of disordered moods as cognitive habits amenable to correction lift the sense of finality associated with much deterministic talk of genetic predispositions? Could the power of expectation be harnessed for more effective self-healing? Is friendship our best bulwark against psychic suffering? Are mood disorders better seen as habits?

Each of these ideas has its supporters today. But let us also credit Robert Burton for entertaining them, and entertaining us with them.

REFERENCES

Addis, D.R., Pan, L., Vu, M.A., Laiser, N. and Schacter, D.L. 2009. Constructive episodic simulation of the future and the past: Distinct subsystems of a core brain network mediate imagining and remembering. *Neuropsychologia* 47(11):2222–2238.

Adriaens, P.R., and De Block, A. 2013. Why we essentialize mental disorders. *Journal of Medicine and Philosophy* 38:107–127.

Akiskal, H.S., and McKinney, W.T. 1973. Depressive disorders: toward a unified hypothesis: clinical, experimental, genetic, biochemical, and neurophysiological data are integrated. *Science* 182:285–305.

Ariely, D. 2008. *Predictably Irrational: The Hidden Forces That Shape Our Decisions.* New York: HarperCollins.

American Psychiatric Association. 1980. *DSM-III-R: Diagnostic and Statistical Manual of Mental Disorders.* Washington DC: American Psychiatric Association.

American Psychiatric Association. 1994. *Diagnostic and Statistical Manual of Mental Disorders.* Fourth Edition. Washington, DC: American Psychiatric Association.

American Psychiatric Association. 2011. *Major Depressive Disorder and the "Bereavement Exclusion."* Washington DC: American Psychiatric Publishing.

American Psychiatric Association. 2013. *Diagnostic and Statistical Manual of Mental Disorders.* Fifth Edition. Washington, DC: American Psychiatric Association.

Anderson, R. J., Dewhurst, S.A. and Nash, R. 2012. Shared cognitive processes underlying past and future thinking: The impact of imagery and concurrent task demands on event specificity. *Journal of Experimental Psychology: Learning, Memory, and Cognition* 38(2): 356–365.

Anderson, B. 2010. Preemption, precaution, preparedness: anticipatory action and future geographies. *Progress in Human Geography* 34:777–798.

Andreason, N.C. 1982. Concepts, diagnosis and classification. In *Handbook of Affective Disorders*, edited by E.S. Paykel. New York: Guilford Press; 22–44.

Andrews, G. 2001. Placebo response in depression: bane of research, boon of therapy. *British Journal of Psychiatry* 178:192–194.

Andrews, P.W., and Thomson, J.A. 2009. Depression's evolutionary roots. *Scientific American*, August 25.

Andrews-Hanna, J.R., Smallwood, J., and Spreng, R.N. 2014. The default network and self-generated thought: component processes, dynamic control, and clinical relevance. *Annals of the New York Academy of Sciences* 1316:29–52. doi: 10.1111/nyas.12360.

Angst, J. 1986. *Schizoaffective Psychoses*. Berlin: Springer.

Angst, J. 1997. Depression and anxiety: implications for nosology, course, and treatment. *Journal of Clinical Psychiatry* 58(Suppl 8):3–10.

Arikha, Noga 2007. *Passions and Tempers: A History of the Humours*. New York: HarperCollins Publishers.

Aristotle. 1985. *Nichomachean Ethics*. Translated with an Introduction by Terence Irwin. Indianapolis and Cambridge: Hackett Publishing Company.

Armitage, R. 2007. Sleep and circadian rhythms in mood disorders. *Acta Psychiatrica Scandinavica* 11(5):104–115.

Aubrey, J. 1949. *Brief Lives*, edited by O.L. Dick. London: Secker & Warburg.

Babb, L. 1959. *Sanity in Bedlam: A Study of Robert Burton's Anatomy of Melancholy*. Westport, CT: Greenwood.

Baird, B., et al. 2012. Inspired by distraction mind wandering facilitates creative incubation. *Psychological Science* 23(10):1117–1122. doi: 10.1177/0956797612446024. Epub 2012 Aug 31

Bakke, A.C., Purtzer, M.Z., and Newton, P. 2002. The effect of hypnotic-guided imagery on psychological well-being and immune function in patients with prior breast cancer. *Journal of Psychosomatic Research* 53:1131–1137.

Baldwin, D.S., et al. 2002. Can we distinguish anxiety from depression? *Psychopharmacology Bulletin* 36:158–165.

Baltussen, H. (ed). 2012. *Greek and Roman Consolations: 8 Studies of a Tradition and its Aftermath*. Swansea: Classical Press of Wales.

Baltzly, D. 2014. Stoicism. In *Stanford Encyclopedia of Philosophy* (Spring 2014 Edition), edited by E.N. Zalta. http://plato.stanford.edu/archives/spr2014/entries/stoicism/

Bamborough, J.B. 1952. *The Little World of Man*. London: Longmans, Green.

Bamborough, J.B. 1989–2000. Introduction to *The Anatomy of Melancholy* by Robert Burton, edited by T. Faulkner, N. Kiessling, and R. Blair. Oxford: Oxford University Press; viii–xxxvi.

REFERENCES

Barlow, D.H., and Campbell, L.A. 2000. Mixed anxiety-depression and its implications for models of mood and anxiety disorders. *Comprehensive Psychiatry* 41(2 Suppl 1):53–60.

Bayne, T., and Pacherie, E. 2005. In defence of the doxastic conception of delusions. *Mind and Language* 20:163–188.

Beard, M. 2014. How stoical was Seneca? *New York Review of Books*, October 9: 31–33.

Beck, A.T., et al. 1979. *Cognitive Therapy of Depression*. New York: Guilford Press.

Beck, A.T., and Alford, B.A. 2009. *Depression: Causes and Treatment*. Philadelphia: University of Pennsylvania Press.

Beck, A.T., Emery, G., and Greenberg, R.L. 2005. *Anxiety Disorders and Phobias: A Cognitive Perspective*. New York: Basic Books.

Beecher, H.K. 1955. The powerful placebo. *Journal of the American Medical Association* 159:1602–1606.

Beer, M.D. 1996. Psychosis: a history of the concept. *Comprehensive Psychiatry* 37:273–291.

Bell, M. 2014. *Melancholia: The Western Malady*. Cambridge: Cambridge University Press.

Bensafi, M., et al. 2003. Olfactomotor activity during imagery mimics that during perception. *Nature Neuroscience* 6(11): 1142–1144.

Bentall, R. 1994. *Madness Explained*. London: Penguin.

Berman, M.G., Jonides, J., and Kaplan, S. 2008. The cognitive benefits of interacting with nature. *Psychological Science* 22: 596–601.

Berrios, G. 1985. The psychopathology of affectivity: conceptual and historical aspects. *Psychological Medicine* 15:745–758.

Berrios, G. 1995. The anhedonias: a conceptual history. *History of Psychiatry* 6:453–470.

Berrios, G. 1996. *The History of Mental Symptoms: Descriptive Psychopathology since the Nineteenth Century*. Cambridge: Cambridge University Press.

Berrios, G. 2011. Preface to *Diseases of the Imagination and Imaginary Disease in the Early Modern Period*, edited by Y. Haskell. Turnhout: Brepols; xv–xxiii.

Berrios, G., and Porter, R. (eds). 1995. *A History of Clinical Psychiatry: The Origin and History of Psychiatric Disorders*. New York: New York University Press.

Berrios, G.E. 1991. Delusions as "wrong beliefs": a conceptual history. *British Journal of Psychiatry* 159:6–13.

Biegler, P. 2011. *The Ethical Treatment of Depression: Autonomy through Psychotherapy*. Cambridge, MA: MIT Press.

Bigelsen, J., and Schupak, C. 2011. Compulsive fantasy: proposed evidence of an under-reported syndrome through a systematic study of 90 self-identified non-normative fantasizers. *Consciousness and Cognition* 20:1634–1648.

Blackburn, I. 1997. Commentary on "The Stoic Conception of Mental Disorder". *Philosophy, Psychiatry, and Psychology* 4:293–294.

REFERENCES

Blackwell, S.E., et al. 2013. Optimism and mental imagery: a possible cognitive marker to promote well-being? *Psychiatry Research* 206.1:56–61.

Blackwood, N.J., et al. 2004. Persecutory delusions and the determination of self-relevance: an fMRI investigation. *Psychological Medicine* 34:591–596.

Block, N. 2010. What was i thinking? *New York Times*, November 26.

Bodeker, G., et al. 2005. *Global Atlas of Traditional, Complementary and Alternative Medicine*. Kobe, Japan: World Health Organization.

Bonanno, G.A. 2004. Loss, trauma, and human resilience: have we underestimated the human capacity to thrive after extremely aversive events? *American Psychologist* 59:20–28.

Bonne, O., et al. 2004. Adaptive and maladaptive psychobiological responses to severe psychological stress: implications for the discovery of novel pharmacotherapy. *Neuroscience and Biobehavioral Reviews* 28:65–94.

Boorde, A. 1547? *The Breviarie of Health*. Bibliographical details of this work are unknown.

Borsboom, D. 2008. Psychometric perspectives on diagnostic systems. *Journal of Clinical Psychology* 64:1089–1108.

Borsboom, D., and Cramer, A.O.J. 2013. Network analysis: an integrative approach to the structure of psychopathology. *Annual Review of Clinical Psychology* 9:91–121.

Bortolotti, L. 2010. *Delusions and Other Irrational Beliefs*. Oxford: Oxford University Press.

Boulenger, J.-P., et al. 1997. Mixed anxiety and depression: from theory to practice. *Journal of Clinical Psychiatry* 58(8 Suppl):27–34.

Boyd, R. 1991. Realism, anti-foundationalism, and the enthusiasm for natural kinds. *Philosophical Studies* 61:127–148.

Brann, E.T.H. 1991. *The World of Imagination: Sum and Substance*. Savage, MD: Rowman & Littlefield.

Bright, T. 1995. *A Treatise of Melancholy*. New York: The Classics of Psychiatry & Behavioral Sciences Library.

Broome, M., and Bortolotti, L. 2009. *Psychiatry as Cognitive Neuroscience: Philosophical Perspectives*. Oxford: Oxford University Press.

Broome, M., and McGuire, P.K. 2009. Imagining and delusions. In *Persecutory Delusions: Assessment, Theory and Treatment*, edited by D. Freeman, R. Bentall, and P. Garety. Oxford: Oxford University Press.

Brown, W. 1998. The placebo effect. *Scientific American* (January):90–95.

Buckner, R.L., and Vincent, J.L. 2007. Unrest at rest: default activity and spontaneous network correlations. *Neuroimage* 37:1091–1096.

Buckner, R.L. and Carroll, D.C. 2007. Self-projection and the brain. *Trends in Cognitive Sciences* 11(2):49–57.

Buhle, J.T., et al. 2014. Cognitive reappraisal of emotion: a meta-analysis of human neuroimaging studies. *Cerebral Cortex* 24:2981–2990.

REFERENCES

Burton, R. 1632/1989–2000. *The Anatomy of Melancholy*. 6 vols. Edited by Thomas Faulkner, Nicolas Kiessling, and Rhonda Blair. Vols. I–III: text; vols. IV–VI: commentary by J.B. Bamborough and Martin Dodsworth. Oxford: Oxford University Press.

Bush, D. 1962. *English Literature in the Seventeenth Century*. New York: Oxford University Press.

Callahan, C.M., and Berrios, G.E. 2005. *Reinventing Depression: A History of the Treatment of Depression in Primary Care, 1940–2004*. Oxford: Oxford University Press.

Carey, B. 2012. Grief could join list of disorders. *New York Times*, January 24.

Carroll, B. et al. 1981. A specific laboratory test for the diagnosis of Melancholia. *British Medical Journal* 2:285–287.

Carter, C.K. 2003. *The Rise of Causal Concepts of Disease*. London: Ashgate.

Chalmers, D. 1996. *The Conscious Mind: In Search of a Fundamental Theory*. Oxford: Oxford University Press.

Charland, L. 2010. Reinstating the passions: arguments from the history of psychopathology. *Oxford Handbook of Philosophy of Emotion*; 237–259.

Collins, M.P., and Dunn, L.F. 2005. The effects of meditation and visual imagery on an immune system disorder: dermatomyositis. *Journal of Alternative and Complementary Medicine* 11:275–284.

Coltheart, M. 2013. On the distinction between monothematic and polythematic delusions. *Mind and Language* 28:103–112.

Cooper, R. 2007. *Psychiatry and Philosophy of Science*. Stocksfield, UK: Acumen.

Cooper, J.M. 2012. *Pursuit of Wisdom: Six Ways of Life in Ancient Philosophy*. London: Princeton University Press.

Cottingham, J. 1998. *Philosophy and the Good Life: Reason and the Passions in Greek, Cartesian and Psychoanalytic Ethics*. Cambridge: Cambridge University Press.

Cramer, A.O.J., et al. 2012. The pathoplasticity of dysphoric episodes: differential impact of stressful life events on the pattern of depressive symptom intercorrelations. *Psychological Medicine* 42:957–965.

Cratsley, K. In press. *The Architecture of Delusion: On Cognitive Models of Pathological Belief*. Cambridge, MA: MIT Press.

Craver, C. 2009. Mechanisms and natural kinds. *Philosophical Psychology* 22:575–594.

Crowther, H.J. 1983. Stress management training and relaxation imagery in the treatment of essential hypertension. *Journal of Behavioral Medicine* 6:169–187.

Cuijpers, P. 1997. Bibliotherapy in unipolar depression. *Journal of Behavior Therapy and Experimental Psychiatry* 28:139–147.

Cuijpers, P., et al. 2012. Preventing depression: a global priority. *Journal of the American Medical Association* 307:1033–1034.

REFERENCES

Culpeper, N. 1985. *Culpeper's Compete Herbal.* Ware, Hertfordshire: Omega Books.

Currie, G. 2000. Imagination, delusion and hallucination. In *Pathologies of Belief*, edited by M. Coltheart and M. Davies. Oxford: Blackwell; 167–182.

Currie, G., and Jureidini, J. 2004. Narrative and coherence. *Mind and Language* 19:409–427.

Currie, G., and Ravenscroft, I. 2002. *Recreative Imagination.* Oxford: Oxford University Press.

Cuthbert, B.N., and Insel, T.R. 2013. Toward precision medicine in psychiatry: the NIMH Research Domain Criteria Project. In *Neurobiology of Mental Illness*, Fourth Edition, edited by D. Charney et al. Oxford: Oxford University Press; 1076–1088.

Damasio, A. 1994. *Descartes' Error: Emotion, Reason, and the Human Brain.* New York: Putnam & Sons.

Damasio, A. 1999. *The Feeling of What Happens: Body and Emotion in the Making of Consciousness.* New York: Harcourt Brace.

Damasio, A. 2012. *Self Comes to Mind: Constructing the Conscious Brain.* New York: Knopf Doubleday Publishing Group.

Darwin, C. 2007. *The Expression of Emotions in Man and Animals.* New York: Filiquarian Publishing.

Davies, A.M.A, et al. 2009. Cognitive and motivational factors in anosognosia. *Delusion and Self-Deception: Affective and Motivational Influences on Belief Formation*, edited by Tim Bayne and Jordi Fernandez. New York: Psychology Press; 187–225.

Davies, M., et al. 2001. Monothematic delusions: towards a two-factor account. *Philosophy, Psychiatry and Psychology* 8:133–158.

Davies, A.M.A. and Davies, M. 2009. Explaining pathologies of belief. *Psychiatry as Cognitive Neuroscience: Philosophical Perspectives.* Oxford: Oxford University Press; 285–326.

Davies, M., and Coltheart, M. 2000. Introduction: pathologies of belief. *Mind and Language* 15(1):1–46.

Day, C., et al. 2015. Impairment and distress patterns distinguishing the melancholic depressive subtype: an iSPOT0D report. *Journal of Affective Disorders* 174:493–502.

Deigh, J. 2010. Concepts of emotion in modern philosophy and psychology. In *The Oxford Handbook of Philosophy of Emotion*, edited by P. Goldie. Oxford: Oxford University Press; 17–40.

Demazeux, S., and Singy, P. (eds). 2015. *The DSM-5 in Perspective: Philosophical Reflections on the Psychiatric Babel.* New York: Springer.

Den Boer, J.A. 1997. Psychopharmacology of comorbid obsessive-compulsive disorder and depression. *Journal of Clinical Psychiatry* 58(Suppl 8):17–19.

Descartes, R. 1961. Passions of the soul. In *Essential Works of Descartes*, translated by Lowell Bair. New York: Bantam Books.

REFERENCES

Descartes, R. 1960 *Discourse on Method and Medititations*. Indianapolis and New York: The Bobbs-Merrill Company Inc.

Descartes, R. 1985. *The World and Treatise of Man*. In *Philosophical Writings of Descartes*, vol. 1, translated by J. Cottingham, R. Stoothoff, and D. Murdock. Cambridge: Cambridge University Press; 79–99.

Diekhof, E.K., et al. 2011. The power of imagination—how anticipatory mental imagery alters perceptual processing of fearful facial expressions. *NeuroImage* 54:1703–1714.

Disner, S.G., et al. 2011. Neural mechanisms of the cognitive model of depression. *Nature Reviews Neuroscience* 12:467–477.

Dixon, T. 2003. *From Passion to Emotion: The Creation of a Secular Psychological Category*. Cambridge: Cambridge University Press.

Dobson, K.S. (ed). 2010. *Handbook of Cognitive Behavioural Therapies*. New York: Guilford Press.

Dobos, G., and Tao, I. 2011. The model of western integrative medicine: the role of Chinese medicine. *Chinese Journal of Integrated Medicine* 17:11–20.

Dowrick, C., and Frances, A. 2013. Medicalising unhappiness: new classification of depression risks more patients being put on drug treatment from which they will not benefit. *British Medical Journal* 347(7): 7140.

DSM-5 Mood Disorders Workgroup. 2010. *Rationale for Anxiety Dimension*. http://www.dsm5.org/Documents/Mood

Du Laurens, A. 1599/1938. *A Discourse of the Preservation of the Sight: of Melancholike Diseases; of Rheumes, and of Old Age*, by M. Andreas Laurentius, translated by Richard Surphlet. London: Humphrey Milford, Oxford University Press, Amen House, Warwick Square, E.C.

Dunning, D., and Story, A.L. 1991. Depression, realism, and the overconfidence effect: are the sadder wiser when predicting future actions and events? *Journal of Personality and Social Psychology* 61:521.

Eardley, S., et al. 2012. A systematic literature review of complementary and alternative medicine prevalence in EU. *Research in Complementary Medicine* 19 (Suppl 2): 18–28.

Egan, A. 2009. Imagination, delusion and self-deception. In *Delusion and Self-Deception: Affective and Motivational Influences on Belief Formation*, edited by T. Bayne and J. Fernandez. New York: Psychology Press; 263–280.

Ehrenberg, A. 2010. *The Weariness of the Self: Diagnosing the History of Depression in the Contemporary Age*. Montreal, Kingston, London, Ithaca: McGill-Queens University Press.

Ellis, B. 2001. *Scientific Essentialism*. Cambridge: Cambridge University Press.

Elster, J., and Loewenstein, G.F. 1992. Utility from memory and anticipation. In *Choice over Time*, edited by G.F. Loewenstein and J. Elster. New York: Russell Sage Foundation; 213–234.

Elyot, T. 1539. *The Castel of Helth*. London.

REFERENCES

Embry, D.D. 2011. Behavioral vaccines and evidence-based kernels: nonpharmaceutical approaches for the prevention of mental, emotional, and behavioural disorders. *Psychiatric Clinics of North America* 34:1–24.

Epictetus. 1926. *The Discourses as Reported by Arrian, the Manual and Fragments.* Translated by W.A. Oldfather. London: William Heinemann.

Erasmus, Desiderius 2004. *The Praise of Folly.* Translated by John Wilson. New York: Barnes & Noble Books.

Evans, B. 1972. *The Psychiatry of Robert Burton.* New York: Octagon Books.

Evans, D. 2001. *Emotion: The Science of Sentiment.* Oxford: Oxford University Press.

Ereshefsky, M. 2009. Defining "health" and "disease." Studies in the History and Philosophy of Biology and Biomedical Sciences 40:221–227.

Fassler, M., et al. 2010. Frequency and circumstances of placebo use in clinical practice—a systematic review of empirical studies. *BMC Medicine* 8:15.

Fava, G., et al. 1990. Prodromal symptoms in primary major depressive disorder. *Journal of Affective Disorders* 19:149–152.

Fava, G.A., and Kellner, R. 1991. Prodromal symptoms in affective disorders. *American Journal of Psychiatry* 148:823–830.

Fava, G.A., and Mangelli, L. 2001. Assessment of subclinical symptoms and psychological well-being in depression. *European Archives of Psychiatry and Clinical Neuroscience* 251(2):47–52.

Fava, G.A., and Tossani, E. 2007. Prodromal stage of major depression. *Early Intervention in Psychiatry* 1(1):9–18.

Ficino, M. 1482/1989. *Three Books on Life.* A critical edition and translation with introduction and notes by C. Kaske and J. Clark. Binghamton, New York: Medieval and Renaissance Texts and Studies, in conjunction with the Renaissance Society of America,

Fine, C. 2006 *A Mind of Its Own: How Your Brain Distorts and Deceives.* New York: Norton.

Fink, M. 2008. The medical evidence-based model for psychiatric syndromes: return to a classical model. *Acta Psychiatrica Scandinavica* 116:81–84.

Finnis, D., et al. 2010. Biological, clinical and ethical advances of placebo effects. *Lancet* 375:686–695.

First, M. 2011. DSM-5 proposals for mood disorders: a cost-benefit analysis [Review]. *Current Opinion in Psychiatry* 24(1):1–9.

Fish, S. 1972. *Self-Consuming Artifacts: The Experience of Seventeenth-Century Literature.* Berkeley: University of California Press.

Flanagan, O. 1998. *Consciousness Reconsidered.* Cambridge: MIT Press.

Fletcher, P.C., and Frith, C.D. 2009. Perceiving is believing: a Baysian approach to explaining the positive symptoms of schizophrenia. *Nature Reviews, Neuroscience* 10:48–54.

Fodor, J.A. 1975. *The Language of Thought.* Vol. 5. Cambridge, MA: Harvard University Press.

Forgas, J. 2007. When sad is better than happy: negative affect can improve the quality and effectiveness of persuasive messages and social influence strategies. *Journal of Experimental Social Psychology* 43:513–528.

Foucault, M. 1965. *Madness and Civilization: A History of Insanity in the Age of Reason*. New York: Vintage.

Foucault, M. 2006 *History of Madness*. Translated by Jonathan Murphy and Jean Khalfa. London and New York: Routledge.

Foucault, M. 1986. *The Care of the Self.* The History of Sexuality, Vol. 3. New York: Pantheon.

Fournier, J.C., et al. 2010. Antidepressant drug effects and depression severity: a patient-level meta-analysis. *Journal of the American Medical Association* 303:47–53.

Fox, R. 1976. *The Tangled Chain: The Structure of Disorder in the Anatomy of Melancholy*. Berkeley: University of California Press.

Frances, A. 2009. Whither DSM-V? *British Journal of Psychiatry* 195:391–392.

Frances, A. 2013. *Saving Normal: An Insider's Look at What Caused the Epidemic of Mental Illness and How to Cure It*. New York: HarperCollins Publishing.

Frass, M., et al. 2012. Use and acceptance of complementary and alternative medicine among the general population and medical personnel: a systematic review. *Ochsner Journal* 12:45–56.

Freeman, D., Bentall, R., and Garety, P. (eds). 2008. *Persecutory Delusions: Assessment, Theory and Treatment*. Oxford: Oxford University Press.

Freud, S. 1957. Mourning and melancholia. *Collected Papers* Vol IV Authorized Translation by Joan Riviere. London: The Hogarth Press; 152–170.

Frith, C.D. 1992. *The Cognitive Neuropsychology of Schizophrenia*. Hillsdale, NJ: Erlbaum.

Galen, 1976. *On the Affected Parts*. Translated and edited by R.E. Seigel. Basel: S. Karger.

Gallagher, S. 2012. Multiple aspects in the sense of agency. *New Ideas in Psychology* 30(1):15–31.

Gallagher, S., and Zahavi, D. 2013. *The phenomenological mind*. London: Routledge.

Gardner, S. 1993. *Irrationality and the Philosophy of Psychoanalysis*. Cambridge: Cambridge University Press.

Garrety, P., and Hemsley, D.R. 1994. *Delusions: Investigations into the Psychology of Delusional Reasoning*. Oxford: Oxford University Press.

Gaukroger, S., Schuster, J., and Sutton, J. (eds). 2000. *Descartes' Natural Philosophy*. New York: Routledge.

Gerrans, P. 2014. *The Measure of Madness: Philosophy of Mind, Cognitive Neuroscience, and Delusional Thought*. Cambridge: MIT Press.

Gert, B. and Culver, G. 2004. Defining mental disorder. In *The Philosophy of Psychiatry: A Companion*, edited by Jennifer Radden. Oxford: Oxford University Press; 415–425.

REFERENCES

Gill, C. 2009. Seneca and selfhood. In *Seneca and the Self*, edited by S. Bartsch and D. Wray. Cambridge: Cambridge University Press; 65–83.

Gill, C. 2010. Stoicism and epicurianism. In *The Oxford Handbook of Philosophy of Emotion*, edited by P. Goldie. Oxford and New York: Oxford University Press; 143–166.

Goddard, G.V., and Douglas, K.M. 1975. Does the engram model of kindling model the engram of long term memory? *Canadian Journal of Neurological Sciences* 2:385–394.

Goldberg, P.D. 1996. A dimensional model for common mental disorders. *British Journal of Psychiatry* 30:44–49.

Goldberg, P.D., et al. 2009. Emotional disorders: cluster 4 of the proposed metastructure for DSM-V and ICD-11. *Psychological Medicine* 39:2043–2059.

Goldie, P. (ed). 2010. *The Oxford Handbook of Philosophy of Emotion*. Oxford: Oxford University Press.

Goodwin, F.K., and Redfield Jamison, K. 2007. *Manic-Depressive Illness: Bipolar Disorders and Recurrent Depression*. Oxford: Oxford University Press.

Gordon, J.S. 2009. *Unstuck: Your Guide to the Seven-Stage Journey out of Depression*. New York: Penguin.

Gotlib, I., and Jammen, C. (eds). 2009. *Handbook of Depression*. Second Edition. New York: Guilford Press.

Gowland, A. 2006. The problem of early modern melancholy. *Past and Present* 191:77–120.

Gowland, A. 2007. *The Worlds of Renaissance Melancholy: Robert Burton in Context*. Cambridge: Cambridge University Press.

Gowland, A. 2014. Melancholy, passions and identity in the renaissance. In *Passions and Subjectivity in Early Modern Culture*, edited by B. Cummings and F. Sierhuis. Farnham: Ashgate; 75–93.

Graham, G. 2010. *The Disordered Mind: An Introduction to Philosophy of Mind and Mental Illness*. London and New York: Routledge.

Griffiths, P.E. 1997. *What Emotions Really Are: The Problem of Psychological Categories*. Chicago: University of Chicago Press.

Griffiths, P.E. 1998. Emotions. In *The Blackwell Guide to Philosophy of Mind* London: Blackwell Publishers; 288–308.

Grimaldi-Bensouda, L., et al. 2012. Who seeks primary care for sleep, anxiety and depressive disorders from physicians prescribing homeopathic and other complementary medicine? Results from the EP13 population survey. *British Medical Journal Open* e001498. doi:10.1136/bmjopen-2012-001498.

Grokroger, S., Shuster, J., and Sutton, J. (eds). 2000. *Descartes' Natural Philosophy*. London and New York: Routledge.

Hacking, I. 1994. The looping effects of human kinds. In *Causal Cognition*, edited by D. Sperber and A.J. Premack. Oxford: Oxford University Press; 351–383.

REFERENCES

Hacking, I. 1995. *Rewriting the Soul: Multiple Personality and the Sciences of Memory*. Princeton: Princeton University Press.

Hacking, I. 1998. *Mad Travelers: Reflections on the Reality of Transient Mental Illnesses*. Charlottesville and London: University Press of Virginia.

Hadas, M. (ed). 1958. *The Stoic Philosophy of Seneca: Essays and Letters*. Translated and with an Introduction. New York: Norton.

Hadot, P. 1995. *Philosophy as a Way of Life: Spiritual Exercises from Socrates to Foucault*. Oxford: Blackwell.

Hahn, R.A. 1999. The nocebo phenomenon: scope and foundations. In *The Placebo Effect: An Interdisciplinary Exploration*, edited by A. Harrington. Cambridge, MA: Harvard University Press; 56–76.

Hammen, C. 2006. Stress generation in depression: reflections on origins, research, and future directions. *Journal of Clinical Psychology* 62:1065–1082.

Harrington, A. (ed). 1999. *The Placebo Effect: An Interdisciplinary Exploration*. Cambridge: Harvard University Press.

Harrington, J.A., and Blankenship, V. 2002. Ruminative thoughts and their relation to depression and anxiety. *Journal of Applied Social Psychology* 32:465–485.

Harris, P.L. 2000. *The Work of the Imagination*. Malden, MA: Blackwell.

Haskell, Y. (ed). 2011. *Diseases of the Imagination and Imaginary Diseases in the Early Modern Period*. Turnhout: Brepols.

Haslan, N. 2002. Kinds of kinds: a conceptual taxonomy of psychiatric categories. *Philosophy, Psychiatry and Psychology* 9:203–217.

Haslan, N. 2014. Natural kinds in psychiatry: conceptually implausible, empirically questionable, and stigmatizing. In *Classifying Psychopathology: Mental Kinds and Natural Kinds*, edited by Harold Kinkaid and J.A. Sullivan. Cambridge, MA: MIT Press; 11–28.

Hassabis, D., Kumaran, D. and Maguire, E.A. 2007. Using imagination to understand the neural basis of episodic memory. *The Journal of Neuroscience* 27(52): 14365–14374.

Hassabis, D. and Maguire, E.A. 2007. Deconstructing episodic memory with construction. *Trends in Cognitive Sciences* 11(7): 299–306.

Healy, D. 1997. *The Anti-Depressant Era*. Cambridge, MA: Harvard University Press.

Heffernan, C.F. 1995. *The Melancholy Muse: Chaucer, Shakespeare and Early Medicine*. Pittsburgh: Duquesne University Press.

Heidegger, M. 1996. *Being and Time*. Translated by J. Stambaugh. New York: SUNY Press.

Helzer, J.E., et al. (eds). 2008. *Dimensional Approaches in Diagnostic Classification: Refining the Research Agenda for DSM-5*. Washington DC: American Psychiatric Association.

REFERENCES

Hippocrates. 1923–31. *Works of Hippocrates*. 4 Vols. Translated and edited by W.H.S. Jones and E.T. Withington. Cambridge, MA: Harvard University Press.

Hippocrates. 1988. *Affections*. Translated by P. Potter. Cambridge, MA: Loeb Classical Library, Harvard University Press.

Hollandare, F., et al. 2011. Randomized trial of Internet-based relapse prevention for partially remitted depression. *Acta Psychiatrica Scandinavica* 124:285–294.

Holmes, E.A. 2013. The powerful impact of mental imagery in changing emotion. *Changing Emotions* 26:187.

Holmes, E.A., Lang, T.J., and Deeprose, C. 2009. Mental imagery and emotion in treatment across disorders: using the example of depression. *Cognitive Behaviour Therapy* 38(S1):21–28.

Holmes, R. 2009. *The Age of Wonder: How the Romantic Generation Discovered the Beauty and Terror of Science*. New York: Vintage.

Horwitz, A. 2002. *Creating Mental Illness*. Chicago: Chicago University Press.

Horwitz, A. 2014. The social functions of natural kinds: the case of major depression. In *Classifying Psychopathology: Mental Kinds and Natural Kinds*, edited by Harold Kinkaid and J.A. Sullivan. Cambridge, MA: MIT Press; 209–226.

Horwitz, A., and Wakefield, J. 2007. *The Loss of Sadness: How Psychiatry Transformed Normal Sorrow into Depressive Disorder*. Oxford: Oxford University Press.

Huet, M.-H. 1993. *Monstrous Imagination*. Cambridge: Harvard University Press.

Huffziger, S., Reinhard, I., and Kuehner, C. 2009. A longitudinal study of rumination and distraction in formerly depressed inpatients and community controls. *Journal of Abnormal Psychology* 118:746.

Iacoviello, B.M., et al. 2013. Patterns of symptom onset and remission in episodes of hopeless depression. *Depression and Anxiety* 30:564–573.

Immordino-Yang, M.H., Christodoulou, J.A., and Singh, V. 2012. Rest is not idleness: implications of the brain's default mode for human development and education. *Perspectives on Psychological Science* 7:352–364.

Insel, T., et al. 2010. Research domain criteria (RDoC): toward a new classification framework for research on mental disorders. *American Journal of Psychiatry* 167:748–751.

Irwin, S., Sheffield, J. and Holland-Thompson, K. 2010. *Essential Skills*. Melbourne: beyondblue.

Izard, C.E. 1991. *The Psychology of Emotions*. New York: Plenum Press.

Jackson, S. 1986. *Melancholia and Depression: From Hippocratic Times to Modern Times*. London: Yale University Press.

Jackson, A., Cavanagh, J., and Scott, J. 2003. A systematic review of manic and depressive prodromes. *Journal of Affective Disorders* 74:209–217.

REFERENCES

Jacob, K.S. 2012. Depression: a major public health problem in need of a multi-sectoral response. *Indian Journal of Medical Research* 136:537.

Jacobs, N. et al. 2006. Stress-related negative affectivity and genetically altered serotonin transporter function. *Archives of General Psychiatry* 63:989–996.

Jacobson, N., and Greenley, D. 2001. What is recovery? A conceptual model and explication. *Psychiatric Services* 52:482–485.

James, S. 1997. *Passion and Action: The Emotions in Seventeenth Century Philosophy.* Oxford: Oxford University Press.

Jaspers, K. 1963. *General Psychopathology.* Toronto: University of Toronto Press.

Johnson, S. 1893. *Letters.* Edited by G.B. Hill. Oxford: Oxford University Press. Vol 1.

Jopling, D. 2008. *Placebos and Placebo Effects.* Oxford: Oxford University Press.

Jorm, A.F. 2014. Why hasn't the mental health of Australians improved? The need for a national prevention strategy. *Australian and New Zealand Journal of Psychiatry* 48:795–801.

Justman, S. 2013. Deceit and transparency in placebo research. *Yale Journal of Biological Medicine* 86:323–331.

Kahneman, D. 2011. *Thinking Fast and Slow.* New York: Penguin.

Kahneman, D., and Tversky, A. 1983. The simulation heuristic. In *Judgement under Uncertainty: Heuristics and Biases*, edited by D. Kahneman, P. Slovic, and A. Tversky. Cambridge: Cambridge University Press; 201–208.

Kam, J.W.Y., and Handy, T.C. 2013. The neurocognitive consequences of the wandering mind: a mechanistic account of sensory-motor decoupling. *Frontiers in Psychology* 4:725–725.

Kapczinski, F., et al. 2008. Increased oxidative stress as a mechanism for decreased BDNF levels in acute manic episodes. *Revista brasileira de psiquiatria*. 30:243–245.

Kaptchuk, T.J., and Miller, F.G. 2015. Placebo Effects in Medicine. *N Engl J Medicine* 373: 8–9.

Kauer-Sant'Anna, M., et al. 2007. Traumatic life events in bipolar disorder: impact on BDNF levels on psychopathology. *Bipolar Disorder* 9:128–135.

Keller, M.C., Neale, M.C., and Kendler, K.S. 2007. Association of different adverse life events with distinct patterns of depressive symptoms. *American Journal of Psychiatry* 164:1521–1529.

Kendler, K.S. 1990. Toward a scientific psychiatric nosology: strengths and limitations. *Archives of General Psychiatry* 47:969–973.

Kendler, K.S. 2010. A statement from Kenneth S. Kendler, MD, on the proposal to eliminate the grief exclusion criterion from major depression, by Kenneth S. Kendler, MD, Member, DSM-5 Mood Disorder Work Group.

Kendler, K.S, Gardner, C.O., and Prescott, C.A. 2002. Toward a comprehensive developmental model for major depression in women. *American Journal of Psychiatry* 159:1133–1145.

REFERENCES

Kendler, K.S., Gardner, C.O., and Prescott, C.A. 2006. Toward a comprehensive developmental model for major depression in men. *American Journal of Psychiatry* 163:115–124.

Kendler, K., Karkowski, L.M., and Prescott, C.A. 1999. Causal relationships between stressful life events and the onset of major depression. *American Journal of Psychiatry* 156:837–842.

Kendler, K.S., Zachar, P., and Craver, C. 2011. What kinds of things are psychiatric disorders? *Psychological Medicine* 41:1143–1150.

Kessing, L.V., et al. 1998. Recurrence in affective disorder. I. Case register study. *British Journal of Psychiatry* 172(1):23–28.

Kessler, R.C. 1997. The effects of stressful life events on depression. *Annual Review of Psychology* 48:191.

Kessler, R.C., et al. 1997. Prevalence, correlates, and course of minor depression and major depression in the National Comorbidity Survey. *Journal of Affective Disorders* 45:19–30.

Kessler, R.C., et al. 2001. Long-term trends in the use of complementary and alternative medical therapies in the United States. *Annual Internal Medicine* 135:262–268.

Kessler, R.C., et al. 2005. Prevalence, severity and comorbidity of 12-month DSM-IV disorders in the National Comorbidity Survey Replication. *Archives of General .Psychiatry* 62:617–627.

Kiessling, N.K. 1988. *The Library of Robert Burton.* Oxford: Oxford Bibliographical Society.

Killingsworth, M.A., and Gilbert, D.T. 2010. A wandering mind is an unhappy mind. *Science* 330:932–932.

Kincaid, H. 2008. Social sciences. *Blackwell Guide to the Philosophy of Science* edited by P. Machamer and M. Silberstein. New York: John Wiley&Sons; 290–311.

Kincaid, H. 2014. Defensible natural kinds. In *Classifying Psychopathology: Mental Kinds and Natural Kinds*, edited by H. Kincaid and J. Sullivan. Cambridge, MA: MIT Press; 145–173.

Kind, A. 2001. Putting the images back in imagination. *Philosophy and Phenomenological Research* 62:85–109.

Kirsch, I. (ed). 1999. *How Expectancies Shape Experience.* Washington DC: American Psychological Association.

Kirsch, I., et al. 2002. The emperor's new drugs: an analysis of antidepressant medication data submitted to the U.S. Food and Drug Administration. *Prevention and Treatment* 5, 23a.

Kirsch, I., et al. 2008. Initial severity and antidepressant benefits: a meta-analysis of data submitted to the Food and Drug Administration. *PLoS Med* 5(2):e45.

Klein, D.F. 1974. Endogenomorphic depression: a conceptual and terminological revision. *Archives of General Psychiatry* 31:447–454.

REFERENCES

Klein, M. 1935. A contribution to the psychogenesis of manic-depressive states. *International Journal of Psychoanalysis* 16;145.

Kocher, P.H. 1953. *Science and Religion in Elizabethan England*. New York: Octagon Books.

Kong, J., et al. 2008. A functional magnetic resonance imaging study on the neural mechanisms of hyperalgesic nocebo effect. *Journal of Neuroscience* 28:13354–13362.

Kosslyn, S.M. et al. 1999. The role of area 17 in visual imagery: convergent evidence from PET and rTMS. *Science* 284(5411): 167–170.

Koster, E.H.W., Fox, E., and MacLeod, C. 2009. Introduction to the special section on cognitive bias modification in emotional disorders. *Journal of Abnormal Psychology* 118(1):1.

Kramer, P. 2005. *Against Depression*. New York: Viking.

Kristellar, P.O. 1088. Humanism. In *The Cambridge History of Renaissance Philosophy*, edited by C.B. Schmitt. Cambridge: Cambridge University Press; 113–137.

Kuehner, C., Holzhauer, S., and Huffziger, S. 2007. Decreased cortisol response to awakening is associated with cognitive vulnerability to depression in a nonclinical sample of young adults. *Psychoneuroendocrinology* 32:199–209.

Kuehner, C., Huffziger, S., and Liebsch, K. 2009. Rumination, distraction and mindful self-focus: effects on mood, dysfunctional attitudes and cortisol stress response. *Psychological Medicine* 39:219–228.

Kupfer, D.J., First, M.D., and Regier, D.A. (eds). 2002. *A Research Agenda for DSM-V*. Washington DC: American Psychiatric Press.

Kupfer, D.J., Frank, E., Perel, J.M. 1989. The advantage of early treatment intervention in recurrent depression. *Archives of General Psychiatry* 46:771–775.

Kuyken, W., et al. 2008. Mindfulness-based cognitive therapy to prevent relapse in depression. *Journal of Consulting and Clinical Psychology* 76:966–978.

Laeng, B., and Teodorescu, D.-S. 2002. Eye scanpaths during visual imagery reenact those of perception of the same visual scene. *Cognitive Science* 26:207–231.

Lakoff, G. and Johnson, M. 1999. *Philosophy in the Flesh: The Embodied Mind and Its Challenges to Western Thought by George Lakoff*. New York: Basic Books.

Lamb, K., Pies, R., and Zisook, S. 2010. The bereavement exclusion for the diagnosis of major depression: to be, or not to be. *Psychiatry* 7:19–25.

Leahy, R.L., and Holland, S. 2012. *Treatment Plans and Interventions for Depression*. New York: Guilford Press.

LeDoux, J. 1996. *The Emotional Brain*. New York: Simon & Schuster.

LeDoux, J. 2000. Emotion circuits in the brain. *Annual Review of Neuroscience* 23:155–184.

LeDoux, J. 2015. Feelings: what are they and how does the brain make them? *American Academy of Arts and Sciences* 144:96–111.

Lee, E. 1838. *A Treatise on Some Nervous Disorders*. London: Churchill.

Lennon, K. 2015. *Imagination and the Imaginary*. New York: Routledge.
Leonhard, K. 1959. *The Classification of the Endogenous Psychoses*. Translated by R. Robins. New York: Wiley & Sons.
Levine, J, et al. 2001a. Symptomatic and syndromal anxiety and depression. *Depression and Anxiety* 14:94–104.
Levine, J., et al. 2001b. Anxiety disorders and major depression: together or apart? *Depression and Anxiety* 14:94–104.
Lewis, A. 1938. States of depression: their clinical and aetiological differentiation. *British Medical Journal* 2:875–878.
Locke, J. 1959. *An Essay Concerning Human Understanding*. Edited by A.C. Fraser. New York: Courier Corporation.
Lokhorst, G. 2015. Descartes and the pineal gland. In Stanford Encyclopedia of Philosophy (Fall 2015 Edition), edited by E.N. Zalta. http://plato.stanford.edu/archives/fall2015/entries/pineal-gland/
Long, A.A. 1986. *Hellenistic Philosophy: Stoics, Epicureans, Sceptics*. Second Edition. Berkeley and Los Angeles: University of California Press.
Lund, M. 2010. *Melancholy, Medicine and Religion in Early Modern England: Reading The Anatomy of Melancholy*. Cambridge: Cambridge University Press.
Lund, M. 2015. Robert Burton, perfect happiness and the *visio dei*. In *The Renaissance of Emotion: Understanding Affect in Shakespeare and His Contemporaries*, edited by R. Meek and E. Sullivan. Manchester: Manchester University Press; 86–105.
Lyons, B. 1971. *Voices of Melancholy: Studies in Literary Treatments of Melancholy in Renaissance England*. London: Routledge & Kegan Paul.
Macdonald, M. 1981a. *Mystical Bedlam: Madness, Anxiety, and Healing in Seventeenth-Century England*. Cambridge: Cambridge University Press.
Macdonald, M. 1981b. Insanity and the realities of history in early modern England. *Psychological Medicine* 11:11–25.
MacLeod, A.K., et al. 1997a. Brief communication: parasuicide, depression and the anticipation of positive and negative future experiences. *Psychological Medicine* 27:973–977.
MacLeod, A.K., et al. 1997b. Retrospective and prospective cognitions in anxiety and depression. *Cognition and Emotion* 11:467–479.
Madan, C., and Singhal, A. 2012. Motor imagery and higher-level cognition: four hurdles before research can spring forward. *Cognitive Processing* 13:211–29.
Maher, B. 1999. Anomalous experience in everyday life. *The Monist* 82: 547–570.
Marchetti, I., et al. 2012. The default mode network and recurrent depression: a neurobiological model of cognitive risk factors. *Neuropsychology Review* 22:229–251.

Marchetti, I., Van de Putte, E., and Koster, E.H.W. 2014. Self-generated thoughts and depression: from daydreaming to depressive symptoms. *Frontiers in Human Neuroscience* 8:1–10.

Margolis, E., Samuels, R., and Stitch, S. (eds). 2012. *The Oxford Handbook of Philosophy of Cognitive Science*. Oxford: Oxford University Press.

Mars, T S., and Abbey, H. 2010. Mindfulness meditation practise as a healthcare intervention: a systematic review. *International Journal of Osteopathic Medicine* 13(2):56–66.

Mathers, C., Fat, D.M., and Boerma, J.T. 2008. *The Global Burden of Disease: 2004 Update*. World Health Organization.

Matthews, A., and Macleod, C. 2005. Cognitive vulnerability to emotional disorders. *Annual Review of Clinical Psychology* 1:167–195.

Mathews, A., Ridgeway, V., and Holmes, E.A. 2013. Feels like the real thing: imagery is both more realistic and emotional than verbal thought. *Cognition and Emotion* 27: 217–229.

Maser, J.D., and Cloninger, C.R. 1990. Comorbidity of anxiety and mood disorders: introduction and overview. *Comorbidity of Mood and Anxiety Disorders* edited by J.D. Maser. New York: American Psychiatric Press; 3–12.

McElroy, S.L., et al. 2001. Axis I psychiatric comorbidity and its relationship to historical illness variables in 288 patients with bipolar disorder. *American Journal of Psychiatry*. 158(3):420–426.

McGinn, C. 2004. *Mindsight: Image, Dream, Meaning*. Cambridge, MA: Harvard University Press.

McGorry, P.D., et al. 2002. Randomized controlled trial of interventions designed to reduce the risk of progression to first-episode psychosis in a clinical sample with subthreshold symptoms. *Archives of General Psychiatry* 59:921–928.

McGuffin, P., et al. 2003. The heritability of bipolar affective disorder and the genetic relationship to unipolar depression. *Archives of General Psychiatry* 60:497–502.

McKay, R.T., and Dennett, D.C. 2009. The evolution of misbelief. *Behavioral and Brain Sciences* 32:493–510.

McLachlan, A. 2014. Preventative therapeutics. *Culture Unbound* 6:815–837.

McLaughlin, K.A. 2011. The public health impact of major depression: a call for interdisciplinary prevention efforts. *Prevention Science* 12:361–371.

Meissner, K., et al. 2011. The placebo effect: advances from different methodological approaches." *Journal of Neuroscience* 31:16117–16124.

Mele, A. 1987. *Irrationality: An Essay on Self-Deception and Self-Control*. New York: Oxford University Press.

Merry, S., et al. 2011. Evidence-based child health. *Cochrane Review Journal* 7:1409–1685.

Mishara, A.L., and Corlett, P. 2009. Are delusions biologically adaptive? Salvaging the doxastic shear pin. *Behavioral and Brain Sciences* 32:530–531.

REFERENCES

Mojtabai, R. 2011. Bereavement-related depressive episodes: characteristics, 3-year course, and implications for the DSM-5. *Archives of General Psychiatry* 68:920–928.

Moncrieff, J., Wessely, S., and Hardy, R. 2004. Active placebo versus antidepressants for depression. *Cochrane Database of Systematic Reviews* 1:1.

Moncrieff, J. 2009. *The Myth of the Chemical Cure: A Critique of Psychiatric Drug Treatment*. Revised Edition. New York: Palgrave.

Montaigne, M. 1957. *The Complete Essays of Montaigne*. Translated by D.M. Frame. Stanford, CA: Stanford University Press.

Montaigne, M. 2003. *The Complete Essays*. Translated by M.A. Screech. London: Penguin Books.

Mora, M.S., Nestoriuc, Y, and Rief, W. 2011. Lessons learned from placebo groups and anti-depressant trials. *Philosophical Transactions: Biological Sciences* 366:1879–1888.

Moran, R 1994. *Authority and Estrangement: An Essay on Self-Knowledge*. Princeton, NJ: Princeton University Press.

Moscovitch, D.A., Chiupka, C.A., and Gavric, D.L. 2013. Within the mind's eye: Negative mental imagery activates different emotion regulation strategies in high versus low socially anxious individuals. *Journal of Behavior Therapy and Experimental Psychiatry* 44:426–432.

Mrazek, P.J., and Haggerty, R.J. (eds). 1994. *Reducing Risks for Mental Disorders: Frontiers for Preventive Intervention Research*. Washington, DC: National Academies Press.

Munafo, M.R., et al. 2009. Gene x environment interactions at the serotonin transporter locus. *Biological Psychiatry* 65:211–219.

Muñoz, R.F., Mrazek, P.J., and Haggerty, R.J. 1996. Institute of Medicine report on prevention of mental disorders: summary and commentary. *American Psychologist* 51:1116.

Munoz, R.F. 2001. On the road to a world without depression. *Journal of Primary Prevention* 21:325–338.

Murphy, D. 2005. *Psychiatry in the Scientific Image*. Cambridge, MA: MIT Press.

Murphy, D. 2015. Concepts of disease and health. *The Stanford Encyclopedia of Philosophy* (Spring 2015 Edition), edited by E.N. Zalta. http://plato.stanford.edu/archives/spr2015/entries/health-disease/

Murphy, S.E., et al. 2015. Imagining a brighter future: the effect of positive imagery training on mood, prospective mental imagery and emotional bias in older adults. *Psychiatry Research* 230(1):36–43.

Murray, C.J.L., and Lopez, A.D. 1997. Alternative projections of mortality and disability and the contribution of risk factors: Global Burden of Disease Study. *Lancet* 349:1436–1442.

National Health Service. 1995. Working Group Report.

Nayak, D., and Patel, P. 2014. Neuronal mechanisms of placebo effects. *Psychiatric Annals* 44(2):74–78.

Nichols, S. (ed). 2006. *The Architecture of the Imagination: New Essays on Pretence, Possibility, and Fiction.* Oxford: Oxford University Press.

Nolen-Hoeksema, S. 1991. Responses to depression and their effects on the duration of depressive episodes. *Journal of Abnormal Psychology* 100:569.

Nolen-Hoeksema, S. 2000. The role of rumination in depressive disorders and mixed anxiety/depressive symptoms. *Journal of Abnormal Psychology* 109:504.

Nolen-Hoeksema, S., Morrow, J., and Fredrickson, B.L. 1993. Response styles and the duration of episodes of depressed mood. *Journal of Abnormal Psychology* 102(1):20.

Nolen-Hoeksema, S., Wisco, S.E., and Lyubomirsky, S. 2008. Rethinking rumination. *Perspectives on Psychological Science* 3:400–424.

Nussbaum, M 1986. *The Fragility of Goodness: Luck and Ethics in Greek Tragedy and Philosophy.* Cambridge: Cambridge University Press.

Nussbaum, M. 1994. *Therapy of Desire: Theory and Practice in Hellenistic Ethics.* Princeton, NJ: Princeton University Press.

Oatley, K., Keltner, D., and Jenkins, J. 2006. *Understanding Emotions.* London: Blackwell.

O'Connell, M.E., Boat, T., and Warner, K.E., (eds). 2009. *Preventing Mental, Emotional and Behavioral Disorders Among Young People: Progress and Possibilities.* National Research Council (US) and Institute of Medicine (US) Committee on the Prevention of Mental Disorders and Substance Abuse Among Children, Youth, and Young Adults: Research Advances and Promising Intervention. Washington, DC: National Academies Press.

Oettingen, G. 2012. Future thought and behavior change. *European Review of Social Psychology* 23:1–63.

Oettingen, G., Mayer, D., and Thorpe, J. 2010. Self-regulation of commitment to reduce cigarette consumption: mental contrasting of future with reality. *Psychological Health* 25:961–977.

Ostler, W. 1922–26. Robert Burton—the man, his book, his library. *Oxford Bibliographical Society Proceedings and Papers.*Oxford: Oxford University Press;163–190.

Palazidou, E. 2012. The neurobiology of depression. *British Medical Bulletin* 101:127–145.

Pampallona, S., et al. 2004. Combined pharmacotherapy and psychological treatment for depression: a systematic review. *Archives of General Psychiatry* 61:714–719.

Panksepp, J. 1998. *Affective Neuroscience: The Foundations of Human and Animal Behavior.* Oxford: Oxford University Press.

REFERENCES

Parker, G. 2007. Defining melancholia: the primacy of psychomotor disturbance. *Acta Psychiatrica Scandinavica* 115(Suppl 433):89–92.

Parker, G., et al. 2010. Issues for DSM-5: whither Melancholia? The case for its classification as a distinct mood disorder. *American Journal of Psychiatry* 167:745–747.

Parker, G., and Hadzi-Pavlovic, D. (eds). 1996. *Melancholia: A Disorder of Movement and Mood: A Phenomenological and Neurobiological Review.* Cambridge: Cambridge University Press.

Parry, R. 2009. Ancient ethical theory. *Stanford Encyclopedia of Philosophy* (Fall 2009 Edition), edited by E.N. Zalta. http://plato.stanford.edu/archives/fall 2014/entries/ethics-ancient/

Paster, G.K. 2004. *Humoring the Body: Emotions and the Shakespearean Stage.* Chicago: University of Chicago Press.

Pearson, D.G., et al. 2013. Assessing mental imagery in clinical psychology: a review of imagery measures and a guiding framework. *Clinical Psychology Review* 33(1):1–23.

Perecman, E. (ed.). 2012. *Cognitive Processing in the Right Hemisphere.* Amsterdam: Elsevier.

Pictet, A, et al. 2011. Fishing for happiness: the effects of generating positive imagery on mood and behaviour. *Behaviour Research and Therapy* 49:885–891.

Pies, R. 2008. The anatomy of sorrow: a spiritual, phenomenological, and neurological perspective. *Philosophy, Ethics and Humanities in Medicine* 3:1–14.

Porter, R. (ed). 2006. *The Cambridge History of Medicine.* Cambridge: Cambridge University Press.

Post, R.M. et al. 1999. Sensitization components of post-traumatic stress disorder: implications for therapeutics. *Seminal Clinical Neuropsychiatry* 4(4): 282–294.

Post, R.M. 2007. Kindling and sensitization as models for affective episode recurrence, cyclicity and tolerance phenomena. *Neuroscience and Biobehavioral Reviews* 31:851–873.

Post, R.M. 2009. Kindling. In *The International Encyclopedia of Depression*, edited by Rich Ingram. New York: Springer; 360–364.

Post, R.M., and Weiss, S.R. 1998a. Kindling: separate vs shared mechanisms in affective disorders and epilepsy. *Neuropsychobiology* 38:167–180.

Post, R.M., and Weiss, S.R. 1998b. Sensitization and kindling phenomena in mood, anxiety, and obsessive-compulsive disorders: the role of serotonergic mechanisms in illness progression. *Biological Psychiatry* 44:193–206.

Prinz, J. 2004. *Gut Feelings: A Perceptual Theory of the Emotions.* Oxford: Oxford University Press.

Radden, J. (ed). 2000. *The Nature of Melancholy: From Aristotle to Kristeva.* New York: Oxford University Press.

REFERENCES

Radden, J. 2003. Is this Dame Melancholy? Equating depression and melancholia. *Psychiatry, Philosophy and Psychology* 10(1):37–52.

Radden, J. 2009. Epidemic depression and Burtonian melancholy. In *Moody Minds Distempered: Essays on Melancholy and Depression*, edited by J. Radden. New York: Oxford University Press; 97–110.

Radden, J. 2013. Shared descriptions: What can be concluded? *Philosophy, Psychiatry & Psychology* 20: 157–159.

Radden, J. 2016. Mental health, public health and depression, a bioethical perspective. *Ethics, Medicine and Public Health* 2:197–204.

Raichle, M., et al. 2001. A default mode of brain function. *Proceedings of the National Academy of Sciences* 98:676–682.

Ratcliffe, M. 2008. *Feelings of Being: Phenomenology, Psychiatry and a Sense of Reality*. Oxford: Oxford University Press.

Ratcliffe, M. Forthcoming. *Verbal Hallucinations, Emotions, and the Interpersonal World*. Cambridge, MA: MIT Press.

Rhead, J.D. 2014. The deeper significance of integrative medicine. *Journal of Alternative and Complementary Medicine* 20:329–329.

Roffe, L., Schmidt, K., and Ernst, E. 2005. A systematic review of guided imagery as an adjuvant cancer therapy. *Psycho-oncology* 14:607–617.

Robinson, H. 2012. Dualism. *Stanford Encyclopedia of Philosophy*, edited by E.N. Zalta. http://plato.stanford.edu/archives/win2012/entries/dualism/

Roberts, C. 2003. *Emotions: An Essay in Aid of Moral Psychology*. Cambridge: Cambridge University Press.

Robertson, D. 2010. *The Philosophy of Cognitive-behavioral Therapy (CBT): Stoic Philosophy as Rational and Cognitive Psychotherapy*. London: Karnac.

Robinson, M.S., and Alloy, L.B. 2003. Negative cognitive styles and stress-reactive rumination interact to predict depression: a prospective study. *Cognitive Therapy and Research* 27:275–291.

Romm, J. 2014. *Dying Every Day: Seneca at the Court of Nero*. New York: Knopf.

Rorty, A. 1982. From passions to emotions and sentiments. *Philosophy* 57:175–188.

Rorty, A. 2010. A plea for ambivalence. In *The Oxford Handbook of Philosophy of Emotion*, edited by P. Goldie. Oxford: Oxford University Press; 425–444.

Roth, M. 1959. The phenomenology of depressive states. *Canadian Psychiatric Association Journal* 4:S32–S53.

Roth, M., and Mountjoy, C.Q. 1982. The Distinction between Anxiety States and Depressive Disorders. In *Handbook of Affective Disorders*, edited by E.S. Paykel. New York: Guilford Press; 70–92.

Sadler, J. 2005. *Values and Psychiatric Diagnosis*. New York and Oxford: Oxford University Press.

Salin-Pascual, R., et al. 2002. Unraveling the diagnostic clues of depression and anxiety: the primary care challenge. *Psychopharmacology Bulletin* 36:150–157.

REFERENCES

Schacter, DL., et al. 2012. The future of memory: remembering, imagining, and the brain. *Neuron* 76:677–694.

Schacter, D.L., and Addis, D.R. 2007. The cognitive neuroscience of constructive memory: remembering the past and imagining the future. *Philosophical Transactions of the Royal Society of London B: Biological Sciences* 362(1481): 773–786.

Schaffner, K. 1993. *Discovery and Explanation in Biology and Medicine*. Chicago: University of Chicago Press.

Schaffner, K. 2002. Neuroethics: reductionism, emergence, and decision-making capacities. In *Descriptions and Prescriptions: Values, Disorders and the DSMs*, edited by J.Z. Sadler. Baltimore: Johns Hopkins Press; 271–290.

Schmidt, J. 2007. *Melancholy and the Care of the Soul: Religious, Moral Philosophy and Madness in Early Modern England*. Aldershot, England: Ashgate.

Schroeder, T., and Matheson, C. 2006. Imagination and emotion. In *Architecture of the Imagination: New Essays on Pretence, Possibility, and Fiction*. edited by S. Nichols. Oxford: Clarendon Press; 19–40.

Schupak, C., and Rosenthal, J. 2009. Excessive daydreaming: a case history and discussion of mind wandering and high fantasy proneness. *Consciousness and Cognition* 18:290–292.

Schwartz, P.H. 2007. Defining dysfunction: natural selection, design, and drawing a line. *Philosophy of Science* 74:364–385.

Scot, R. 1586/1989. *The Discovery of Witchcraft*. New York: Dover.

Scull, A. 2009. *Hysteria: A Biography*. Oxford: Oxford University Press.

Seeley, W.W., et al. 2007. Dissociable intrinsic connectivity networks for salience processing and executive control. *Journal of Neuroscience* 27:2349–2356.

Segal, S.J. (ed.). 2014. *Imagery: Current Cognitive Approaches*. New York: Academic Press.

Shapiro, A.K. 1969. Iatroplacebogenics. *International Psychopharmacology* 2:215–248.

Shear, M.K., et al. 2011. Complicated grief and related bereavement issues for DSM-V. *Depression and Anxiety* 28:103–117.

Shields, C. 2008. Aristotle. *Stanford Encyclopedia of Philosophy* (Spring 2014 Edition), edited by E.N. Zalta. http://plato.stanford.edu/archives/spr2014/entries/aristotle/

Shorter, A. 1992. *From Paralysis to Fatigue: A History of Psychosomatic Illness in the Modern Era*. New York: Free Press.

Shorter, A. 2007. The doctrine of the two depressions in historical perspective. *Acta Psychiatrica Scandinavica* 115(Suppl 433):5–13.

Shorter, A. 2013. *How Everyone Became Depressed: The Rise and Fall of the Nervous Breakdown*. Oxford and New York: Oxford University Press.

Shorter, A., and Fink, M. 2010. *Endocrine Psychiatry: Solving the Riddle of Melancholia*. New York: Oxford University Press.

Skultans, V. 1979. *English Madness: Ideas on Insanity, 1580–1890*. London: Routledge.

Smallwood, J., and Andrews-Hanna, J. 2013. Not all minds that wander are lost: the importance of a balanced perspective on the mind-wandering state. *Frontiers in Psychology* 4:1–6.

Smallwood, J., and O'Connor, R.C. 2011. Imprisoned by the past: unhappy moods lead to a retrospective bias to mind wandering. *Cognition and Emotion* 25:1481–1490.

Smallwood, J., and Schooler, J.W. 2006. The restless mind. *Psychological Bulletin* 132:946.

Smallwood, J., Schooler, J., and Handy, T. 2008. Going AWOL in the brain: mind wandering reduces cortical analysis of external events. *Journal of Cognitive Neuroscience* 20:747–752.

Solomon, R. 1976. *The Passions.* New York: Doubleday.

Solomon, R. 2004. *In Defense of Sentimentality.* Oxford and New York: Oxford University Press.

Sorabji, R. 2002. *Emotion and Peace of Mind: From Stoic Agitation to Christian Temptation.* Oxford: Oxford University Press.

Spasojević, J., and Alloy, L.B. 2001. Rumination as a common mechanism relating depressive risk factors to depression. *Emotion* 1:25.

Spaulding, W.D., Sullivan, M.E., and Poland, J. 2003. *Treatment and Rehabilitation of Severe Mental Illness.* New York: Guilford Press.

Spreng, R.N., Mar, R.A. and Kim, A.S. 2009. The common neural basis of autobiographical memory, prospection, navigation, theory of mind, and the default mode: a quantitative meta-analysis. *Journal of Cognitive Neuroscience* 21(3):489–510.

Stahl, S.M. 1997. Mixed depression and anxiety: seratonin receptors as a common pharmacologic link. *Journal of Clinical Psychiatry* 58(Suppl 8):20–26.

Stahl, S.T., et al. 2014. Coaching in healthy dietary practices in at-risk older adults: a case of indicated depression prevention. *American Journal of Psychiatry* 171:499–505.

Stetter, F., and Kupper, S. 2002. Autogenic training: a meta-analysis of clinical outcome studies. *Applied Psychophysiological Biofeedback* 27:45–98.

St Ignatius. 1964. *Spiritual Exercises.* New York: Image Books.

Stix, G. 2011. The Neuroscience of True Grit-When tragedy strikes, most of us ultimately rebound surprisingly well. Where does such resilience come from? *Scientific American* 304(3):28–33.

Stroebe, M.S., et al. (eds). 2008. *Handbook of Bereavement Research and Practice: Advances in Theory and Intervention.* Washington DC: American Psychological Association.

Summerfield, J.J. Hassabis, D. and Maguire, E.A. 2010. Differential engagement of brain regions within a 'core'network during scene construction. *Neuropsychologia* 48(5):1501–1509.

REFERENCES

Swan, J. (ed). 1742. *The Entire Works of Dr Thomas Sydenham, Newly Made English from the originals: Wherein The History of acute and chronic Diseases, and the safest and most effectual Methods of treating them, are faithfully, clearly, and accurately delivered. To which are added, explanatory and practical notes, from the best medical writers*. London: Cave.

Sydenham, R. 1979. *The Works of Thomas Sydenham*. Edited by R.G. Latham. New York: Classics of Medicine Library.

Takano, K., and Tanno, Y. 2009. Self-rumination, self-reflection, and depression: self-rumination counteracts the adaptive effect of self-reflection. *Behaviour Research and Therapy* 47:2602–64.

Tauber, A. 2010. *Freud: The Reluctant Philosopher*. Princeton, NJ: Princeton University Press.

Taylor, M.A., and Fink, M. 2006. *Melancholia: The Diagnosis, Pathophysiology, and Treatment of Depressive Illness*. Cambridge: Cambridge University Press.

Taylor, M.A., and Fink, M. 2008. The medical evidence-based model for psychiatric syndromes: return to a classical paradigm. *Acta Psychiatrica Scandinavica* 117:81–84.

Tekin, S. 2011. Self-concepts through the diagnostic looking glass: narratives and mental disorder. *Philosophical Psychology* 24:357–380.

Tekin, S. 2013. The missing self in hacking's looping effects. In *Mental Kinds and Natural Kinds*, edited by H. Kincaid and J. A. Sullivan. Cambridge, MA: MIT Press.

Tekin, S. 2014. Self-insight in the time of mood disorders: after the diagnosis, beyond the treatment. *Philosophy, Psychiatry, and Psychology* 21:139–155.

Tekin, S. 2015. Against hyponarrating grief: incompatible research and treatment interests in the DSM-5. In *The DSM-5 in Perspective*. Netherlands: Springer; 179–197.

Thagard, P. 1999. *How Scientists Explain Disease*. Princeton, NJ: Princeton University Press.

Thiher, A. 1999. *Revels in Madness: Insanity in Medicine and Literature*. Ann Arbor: University of Michigan Press.

Thomas, K. 1971. *Religion and the Decline of Magic*. Oxford: Oxford University Press.

Tillyard, E.M.W. 1963. *The Elizabethan World Picture*. Harmondsworth, Middlesex: Penguin Books.

Tilmouth, C. 2005. Burton's "Turning Picture": argument and anxiety in the *Anatomy of Melancholy*. *Review of English Studies* n.s., 56:524–549.

Trapnell, P.D., and Campbell, J.D. 1999. Private self-consciousness and the five-factor model of personality: distinguishing rumination from reflection. *Journal of Personality and Social Psychology* 76:284.

Treynor, W., Gonzalez, R., and Nolen-Hoeksema, S. 2003. Rumination reconsidered: a psychometric analysis. *Cognitive Therapy and Research* 27:247–259.

REFERENCES

Tsuang, M.T., and Marneros, A. 1986. Schizoaffective psychosis: questions and directions. In *Schizoaffective Psychoses*, edited by A. Marneros and M.T. Tsuang. Berlin: Springer Verlag; 1–7.

Turner, E.H., et al. 2008. Selective publication of antidepressant trials and its influence on apparent efficacy. *New England Journal of Medicine* 358:252–260.

Tversky, A., and Kahneman, D. 1974. Judgment under uncertainty: heuristics and biases. *Science* 185:1124–1131.

Uhlhaas, P.J., and Mishara, A.L. 2007. Perceptual anomalies in schizophrenia: integrating phenomenology and cognitive neuroscience. *Schizophrenia Bulletin* 33:142–156.

Välimäki, M., et al. 2012. Developing an Internet-based support system for adolescents with depression. *Journal of Medical Internet Research Research Protocols* 1(2):e22–e22.

Van Straten, A., Cuijpers, P., and Smits, N. 2008. Effectiveness of a Web-based self-help intervention for the symptoms of depression, anxiety, and stress: randomized controlled trial. *Journal of Medical Internet Research* 10:e7 doi:10.2196/jmir.954

Van Voorhees, B.W., et al. 2011. Internet-based depression prevention over the life course: a call for behavioral vaccines. *Psychiatric Clinics of North America* 34:167–183.

Van Zoonen, K., et al. 2014. Preventing the onset of major depressive disorder: a meta-analytic review of psychological interventions. *International Journal of Epidemiology* 43:318–329.

Varela, F.J., Thompson, E., Rosch, E. 1993. *The Embodied Mind*. Cambridge, MA: MIT Press.

Varga, S. 2012a. Cognitive theory, mental representations and emotions philosophy and therapeutic practice. *Deutsche Zeitschrift für Philosophie* 60:937–954.

Varga, S. 2012b. Evolutionary psychiatry and depression: testing two hypotheses. *Medicine, Health Care and Philosophy* 15(1):41–52.

Varga, S. 2013. From melancholia to depression: ideas on a possible continuity. *Philosophy, Psychiatry, and Psychology* 20:141–155.

Vaughn, L.A., and Weary, G. 2002. Roles of the availability of explanations, feelings of ease, and dysphoria in judgments about the future. *Journal of social and clinical psychology* 21.6:686–704.

Vicari, E.P. 1989. *The View from Minerva's Tower: Learning and Imagination in the Anatomy of Melancholy*. Toronto: University of Toronto Press.

Vogt, K. 2015. Seneca. *Stanford Encyclopedia of Philosophy* (Spring 2015 Edition), edited by E.N. Zalta. http://plato.stanford.edu/archives/spr2015/entries/seneca/

Volz, M.S., et al. 2015. Mental imagery-induced attention modulates pain perception and cortical excitability. *BMC Neuroscience* 16(1):15.

Von Eckardt, B. 1995. *What Is Cognitive Science?* Cambridge: Bradford Books.

REFERENCES

Von Zoonen, L., et al. 2014. Preventing the onset of major depressive disorder: a meta-analytic review of psychological interventions. *International Journal of Epidemiology* 43:318–329.

Wakefield, J.C. 1992. Disorder as harmful dysfunction: a conceptual critique of DSM-III-R's definition of mental disorder. *Psychological Review* 99:232.

Wakefield, J.C. 2012. Editorial: DSM-5: proposed changes to depressive disorders. *Current Medical Research and Opinion* 28:335–343.

Wakefield, J.C., and Schmitz, M.F. 2012. Recurrence of depression after bereavement-related depression: evidence for the validity of DSM-IV bereavement exclusion from the Epidemiologic Catchment Area Study. *Journal of Nervous and Mental Disease* 200:480–485.

Walsh, R. 2011. Lifestyle and mental health. *American Psychologist* 66:579–592.

Walton, K.L. 1990. *Mimesis as Make-Believe: On the Foundations of the Representational Arts.* Cambridge, MA: Harvard University Press.

Watkins, E., and Brown, R.G. 2002. Rumination and executive function in depression: an experimental study. *Journal of Neurology, Neurosurgery and Psychiatry* 72:400–402.

Watkins, E., and Moulds, M. 2005. Distinct modes of ruminative self-focus: impact of abstract versus concrete rumination on problem solving in depression. *Emotion* 5:319.

Watkins, E. and Teasdale, D.J. 2001. Rumination and overgeneral memory in depression: effects of self-focus and analytic thinking. *Journal of Abnormal Psychology* 110:353.

Watkins, P.C., et al. 1996. Unconscious mood-congruent memory bias in depression. *Journal of Abnormal Psychology* 105:34–41.

Wear, A. 1985. Explorations in Renaissance writings on the practice of medicine. In *The Medical Renaissance of the Sixteenth Century,* edited by A. Wear, R.K. French, and I.M. Lonie. Cambridge: Cambridge University Press; 118–145.

Wear, A., French, R.K., and Lonie, I.M. (eds). 1985. *The Medical Renaissance of the Sixteenth Century.* Cambridge: Cambridge University Press.

Weydert, J.A., et al. 2006. Evaluation of guided imagery as treatment for recurrent abdominal pain in children: a randomized controlled trial. *BMC Pediatrics* 6(1):29.

Whitfield-Gabrieli, S., et al. 2009. Hyperactivity and hyperconnectivity of the default network in schizophrenia and in first-degree relatives of persons with schizophrenia. *Proceedings of the National Academy of Sciences* 106:1279–1284.

Wichers, M. 2014. The dynamic nature of depression: a new micro-level perspective of mental disorder that meets current challenges. *Psychological Medicine* 44:1349–1360.

Williams, H. 2003. Resisting the Psychotic Library: Periphrasis and Paranoia in Burton's *Anatomy of Melancholy. Exemplaria: A Journal of Theory in Medieval and Renaissance Studies* 15:202.

REFERENCES

Williams, M., and Kabat-Zinn, J. (eds). 2013. Mindfulness: Diverse Perspectives on Its Meaning, Origins and Applications. London: Routledge.

Williams, R.G. 2001. Disfiguring the body of knowledge: anatomical discourse and Robert Burton's The Anatomy of Melancholy. *English Literary History* 68(3): 593–613.

Wilson, A. 2000. On the history of disease-concepts: the case of pleurisy. *History of Science* 38:271–319.

Wilson, E. 2014. *The Greatest Empire: A Life of Seneca*. Oxford: Oxford University Press.

Wilson, R.A., and Foglia, L. 2011. Embodied cognition. *Stanford Encyclopedia of Philosophy*. http://plato.stanford, edu/entries/embodied-cognition

Winkelman, P., et al. 2015. Chapter 4. In *APA Handbook of Personality and Social Psychology* edited by M. Mikulincer and P.R. Shaver. Washington, DC: American Psychological Press; 151–175.

Woese, C.R. 2004. A new biology for the new century. *Microbiology and Molecular Biology Reviews* 68:173–186.

World Health Organization (WHO). 1992. *The ICD-10 Classification of Mental And Behavioural Disorders: Clinical Descriptions and Diagnostic Guidelines*. Geneva: World Health Organization.

World Medical Association. 2001. World Medical Association Declaration of Helsinki: ethical principles for medical research involving human subjects. *Bulletin of the World Health Organization* 79:373.

Wright, T. 1986. *The Passions of the Mind in General*. Edited by W.W. Newbold. New York and London: Garland.

Yoo, H.J., et al. 2003. Neural substrates of tactile imagery: a functional MRI study. *Neuroreport* 14:581–585.

Yoo, H.J., et al. 2005. Efficacy of progressive muscle relaxation training and guided imagery in reducing chemotherapy side effects in patients with breast cancer and in improving their quality of life. *Support Care Cancer* 13:826–833.

Young, G. 2011. Beliefs, experiences, and misplaced being: an interactionist account of delusional misidentification. *Phenomenology and the Cognitive Sciences* 10:195–215.

Young, G. 2008. Capgras delusion: an interactionist model. *Consciousness and Cognition* 17:863–876.

Zachar, P. 2014. *A Metaphysics of Psychopathology*. Cambridge, MA: MIT Press.

Zisook, S., and Kendler, K.S. 2007. Is bereavement-related depression different than non-bereavement related depression? *Psychological Medicine* 37:779–794.

Zisook, S., Shear, K., and Kendler, K.S. 2007. Validity of the bereavement exclusion criterion for the diagnosis of major depressive episode. *World Psychiatry (WPA)* 6:102–107.

INDEX OF NAMES

Aristotle 19, 24, 35, 51–52, 155–157, 229, 231
Avicenna 19, 191

Babb, L. 74–75, 77
Bamborough, J.B. 25
Barlow, H.D. and Campbell L.A. 138
Beck, A. 275
Berrios, G. 101–102, 183
Biegler, P. 238–239
Borsboom, D. and Cramer, A. 137, 288
Boyle, R. 20
Bright, T. 54, 90, 124, 130–131

Carter, C. 99–100
Cartesianism 32–33, 40, 126
Chalmers, D. 70
Charland, L. 140
Chrysippus 151, 153, 159, 257
Cottingham, J. 160
Currie, G. 195–198

Damasio, A. 41–47, 161
Darwin, C. 137
Descartes, R. 10, 29–41, 119, 139–140
Du Laurens, A. 53, 55, 68, 85, 90, 96, 124, 193, 196, 197, 208

Egan, A. 195–197
Ehrenberg, A. 113
Elyot, T. 253
Epictetus 151, 246, 257–258, 260

Fallopio 20
Ficino 7–8, 54, 127, 231
Foucault, M. 9, 246

Galen 19–22, 30, 85, 87–93, 146–148, 253–265, 268, 288
Gerrans, P. 64, 205–209
Gowland, A. 13, 221

Hadot, P. 150, 224, 259
Harvey, W. 20
Haskell, Y. 57
Hercules de Saxonia 133
Hippocrates 90, 94
Horwitz, A. 145, 224
Horwitz, A. and Wakefield, J. 224–225, 227

James, S. 157
James, W. 45, 230
Jopling, D. 80

Kahneman, D. 174–175, 234–237
Kam, J.W.Y. and Handy, T.C. 170–171

321

INDEX OF NAMES

Kendler, K. 83, 109, 288
Kind, A. 61
Kramer, P. 230
Lakoff, G. and Johnson, M. 41
LeDoux, J. 41–48, 161
Lewis, A. 104, 142
Lipsius, J. 120, 152, 217
Lucretius 51

Marcus Aurelius 151, 246, 257
McGinn, C. 197–198
Melancthon, P. 122, 127–128
Montaigne, M. 70, 72
Moran, R. 67

Napier, R. 122, 132, 221
Nayak, D. and Patel, P. 78
Nichols, S. 59

Paracelsus 21, 54, 222
Paré 20
Parker, G. 143
Philo Judaeus 95
Plater, F. 8, 52–53
Post, R.M. 178

Ratcliffe, M. 197
Rhazes 19, 51
Rorty, A. 65
Rufus 19

Scot, R. 75
Seneca 11, 121, 152–153, 155, 168, 217–218, 232, 246, 257
Shorter, E. 131, 142, 145
Sydenham, T. 91, 98

Taylor, M.A. and Fink, M. 143, 145
Thomas, K. 248
Tilmouth, C. 14, 36, 162, 187
Tversky, A. *See* Kahneman

Vaughn, L.A. and Weary, G. 176
Versalius, A. 20

Weyer, J. 8, 52, 74, 245
Whitfield-Gabrieli, S. 206
Wichers, M. 110
Wright, T. 35, 120–122, 191

Zachar, P. 103, 109–110, 116

TOPICAL INDEX

adustion. *See* melancholy: adusted
agency. *See* self care and self healing
akrasia, 157–162
  and melancholising, 162–167
anxiety and depression
  comorbidity of, 118–119, 136–138
  parallels with fear and sadness,
    135–136, 148
Aristotelianism, 23, 48, 155
"as if" loops, 43–46
astrology, 54, 270

bereavement. *See* normal sadness and
  sorrow: contemporary debates
black bile. *See* humors

Cartesianism, 32–33, 40, 126
cognitive behavioral therapy (CBT),
  276, 281
cognitivism
  as cognitive psychology, 41, 48, 179, 273
  as theories of emotion, 122, 133,
    141, 152
continuity mirage (Berrios), 102, 117

Declaration of Helsinki, 80
default attentional system, 63, 81, 210
  as mind wandering, 63–67, 150–151,
    169–176, 244

delusional thought, 9–10, 19, 25, 50–66,
  115, 163, 180–183, 186–187, 191–193
  as mind science, 194–208
  as psychosis today, 146–147
  and two-factor theorizing, 200–210
demonic influence, 50, 92, 257
disease
  as habit, 92–111, 122–126, 134,
    146–147, 150, 167, 171–178, 180–187,
    213–227
  as progressive, 110, 178–179, 263, 287
disease models
  common cause (etiological), 83,
    103–125, 137–148, 266–267,
    288–289
  habituation (*see* disease: as habit)
  network, 63, 83, 107–117, 271, 289
  syndromal, 97–99, 108–112, 148
dualism, 29–41, 274

early prevention. *See* prevention
eclectic (multifactorial) treatment, 274,
  276–278
embodiment
  as embodied cognition, 39
  and interactionism, 23–32
Empiricists (Empirics) and Dogmatists,
  21–22, 88
etiological stance. *See* disease models

323

TOPICAL INDEX

expectation
 science of, 77–80
 in self healing, 71–76

faculty psychology, 22–32
fear and sadness. *See* passions

Galenic nonnaturals. *See* self care and self healing
germ theory of disease, 97, 99, 115

habituation. *See* disease: as habit
"harmful dysfunction" analysis of mental disorder, 103
Hellenistic philosophy. *See* Stoics
humors (humours), 13, 19
 as metaphors, 19–21
 as robust causes, 13, 21–37

imagination (*phantasia*)
 as cause of melancholy, 36–77
 definition of, 56–67
 as imagery, 62, 67

kindling. *See* sensitization
kinds
 categorical and dimensional, 82, 96, 108, 115–117, 227, 287
 practical, 116–117

madness
 as delusional states in the early modern period, 181–182
 as normalized during renaissance, 9
 in relation to melancholy, 10–11, 84–85, 133–134, 181
magic bullets, 113–115, 277
melancholic depression, 119, 142–148, 267, 287–288
melancholising (melancholizing), 151, 162–167
 and depressive rumination, 171–184
 as a habit, 163–184
melancholy
 adusted, 19, 115, 191, 213–214
 in disposition and habit, 116, 126, 183–185, 211, 215
 habituation model of (*see* disease: as habit)

mind wandering. *See* default attentional system

natural history. *See* symptoms
Neoplatonist ideas, 73
networks. *See* disease models
nocebo. *See* expectation
nonnaturals. *See* self care and self healing
normal sadness and sorrow, 217, 222, 227, 241
 contemporary debates, 213, 222–227
 as an unavoidable issue for mind science, 290

original sin, 54, 92, 151

passions, 121
 and imagination, 35–39, 123–126
 reduced to emotions, 139–140
 regulation of, 151–156, 244–265
 in today's mind sciences, 44–50
placebo effect. *See* expectation
prevention, 178, 263–271, 280–286, 291
 "beyond blue" program, 281
 as public health, 282–283
 as self care, 283–286
psychopharmacology. *See* magic bullets
psychosis. *See* delusional thought

reasoning bias, 10, 80, 174–177, 200–205, 232–241, 244
rumination
 and depression, 151, 171–178

self care and self healing, 155–156, 246–252
 attitudes underlying, 246
 as a criterion of severity, 188, 190
 daily regimen of, 254–264
 imagination in, 72, 76, 188
 limits to, 267–272
 with today's mood disorders, 268–269, 282
self governance. *See* self care and self healing
sensitization, 178
simulation. *See* imagination

324

TOPICAL INDEX

soul, 16
  divisions of, 23–32
  relation to body, 32–37
Stoicism and the Stoics, 122, 150–156, 207, 217, 233, 255–259
symptoms, 3, 5, 83–84, 93
  emphasis on, 5
  in chronic disease, 14
  fear and sadness as, 42, 111, 124
  as causes, 22, 86, 106, 289
  in conceptions of disease, 97–117
  as rumination, 171
  as making up Melancholy, 262–266, 289

syndrome. *See* disease models

temperament
  as a diathesis, 48, 90, 96, 101, 147, 179, 183–184, 213, 264, 269–271
  as a genetic risk factor for mood disorder, 284
  humoral, 10, 19, 184
  two-factor theorizing. *See* delusional thought

will. *See* soul: divisions of

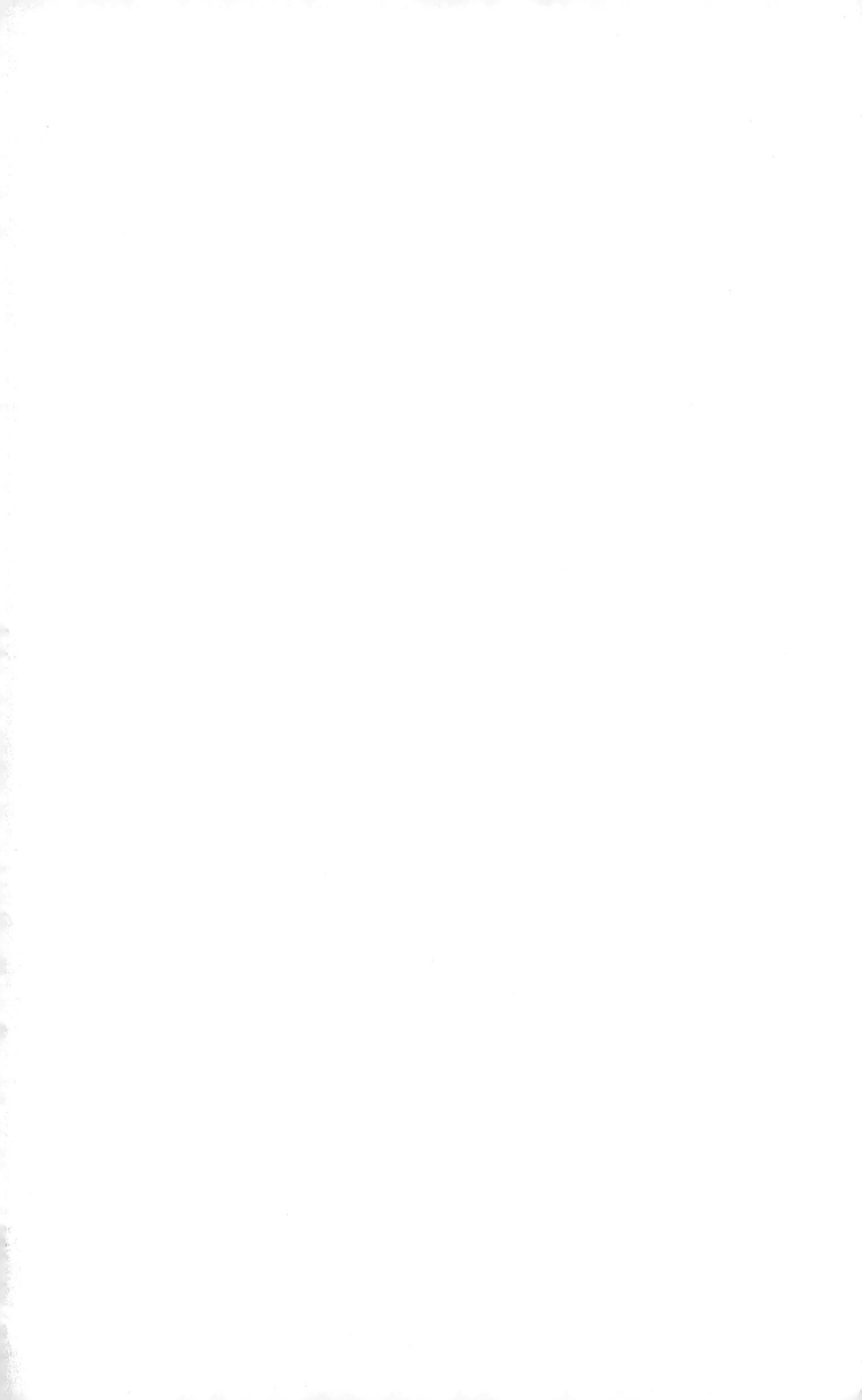